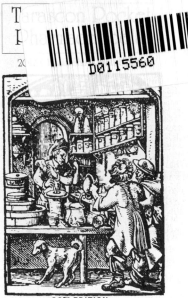

26TH EDITION

"Desire to take medicines ... distinguishes man from animals."
—Sir William Osler

Editor in Chief
Richard J. Hamilton, MD, FAAEM, FACMT
Professor and Chair, Department of Emergency Medicine
Drexel University College of Medicine
Philadelphia, PA

JONES & BARTLETT
LEARNING

World Headquarters
Jones & Bartlett Learning
5 Wall Street
Burlington, MA 01803
978-443-5000
info@jblearning.com
www.jblearning.com

Jones & Bartlett Learning books and products are available through most bookstores and online booksellers. To contact Jones & Bartlett Learning directly, call 800-832-0034, fax 978-443-8000, or visit our website www.jblearning.com.

ISSN: 1945-9076
ISBN: 978-1-4496-2424-8
6048
Printed in the United States of America
15 14 13 12 11   10 9 8 7 6 5 4 3 2 1

Production Credits

Chief Executive Officer: Ty Field
President: James Homer
SVP, Chief Operating Officer: Don Jones, Jr.
SVP, Chief Technology Officer: Dean Fossella
SVP, Chief Marketing Officer: Alison M. Pendergast
SVP, Chief Financial Officer: Ruth Siporin
V.P., Design and Production: Anne Spencer
V.P., Manufacturing and Inventory Control: Therese Connell
Manufacturing and Inventory Control Supervisor: Amy Bacus

Executive Publisher: Christopher Davis
Senior Acquisitions Editor: Nancy Anastasi Duffy
Managing Editor: Kathy Richardson
Associate Editor: Laura Burns
Production Editor: Daniel Stone
Medicine Marketing Manager: Rebecca Rockel
Composition: Newgen
Text and Cover Design: Anne Spencer
Printing and Binding: Cenveo
Cover Printing: Cenveo

If you obtained your *Pocket Pharmacopoeia* from a bookstore, please send your address to info@tarascon.com. This allows you to be the first to hear of updates! (We don't sell or distribute our mailing lists, by the way.)

The cover woodcut is The *Apothecary* by Jost Amman, Frankfurt, 1574.

For those of you still trying to solve last year's puzzle, here is the answer:

To solve it, you let x equal the volume of the infusion. For the first bag, the ratio of volumes is x-72:72. For the second bag the ratio of volumes is 2x-40:x+40. This is the ratio of the rates of infusions for each patient and they are equal, and so they can be solved for x. Thus each bag has 176 mLs. This puzzle was adapted from Martin Gardner's "The colossal book of short puzzles and problems", 2006, page 91.

This year's puzzle should appeal to the topologists amongst our readers and best of all there is no arithmetic involved.

Grab the opposite corners of a hospital bed sheet, one corner in each hand. Now tie a knot in it without letting go of the corners. We will send a free copy of next year's edition to the first 25 readers who can correctly tell us how they did it!

CONTENTS

ANALGESICS.....................1
Antirheumatic Agents.....1
Muscle Relaxants.............2
Non-Opioid Analgesic
Combinations................2
Non-Steroidal Anti-
Inflammatories..............4
Opioid Agonist-
Antagonists..................6
Opioid Agonists..............7
Opioid Analgesic
Combinations................9
Opioid Antagonists........11
Other Analgesics...........12
ANESTHESIA....................12
Anesthetics and
Sedatives...................12
Local Anesthetics..........13
Neuromuscular
Blockers.....................13
ANTIMICROBIALS...........13
Aminoglycosides............13
Antifungal Agents..........14
Antimalarials................16
Antimycobacterial
Agents.......................17
Antiparasitics...............18
Antiviral Agents............19
Carbapenems................29
Cephalosporins.............29
Macrolides...................31
Penicillins...................34
Quinolones...................37
Sulfonamides...............37
Tetracyclines...............38
Other Antimicrobials......39
CARDIOVASCULAR..........41
ACE Inhibitors..............41
Aldosterone
Antagonists................43
Angiotensin Receptor
Blockers (ARBs)...........43
Antiadrenergic Agents....44
Anti-Dysrhythmics/
Cardiac Arrest.............46
Anti-Hyperlipidemic
Agents.......................49
Antihypertensive
Combinations..............54
Antihypertensives.........55

Antiplatelet Drugs.........56
Beta-Blockers...............57
Calcium Channel
Blockers (CCBs)...........59
Diuretics.....................61
Nitrates......................62
Pressors/Inotropes........63
Pulmonary Arterial
Hypertension...............64
Thrombolytics..............64
Volume Expanders.........65
Other.........................65
CONTRAST MEDIA..........66
MRI Contrast................66
Radiography Contrast.....67
DERMATOLOGY..............67
Acne Preparations.........67
Actinic Keratosis
Preparations...............69
Antibacterials (Topical)...69
Antifungals (Topical)......70
Antiparasitics (Topical)...71
Antipsoriatics..............72
Antivirals (Topical)........72
Atopic Dermatitis
Preparations...............73
Corticosteroid/
Antimicrobial
Combinations..............73
Hemorrhoid Care..........75
Other Dermatologic
Agents.......................75
**ENDOCRINE AND
METABOLIC**...............77
Androgens / Anabolic
Steroids.....................77
Bisphosphonates..........77
Corticosteroids............78
Diabetes-Related..........80
Gout-Related...............86
Minerals.....................86
Nutritionals.................89
Phosphate Binders........90
Thyroid Agents.............90
Vitamins.....................90
Other.........................93
ENT..............................94
Antihistamines.............94
Antitussives /
Expectorants..............95

Decongestants..............96
Ear Preparations...........96
Mouth and Lip
Preparations...............98
Nasal Preparations........99
GASTROENTEROLOGY....100
Antidiarrheals.............100
Antiemetics................101
Antiulcer...................103
Laxatives...................107
Ulcerative Colitis.........109
Other GI Agents...........110
HEMATOLOGY...............112
Anticoagulants............112
Colony Stimulating
Factors.....................115
Other Hematological
Agents......................115
**HERBAL & ALTERNATIVE
THERAPIES**...............116
IMMUNOLOGY...............123
Immunizations.............123
Immunoglobulins..........124
Immunosuppression......126
Other.........................126
NEUROLOGY.................127
Alzheimer's Disease......127
Anticonvulsants...........127
Migraine Therapy..........130
Multiple sclerosis........132
Myasthenia Gravis........132
Parkinsonian Agents......132
Other Agents...............135
OB/GYN.......................135
Contraceptives............135
Estrogens...................136
Hormone
Combinations.............137
Labor Induction /
Cervical Ripening........138
Ovulation Stimulants.....138
Progestins..................138
Selective Estrogen
Receptor Modulators....140
Uterotonics................140
Vaginitis
Preparations..............140
Other OB/GYN
Agents......................142
ONCOLOGY...................142

OPHTHALMOLOGY............144
Antiallergy.......................144
Antibacterials.................145
Antiviral Agents.............146
Corticosteroid &
 Antibacterial
 Combinations 146
Corticosteroids..............147
Glaucoma Agents 148
Mydriatics & Cycloplegics..149
Non-Steroidal
 Anti-Inflammatories ...150
Other Ophthalmologic
 Agents 150

PSYCHIATRY..................151
Antidepressants 151
Antimanic (Bipolar)
 Agents 154
Antipsychotics................155
Anxiolytics/
 Hypnotics...................159
Combination Drugs 161
Drug Dependence
 Therapy......................161
Stimulants/ADHD/
 Anorexiants................162
PULMONARY..................164
Beta Agonists................164

Combinations.................165
Inhaled Steroids............165
Leukotriene
 Inhibitors...................167
Other Pulmonary
 Medications................168
TOXICOLOGY..................169
Toxicology......................169
UROLOGY......................170
Benign Prostatic
 Hyperplasia................170
Bladder Agents..............170
Erectile Dysfunction 172
Nephrolithiasis..............172

PAGE INDEX FOR TABLES

GENERAL
Abbreviations ix
Therapeutic drug
 levels ix
Pediatric drugs.................. x
Pediatric vital signs and
 IV drugs xi
Conversions..................... xii
Drug therapy reference
 websites......................xii
Adult emergency drugs ..200
Cardiac dysrhythmia
 protocols...................201
Antiviral drugs for
 Influenza....................202
ANALGESICS
NSAIDs.............................5
Opioid equivalency............8
Fentanyl transdermal 9
ANTIMICROBIALS
Bacterial pathogens.........26
Cephalosporins 31
STDs/vaginitis.................32
SBE prophylaxis...............36
Penicillins 36

Quinolones 37
C. difficile infection in
 adults.........................40
CARDIOVASCULAR
ACE inhibitors 42
HTN therapy....................44
QT interval drugs.............47
Lipid reduction by
 class/agent..................50
LDL goals 52
Statins lipid
 response......................53
Cardiac parameters..........64
Thrombolysis in MI 65
DERMATOLOGY
Topical steroids 74
ENDOCRINE
Corticosteroids 79
Diabetes numbers............81
Injectable insulins...........83
Fluoride dose..................87
IV solutions....................87
Potassium forms..............88
ENT
ENT combinations 97

GASTROENTEROLOGY
H pylori treatment 105
HEMATOLOGY
Heparin dosing for ACS ..114
Weight-Based heparin......114
Therapeutic goals for
 anticoagulation 115
IMMUNOLOGY
Child immunizations......125
Tetanus 126
NEUROLOGY
Dermatomes...................134
OB/GYN
Emerg contraception 138
Oral contraceptives 139
Drugs in pregnancy........141
PSYCHIATRY
Antipsychotics................158
Body mass index 163
PULMONARY
Peak flow......................165
Inhaled steroids 166
Inhaler colors 167
TOXICOLOGY
Antidotes.......................169

*Affiliations are given for information purposes only, and no affiliation sponsorship is claimed.

PREFACE TO THE TARASCON POCKET PHARMACOPOEIA®

The *Tarascon Pocket Pharmacopoeia®* arranges drugs by clinical class with a comprehensive index in the back. Trade names are italicized and capitalized. Drug doses shown in mg/kg are generally intended for children, while fixed doses represent typical adult recommendations. Brackets indicate currently available formulations, although not all pharmacies stock all formulations. The availability of generic, over-the-counter, and scored formulations is mentioned. We have underlined the disease or indication for the pharmaceutical agent. It is meant to function as an aid to find information quickly. Codes are as follows:

▶ **METABOLISM & EXCRETION:** **L** = primarily liver, **K** = primarily kidney, **LK** = both, but liver > kidney, **KL** = both, but kidney > liver.

♀ **SAFETY IN PREGNANCY:** **A** = Safety established using human studies, **B** = Presumed safety based on animal studies, **C** = Uncertain safety; no human studies and animal studies show an adverse effect, **D** = Unsafe - evidence of risk that may in certain clinical circumstances be justifiable, **X** = Highly unsafe - risk of use outweighs any possible benefit. For drugs that have not been assigned a category: **+** Generally accepted as safe, **?** Safety unknown or controversial, **−** Generally regarded as unsafe.

▶ **SAFETY IN LACTATION:** **+** = Generally accepted as safe, **?** Safety unknown or controversial, **−** Generally regarded as unsafe. Many of our "+" listings are from the AAP policy "The Transfer of Drugs and Other Chemicals Into Human Milk" (see www.aap.org) and may differ from those recommended by the manufacturer.

© **DEA CONTROLLED SUBSTANCES:** **I** = High abuse potential, no accepted use (eg, heroin, marijuana), **II** = High abuse potential and severe dependence liability (eg, morphine, codeine, hydromorphone, cocaine, amphetamines, methylphenidate, secobarbital). Some states require triplicates. **III** = Moderate dependence liability (eg, *Tylenol #3, Vicodin*), **IV** = Limited dependence liability (benzodiazepines, propoxyphene, phentermine), **V** = Limited abuse potential (eg, *Lomotil*).

$ **RELATIVE COST:** Cost codes used are "per month" of maintenance therapy (eg, antihypertensives) or "per course" of short-term therapy (eg, antibiotics). Codes are calculated using average wholesale prices (at press time in US dollars) for the most common indication and route of each drug at a typical adult dosage. For maintenance therapy, costs are calculated based upon a 30-day supply or the quantity that might typically be used in a given month. For short-term therapy (ie, 10 days or less), costs are calculated on a single treatment course. When multiple forms are available (eg,

Code	Cost
$	< $25
$$	$25 to $49
$$$	$50 to $99
$$$$	$100 to $199
$$$$$	≥ $200

generics), these codes reflect the least expensive generally available product. When drugs don't neatly fit into the classification scheme above, we have assigned codes based upon the relative cost of other similar drugs. *These codes should be used as a rough guide only,* as (1) they reflect cost, not charges, (2) pricing often varies substantially from location to location and time to time, and (3) HMOs, Medicaid, and buying groups often negotiate quite different pricing. Check with your local pharmacy if you have any questions.

🍁 **CANADIAN TRADE NAMES:** Unique common Canadian trade names not used in the US are listed after a maple leaf symbol. Trade names used in both nations or only in the US are displayed without such notation.

■ **BLACK BOX WARNINGS:** This icon indicates that there is a black box warning associated with this drug. Note that the warning itself is not listed.

ABBREVIATIONS IN TEXT

AAP – American Academy of Pediatrics
ACCP – American College of Chest Physicians
ACT – activated clotting time
ADHD – attention deficit hyperactivity disorder
AHA – American Heart Association
Al – aluminum
ANC – absolute neutrophil count
ASA – aspirin
BP – blood pressure
BPH – benign prostatic hyperplasia
BUN – blood urea nitrogen
Ca – calcium
CAD – coronary artery disease
cap – capsule
cm – centimeter
CMV – cytomegalovirus
CNS – central nervous system
COPD – chronic obstructive pulmonary disease
CrCl – creatinine clearance
CVA – stroke

CYP – cytochrome P450
D5W – 5% dextrose
dL – deciliter
DM – diabetes mellitus
DPI – dry powder inhaler
ECG – electrocardiogram
EPS – extrapyramidal symptoms
ET – endotracheal
g – gram
GERD – gastroesophageal reflux disease
gtts – drops
GU – genitourinary
h – hour
HAART – highly active antiretroviral therapy
Hb – hemoglobin
HCTZ – hydrochlorothiazide
HIT – heparin-induced thrombocytopenia
HSV – herpes simplex virus
HTN – hypertension
IM – intramuscular
INR – international normalized ratio
IU – international units
IV – intravenous
JRA – juvenile rheumatoid arthritis

kg – kilogram
lbs – pounds
LFT – liver function test
LV – left ventricular
LVEF – left ventricular ejection fraction
m² – square meters
MAOI – monoamine oxidase inhibitor
mcg – microgram
MDI – metered dose inhaler
mEq – milliequivalent
mg – milligram
Mg – magnesium
MI – myocardial infarction
min – minute
mL – milliliter
mm – millimeter
mo – months old
MRSA – methicillin-resistant Staphylococcus aureus
ng – nanogram
NHLBI – National Heart, Lung, and Blood Institute
NPH – neutral protamine hagedorn
NS – normal saline
N/V – nausea/vomiting

NYHA – New York Heart Association
OA – osteoarthritis
oz – ounces
pc – after meals
PO – by mouth
PR – by rectum
prn – as needed
PTT – partial thromboplastin time
q – every
RA – rheumatoid arthritis
RSV – respiratory synctial virus
SC – subcutaneous
sec – second
soln – solution
supp – suppository
susp – suspension
tab – tablet
TB – tuberculosis
TCA – tricyclic antidepressant
TNF – tumor necrosis factor
TPN – total parenteral nutrition
UTI – urinary tract infection
wt – weight
y – year
yo – years old

THERAPEUTIC DRUG LEVELS

Drug	Level	Optimal Timing
amikacin peak	20–35 mcg/mL	30 minutes after infusion
amikacin trough	<5 mcg/mL	Just prior to next dose
carbamazepine trough	4–12 mcg/mL	Just prior to next dose
cyclosporine trough	50–300 ng/mL	Just prior to next dose
digoxin	0.8–2.0 ng/mL	Just prior to next dose
ethosuximide trough	40–100 mcg/mL	Just prior to next dose
gentamicin peak	5–10 mcg/mL	30 minutes after infusion
gentamicin trough	<2 mcg/mL	Just prior to next dose
lidocaine	1.5–5 mcg/mL	12–24 hours after start of infusion
lithium trough	0.6–1.2 meq/l	Just prior to first morning dose
NAPA	10–30 mcg/mL	Just prior to next procainamide dose
phenobarbital trough	15–40 mcg/mL	Just prior to next dose
phenytoin trough	10–20 mcg/mL	Just prior to next dose
primidone trough	5–12 mcg/mL	Just prior to next dose
procainamide	4–10 mcg/mL	Just prior to next dose
quinidine	2–5 mcg/mL	Just prior to next dose
theophylline	5–15 mcg/mL	8–12 hours after once daily dose
tobramycin peak	5–10 mcg/mL	30 minutes after infusion
tobramycin trough	<2 mcg/mL	Just prior to next dose
valproate trough (epilepsy)	50–100 mcg/mL	Just prior to next dose
valproate trough (mania)	45–125 mcg/mL	Just prior to next dose
vancomycin trough[1]	10–20 mg/L	Just prior to next dose
zonisamide[2]	10–40 mcg/mL	Just prior to dose

[1]Maintain trough >10 mg/L to avoid resistance; optimal trough for complicated infections is 15–20 mg/L
[2]Ranges not firmly established but supported by clinical trial results

PEDIATRIC DRUGS		*Age*	2mo	4mo	6mo	9mo	12mo	15mo	2yo	3yo	5yo
		kg	5	6½	8	9	10	11	13	15	19
		lbs	11	15	17	20	22	24	28	33	42
med	***strength***	***freq***	***teaspoons of liquid per dose*** *(1 tsp = 5 mL)*								
Tylenol (mg)		q4h	80	80	120	120	160	160	200	240	280
Tylenol (tsp)	160/t	q4h	½	½	¾	¾	1	1	1¼	1½	1¾
ibuprofen (mg)		q6h	--	--	75†	75†	100	100	125	150	175
ibuprofen (tsp)	100/t	q6h	--	--	¾†	¾†	1	1	1¼	1½	1¾
amoxicillin or	125/t	bid	1	1¼	1½	1¾	1¾	2	2¼	2¾	3½
Augmentin	200/t	bid	½	¾	1	1	1¼	1¼	1½	1¾	2¼
(not otitis media)	250/t	bid	½	½	¾	¾	1	1	1¼	1¼	1¾
	400/t	bid	¼	½	½	½	¾	¾	¾	1	1
amoxicillin,	200/t	bid	1	1¼	1¾	2	2	2¼	2¾	3	4
(otitis media)‡	250/t	bid	¾	1¼	1½	1½	1¾	1¾	2¼	2½	3¼
	400/t	bid	½	¾	¾	1	1	1¼	1½	1½	2
Augmentin ES‡	600/t	bid	?	½	½	¾	¾	¾	1	1¼	1½
azithromycin*§	100/t	qd	¼†	½†	½	½	½	½	¾	¾	1
(5-day Rx)	200/t	qd	--	¼†	¼	¼	¼	¼	½	½	½
Bactrim/Septra	---	bid	½	¾	1	1	1	1¼	1½	1½	2
cefaclor*	125/t	bid	1	1	1¼	1½	1½	1¾	2	2½	3
"	250/t	bid	½	½	¾	¾	¾	1	1	1¼	1½
cefadroxil	125/t	bid	½	¾	1	1	1¼	1¼	1½	1¾	2¼
"	250/t	bid	¼	½	½	½	¾	¾	¾	1	1
cefdinir	125/t	qd	--	¾†	1	1	1	1¼	1½	1¾	2
cefixime	100/t	qd	½	½	¾	¾	¾	1	1	1¼	1½
cefprozil*	125/t	bid	--	¾†	1	1	1¼	1½	1½	2	2¼
"	250/t	bid	--	½†	½	½	¾	¾	¾	1	1¼
cefuroxime	125/t	bid	--	¾	¾	1	1	1	1½	1¾	2¼
cephalexin	125/t	qid	--	½	¾	¾	1	1	1¼	1½	1¾
"	250/t	qid	--	¼	¼	½	½	½	¾	¾	1
clarithromycin	125/t	bid	½†	½†	½	½	¾	¾	¾	1	1¼
"	250/t	bid	--	--	--	¼	½	½	½	½	¾
dicloxacillin	62½/t	qid	½	¾	1	1	1¼	1¼	1½	1¾	2
nitrofurantoin	25/t	qid	¼	½	½	½	½	¾	¾	¾	1
Pediazole	---	tid	½	½	¾	¾	1	1	1	1¼	1½
penicillin V**	250/t	bid-tid	--	1	1	1	1	1	1	1	1
cetirizine	5/t	qd	--	--	½	½	½	½	½	½	½
Benadryl	12.5/t	q6h	½	½	¾	¾	1	1	1¼	1½	2
prednisolone	15/t	qd	¼	½	½	¾	¾	¾	1	1	1¼
prednisone	5/t	qd	1	1¼	1½	1¾	2	2¼	2½	3	3¾
Robitussin	---	q4h	--	--	¼†	¼†	½	½	¾	¾	1
Tylenol w/ codeine		q4h	--	--	--	--	--	--	--	1	1

*Dose shown is for otitis media only; see dosing in text for alternative indications.
†Dosing at this age/weight not recommended by manufacturer.
‡AAP now recommends high dose (80-90 mg/kg/d) for all otitis media in children; with Augmentin used as ES only.
§Give a double dose of azithromycin the first day.
**AHA dosing for streptococcal pharyngitis. Treat for 10 days.
tsp=teaspoon; t=teaspoon; q=every; h=hour; kg=kilogram; Lbs=pounds; ml=mililiter; bid=two times per day; tid=three times per day; qid=four times per day; qd=every day.

PEDIATRIC VITAL SIGNS AND INTRAVENOUS DRUGS

Age		Pre-matr	New-born	2m	4m	6m	9m	12m	15m	2y	3y	5y
Weight	(kg)	2	3½	5	6½	8	9	10	11	13	15	19
	(lbs)	4½	7½	11	15	17	20	22	24	28	33	42
Maint fluids	(mL/h)	8	14	20	26	32	36	40	42	46	50	58
ET tube	(mm)	2½	3/3½	3½	3½	3½	4	4	4½	4½	4½	5
Defib	(Joules)	4	7	10	13	16	18	20	22	26	30	38
Systolic BP	(high)	70	80	85	90	95	100	103	104	106	109	114
	(low)	40	60	70	70	70	70	70	70	75	75	80
Pulse rate	(high)	145	145	180	180	180	160	160	160	150	150	135
	(low)	100	100	110	110	110	100	100	100	90	90	65
Resp rate	(high)	60	60	50	50	50	46	46	30	30	25	25
	(low)	35	30	30	30	24	24	20	20	20	20	20
adenosine	(mg)	0.2	0.3	0.5	0.6	0.8	0.9	1	1.1	1.3	1.5	1.9
atropine	(mg)	0.1	0.1	0.1	0.13	0.16	0.18	0.2	0.22	0.26	0.30	0.38
Benadryl	(mg)	-	-	5	6½	8	9	10	11	13	15	19
bicarbonate	(meq)	2	3½	5	6½	8	9	10	11	13	15	19
dextrose	(g)	1	2	5	6½	8	9	10	11	13	15	19
epinephrine	(mg)	.02	.04	.05	.07	.08	.09	0.1	0.11	0.13	0.15	0.19
lidocaine	(mg)	2	3½	5	6½	8	9	10	11	13	15	19
morphine	(mg)	0.2	0.3	0.5	0.6	0.8	0.9	1	1.1	1.3	1.5	1.9
mannitol	(g)	2	3½	5	6½	8	9	10	11	13	15	19
naloxone	(mg)	.02	.04	.05	.07	.08	.09	0.1	0.11	0.13	0.15	0.19
diazepam	(mg)	0.6	1	1.5	2	2.5	2.7	3	3.3	3.9	4.5	5
fosphenytoin*	(PE)	40	70	100	130	160	180	200	220	260	300	380
lorazepam	(mg)	0.1	0.2	0.3	0.35	0.4	0.5	0.5	0.6	0.7	0.8	1.0
phenobarb	(mg)	30	60	75	100	125	125	150	175	200	225	275
phenytoin*	(mg)	40	70	100	130	160	180	200	220	260	300	380
ampicillin	(mg)	100	175	250	325	400	450	500	550	650	750	1000
ceftriaxone	(mg)	-	-	250	325	400	450	500	550	650	750	1000
cefotaxime	(mg)	100	175	250	325	400	450	500	550	650	750	1000
gentamicin	(mg)	5	8	12	16	20	22	25	27	32	37	47

*Loading doses; fosphenytoin dosed in "phenytoin equivalents."

CONVERSIONS

Temperature:	Liquid:	Weight:
F = (1.8) C + 32	1 fluid ounce = 30 mL	1 kilogram = 2.2 lbs
C = (F – 32)/1.8	1 teaspoon = 5 mL	1 ounce = 30 g
	1 tablespoon = 15 mL	1 grain = 65 mg

DRUG THERAPY REFERENCE WEBSITES (selected)

Professional societies or governmental agencies with drug therapy guidelines

AAP	American Academy of Pediatrics	www.aap.org
ACC	American College of Cardiology	www.acc.org
ACCP	American College of Chest Physicians	www.chestnet.org
ACCP	American College of Clinical Pharmacy	www.accp.com
ADA	American Diabetes Association	www.diabetes.org
AHA	American Heart Association	www.heart.org
AHRQ	Agency for Healthcare Research and Quality	www.ahcpr.gov
AMA	American Medical Association	www.ama-assn.org
APA	American Psychiatric Association	www.psych.org
APA	American Psychological Association	www.apa.org
ASHP	Amer. Society Health-Systems Pharmacists	www.ashp.org
ATS	American Thoracic Society	www.thoracic.org
CDC	Centers for Disease Control and Prevention	www.cdc.gov
CDC	CDC bioterrorism and radiation exposures	www.bt.cdc.gov
IDSA	Infectious Diseases Society of America	www.idsociety.org
MHA	Malignant Hyperthermia Association	www.mhaus.org
NHLBI	National Heart, Lung, and Blood Institute	www.nhlbi.nih.gov

Other therapy reference sites

Cochrane library	www.cochrane.org
Emergency Contraception Website	www.not-2-late.com
Immunization Action Coalition	www.immunize.org
Int'l Registry for Drug-Induced Arrhythmias	www.qtdrugs.org
Managing Contraception	www.managingcontraception.com

ANALGESICS

Antirheumatic Agents—Biologic Response Modifiers

NOTE: *Death, sepsis, and serious infections (eg, TB and invasive fungal infections) have been reported.*

ADALIMUMAB (*Humira*) RA, psoriatic arthritis, ankylosing spondylitis: 40 mg SC every 2 weeks, alone or in combination with methotrexate or other disease-modifying antirheumatic drugs (DMARDs). May increase frequency to once a week if not on methotrexate. Crohn's disease: 160 mg SC at week 0, 80 mg at week 2, then 40 mg every other week starting with week 4. [Trade only: 40 mg prefilled glass syringes or vials with needles, 2 per pack.] ▶Serum ♀B ▶ $$$$$ ■

ANAKINRA (*Kineret*) RA: 100 mg SC daily. [Trade only: 100 mg prefilled glass syringes with needles, 7 or 28 per box.] ▶K ♀B ▶? $$$$$

ETANERCEPT (*Enbrel*) RA, psoriatic arthritis, ankylosing spondylitis: 50 mg SC once a week. Plaque psoriasis: 50 mg SC 2 times per week for 3 months, then 50 mg SC once a week. JRA age 4 to 17 yo: 0.8 mg/kg SC once a week, to max single dose of 50 mg. Max dose per injection site is 25 mg. [Supplied in a carton containing four dose trays and as single-use prefilled syringes. Each dose tray contains one 25 mg single-use vial of etanercept, one syringe (1 mL sterile bacteriostatic water for injection, containing 0.9% benzyl alcohol), one plunger, and two alcohol swabs. Single-use syringes contain 50 mg/mL.] ▶Serum ♀B ▶– $$$$$ ■

INFLIXIMAB (*Remicade*) RA: 3 mg/kg IV in combination with methotrexate at 0, 2, and 6 weeks. Ankylosing spondylitis: 5 mg/kg IV al 0, 2, and 6 weeks. Plaque psoriasis, psoriatic arthritis, moderately to severely active Crohn's disease, ulcerative colitis, or fistulizing disease: 5 mg/kg IV infusion at 0, 2, and 6 weeks, then q 8 weeks. ▶Serum ♀B ▶? $$$$$ ■

Antirheumatic Agents—Disease Modifying Antirheumatic Drugs (DMARDs)

AZATHIOPRINE (*Azasan, Imuran*) RA: Initial dose 1 mg/kg (50 to 100 mg) PO daily or divided two times per day. Increase after 6 to 8 weeks. [Generic/Trade: Tabs 50 mg, scored. Trade only (Azasan): 75, 100 mg, scored.] ▶LK ♀D ▶– $$$ ■

HYDROXYCHLOROQUINE (*Plaquenil*) RA: Start 400 to 600 mg PO daily, then taper to 200 to 400 mg daily. SLE: 400 PO one to two times per day to start, then taper to 200 to 400 mg daily. [Generic/Trade: Tabs 200 mg, scored.] ▶K ♀C ▶+ $$ ■

LEFLUNOMIDE (*Arava*) RA: Loading dose: 100 mg PO daily for 3 days. Maintenance dose: 10 to 20 mg PO daily. [Generic/Trade: Tabs 10, 20 mg. Trade only: Tabs 100 mg.] ▶LK ♀X ▶– $$$$$ ■

METHOTREXATE (*Rheumatrex, Trexall*) RA, psoriasis: Start with 7.5 mg PO single dose once a week or 2.5 mg PO q 12 h for 3 doses given once a week. Max dose 20 mg/week. Supplement with 1 mg/day of folic acid. Chemotherapy doses vary by indication. [Trade only (Trexall): Tabs 5, 7.5, 10, 15 mg. Dose Pak (Rheumatrex) 2.5 mg (# 8, 12, 16, 20, 24). Generic/Trade: Tabs 2.5 mg, scored.] ▶LK ♀X ▶– $$ ■

Muscle Relaxants

BACLOFEN (*Lioresal, Kemstro*) <u>Spasticity related to MS or spinal cord disease/injury</u>: Start 5 mg PO three times per day, then increase by 5 mg/dose q 3 days until 20 mg PO three times per day. Max dose 20 mg four times per day. [Generic only: Tabs 10, 20 mg. Trade only (Kemstro): Tabs, orally disintegrating 10, 20 mg.] ▶K ♀C ▶+ $$

CARISOPRODOL (*Soma*) <u>Acute musculoskeletal pain</u>: 350 mg PO three to four times per day. Abuse potential. [Generic/Trade: Tabs 350 mg. Trade only: Tabs 250 mg.] ▶LK ♀? ▶– $

CHLORZOXAZONE (*Parafon Forte DSC*) <u>Musculoskeletal pain</u>: 500 to 750 mg PO three to four times per day. Decrease to 250 mg three to four times per day if necessary. [Generic/Trade: Tabs 250, 500 mg (Parafon Forte DSC 500 mg tabs, scored).] ▶LK ♀C ▶? $

CYCLOBENZAPRINE (*Amrix, Flexeril, Fexmid*) <u>Musculoskeletal pain</u>: Start 5 to 10 mg PO three times per day, max 30 mg/day or 15 to 30 mg (extended-release) PO daily. Not recommended in elderly. [Generic/Trade: Tab 5, 10 mg. Generic only: Tabs 7.5 mg. Trade only: (Amrix $$$$$): Extended-release caps 15, 30 mg.] ▶LK ♀B ▶? $

DANTROLENE (*Dantrium*) <u>Chronic spasticity related to spinal cord injury, CVA, cerebral palsy, MS</u>: 25 mg PO daily to start, up to max of 100 mg two to four times per day. <u>Malignant hyperthermia</u>: 2.5 mg/kg rapid IV push q 5 to 10 min continuing until symptoms subside or to a maximum total dose of 10 mg/kg. [Generic/Trade: Caps 25, 50, 100 mg.] ▶LK ♀C ▶– $$$$ ■

METAXALONE (*Skelaxin*) <u>Musculoskeletal pain</u>: 800 mg PO three to four times per day. [Generic/Trade: Tabs 800 mg, scored.] ▶LK ♀? ▶? $$$$

METHOCARBAMOL (*Robaxin, Robaxin-750*) <u>Acute musculoskeletal pain</u>: 1500 mg PO four times per day or 1000 mg IM/IV three times per day for 48 to 72 h. Maintenance: 1000 mg PO four times per day, 750 mg PO q 4 h, or 1500 mg PO three times per day. <u>Tetanus</u>: Specialized dosing. [Generic/Trade: Tabs 500 and 750 mg. OTC in Canada.] ▶LK ♀C ▶? $$

ORPHENADRINE (*Norflex*) <u>Musculoskeletal pain</u>: 100 mg PO two times per day. 60 mg IV/IM two times per day. [Generic only: 100 mg extended-release. OTC in Canada.] ▶LK ♀C ▶? $$

TIZANIDINE (*Zanaflex*) <u>Muscle spasticity due to MS or spinal cord injury</u>: 4 to 8 mg PO q 6 to 8 h prn, max 36 mg/day. [Generic/Trade: Tabs 4 mg, scored. Trade only: Caps 2, 4, 6 mg. Generic only: Tabs 2 mg.] ▶LK ♀C ▶? $$$$

Non-Opioid Analgesic Combinations

ASCRIPTIN (acetylsalicylic acid + aluminum hydroxide + magnesium hydroxide + calcium carbonate, *Aspir-Mox*) Multiple strengths. 1 to 2 tabs PO q 4 h. [OTC Trade only: Tabs 325 mg aspirin/50 mg Mg hydroxide/50 mg Al hydroxide/50 mg Ca carbonate (Ascriptin and Aspir-Mox). 500 mg aspirin/33 mg Mg hydroxide/33 mg Al hydroxide/ 237 mg Ca carbonate (Ascriptin Maximum Strength).] ▶K ♀D ▶? $

BUFFERIN (acetylsalicylic acid + calcium carbonate + magnesium oxide + magnesium carbonate) 1 to 2 tabs/caps PO q 4 h. Max 12 in 24 h. [OTC Trade only: Tabs/caps 325 mg aspirin/158 mg Ca carbonate/63 mg of Mg oxide/34 mg of Mg carbonate. Bufferin ES: 500 mg aspirin/222.3 mg Ca carbonate/88.9 mg of Mg oxide/55.6 mg of Mg carbonate.] ▶K ♀D ▶? $

ESGIC (acetaminophen + butalbital + caffeine) 1 to 2 tabs or caps PO q 4 h. Max 6 in 24 h. [Generic only: Tabs/caps, 325 mg acetaminophen/50 mg butalbital/40 mg caffeine. Oral soln 325/50/40 mg per 15 mL. Generic/Trade: Tabs, Esgic Plus is 500/50/40 mg.] ▶LK ♀C ▶? $

EXCEDRIN MIGRAINE (acetaminophen + acetylsalicylic acid + caffeine) 2 tabs/caps/geltabs PO while symptoms persist. Max 8 tabs/caps/geltabs in 24 h. [OTC Generic/Trade: Tabs/caps/geltabs 250 mg acetaminophen/250 mg aspirin/65 mg caffeine.] ▶LK ♀D ▶? $

FIORICET (acetaminophen + butalbital + caffeine) 1 to 2 caps PO q 4 h. Max 6 caps in 24 h. [Generic/Trade: Tabs 325 mg acetaminophen/50 mg butalbital/40 mg caffeine.] ▶LK ♀C ▶? $

FIORINAL (acetylsalicylic acid + butalbital + caffeine, ◆ *Trianal*) 1 to 2 tabs PO q 4 h. Max 6 tabs in 24 h. [Generic/Trade: Caps 325 mg aspirin/ 50 mg butalbital/40 mg caffeine.] ▶KL ♀D ▶–©III $

GOODY'S EXTRA STRENGTH HEADACHE POWDER (acetaminophen + acetylsalicylic acid + caffeine) 1 powder PO followed with liquid, or stir powder into a glass of water or other liquid. Repeat in 4 to 6 h prn. Max 4 powders in 24 h. [OTC trade only: 260 mg acetaminophen/520 mg aspirin/32.5 mg caffeine per powder paper.] ▶LK ♀D ▶? $

NORGESIC (orphenadrine + acetylsalicylic acid + caffeine) Multiple strengths; write specific product on Rx. Norgesic: 1 to 2 tabs PO three to four times per day. Norgesic Forte, 1 tab PO three to four times per day. [Generic/Trade: Tabs Norgesic 25 mg orphenadrine/385 mg aspirin/30 mg caffeine. Norgesic Forte 50/770/60 mg.] ▶KL ♀D ▶? $$

PHRENILIN (acetaminophen + butalbital) <u>Tension or muscle contraction headache</u>: 1 to 2 tabs PO q 4 h. Max 6 in 24 h. [Generic/Trade: Tabs, Phrenilin 325 mg acetaminophen/50 mg butalbital. Caps, Phrenilin Forte 650/50 mg.] ▶LK ♀C ▶? $

SEDAPAP (acetaminophen + butalbital) 1 to 2 tabs PO q 4 h. Max 6 tabs in 24 h. [Generic only: Tabs 650 mg acetaminophen/50 mg butalbital.] ▶LK ♀C ▶? $

SOMA COMPOUND (carisoprodol + acetylsalicylic acid) 1 to 2 tabs PO four times per day. Abuse potential. [Generic/Trade: Tabs 200 mg carisoprodol/325 mg aspirin.] ▶LK ♀D ▶– $$$

ULTRACET (tramadol + acetaminophen, ◆ *Tramacet*) <u>Acute pain</u>: 2 tabs PO q 4 to 6 h prn, (up to 8 tabs/day for no more than 5 days). Adjust dose in elderly and renal dysfunction. Avoid in opioid-dependent patients. Seizures may occur if concurrent antidepressants or seizure disorder. [Generic/Trade: Tabs 37.5 mg tramadol/ 325 mg acetaminophen.] ▶KL ♀C ▶– $$

Non-Steroidal Anti-Inflammatories—COX-2 Inhibitors

CELECOXIB (*Celebrex*) OA, ankylosing spondylitis: 200 mg PO daily or 100 mg PO two times per day. RA: 100 to 200 mg PO two times per day. Familial adenomatous polyposis: 400 mg PO two times per day with food. Acute pain, dysmenorrhea: 400 mg single dose, then 200 mg two times per day prn. An additional 200 mg dose may be given on day 1 if needed. JRA: Give 50 mg PO two times per day for age 2 to 17 yo and wt 10 to 25 kg, give 100 mg PO two times per day for wt greater than 25 kg. Contraindicated in sulfonamide allergy. [Trade only: Caps 50, 100, 200, 400 mg.] ▶L ♀C (D in 3rd trimester) ▶? $$$$$ ■

Non-Steroidal Anti-Inflammatories—Salicylic Acid Derivatives

ACETYLSALICYLIC ACID (*Ecotrin, Empirin, Halfprin, Bayer, Anacin, Zorprin, Aspirin,* ✦*Asaphen, Entrophen, Novasen*) Analgesia: 325 to 650 mg PO/PR q 4 to 6 h. Platelet aggregation inhibition: 81 to 325 mg PO daily. [Generic/Trade (OTC): Tabs, 325, 500 mg; chewable 81 mg; enteric-coated 81, 162 mg (Halfprin), 81, 325, 500 mg (Ecotrin), 650, 975 mg. Trade only: Tabs, controlled-release 650, 800 mg (ZORprin, Rx). Generic only (OTC): Supps 60, 120, 200, 300, 600 mg.] ▶K ♀D ▶? $

CHOLINE MAGNESIUM TRISALICYLATE (*Trilisate*) RA/OA: 1500 mg PO two times per day. [Generic only: Tabs 500, 750, 1000 mg. Soln 500 mg/5 mL.] ▶K ♀C (D in 3rd trimester) ▶? $$

DIFLUNISAL (*Dolobid*) Pain: 500 to 1000 mg initially, then 250 to 500 mg PO q 8 to 12 h. RA/OA: 500 mg to 1 g PO divided two times per day. [Generic/Trade: Tabs 250, 500 mg.] ▶K ♀C (D in 3rd trimester) ▶– $$$ ■

SALSALATE (*Salflex, Disalcid, Amigesic*) RA/OA: 3000 mg/day PO divided q 8 to 12 h. [Generic only: Tabs 500, 750 mg, scored.] ▶K ♀C (D in 3rd trimester) ▶? $$ ■

Non-Steroidal Anti-Inflammatories—Other

ARTHROTEC (diclofenac + misoprostol) OA: One 50/200 tab PO three times per day. RA: One 50/200 tab PO three to four times per day. If intolerant, may use 50/200 or 75/200 PO two times per day. Misoprostol is an abortifacient. [Trade only: Tabs 50 mg/200 mcg, 75 mg/200 mcg, diclofenac/misoprostol.] ▶LK ♀X ▶– $$$$$ ■

DICLOFENAC (*Voltaren, Voltaren XR, Cataflam, Flector, Zipsor, Cambia,* ✦*Voltaren Rapide*) Multiple strengths; write specific product on Rx. Immediate- or delayed-release 50 mg PO two to three times per day or 75 mg PO two times per day. Extended-release (Voltaren XR): 100 to 200 mg PO daily. Patch (Flector): apply 1 patch to painful area two times per day. Gel: 2 to 4 g to affected area four times per day. Acute migraine with or without aura: 50 mg single dose (Cambia) [Generic/Trade: Tabs, immediate-release (Cataflam) 50 mg, extended-release (Voltaren XR) 100 mg. Generic only: Tabs, delayed-release 25, 50, 75 mg. Trade only: Patch (Flector) 1.3% diclofenac epolamine.

(cont.)

Topical gel (Voltaren) 1% 100 g tube. Trade only: Caps, liquid-filled (Zipsor) 25 mg. Trade only: Powder for oral soln (Cambia) 50 mg.] ▶L ♀B (D in 3rd trimester) ▶– $$$ ■

ETODOLAC Multiple strengths; write specific product on Rx. Immediate-release 200 to 400 mg PO two to three times per day. Extended-release: 400 to 1200 mg PO daily. [Generic only: Caps immediate-release 200, 300 mg, Tabs immediate-release 400, 500 mg, Tabs extended-release 400, 500, 600 mg.] ▶L ♀C (D in 3rd trimester) ▶– $$$ ■

FLURBIPROFEN (*Ansaid*) 200 to 300 mg/day PO divided two to four times per day. [Generic/Trade: Tabs immediate-release 50, 100 mg.] ▶L ♀B (D in 3rd trimester) ▶+ $$$ ■

IBUPROFEN (*Motrin, Advil, Nuprin, Rufen, NeoProfen, Caldolor*) 200 to 800 mg PO four to four times per day. Peds older than 6 mo: 5 to 10 mg/kg PO q 6 to 8 h. GI perforation and necrotizing enterocolitis has been reported with NeoProfen. [OTC: Caps/Liqui-Gel Caps 200 mg. Tabs 100, 200 mg. Chewable tabs 50, 100 mg. Susp (infant gtts) 50 mg/1.25 mL (with calibrated dropper), 100 mg/5 mL. Rx Generic/Trade: Tabs 300, 400, 600, 800 mg. Vials: 400 mg/4 mL or 800 mg/8 mL.] ▶L ♀B (D in 3rd trimester) ▶+ $ ■

INDOMETHACIN (*Indocin, Indocin SR, Indocin IV, ✦ Indocid-P.D.A.*) Multiple strengths; write specific product on Rx. Immediate-release preparations 25 to 50 mg cap PO three times per day. Sustained-release: 75 mg cap PO one to two times per day. [Generic/Trade: Caps, sustained-release 75 mg. Generic only: Caps, immediate-release 25, 50 mg. Suppository 50 mg. Trade only: Oral susp 25 mg/5 mL (237 mL).] ▶L ♀B (D in 3rd trimester) ▶+ $ ■

KETOPROFEN (*Orudis, Orudis KT, Actron, Oruvail*) Immediate-release: 25 to 75 mg PO three to four times per day. Extended-release: 100 to 200 mg cap PO daily. [OTC: Tabs, immediate-release 12.5 mg. Rx Generic only: Caps, extended-release 100, 150, 200 mg. Caps, immediate-release 25, 50, 75 mg.] ▶L ♀B (D in 3rd trimester) ▶– $$$ ■

KETOROLAC (*Toradol*) Moderately severe acute pain: 15 to 30 mg IV/IM q 6 h or 10 mg PO q 4 to 6 h prn. Combined duration IV/IM and PO is not to exceed 5 days. [Generic only: Tabs 10 mg.] ▶L ♀C (D in 3rd trimester) ▶+ $ ■

MECLOFENAMATE Mild to moderate pain: 50 mg PO q 4 to 6 h prn. Max dose 400 mg/day. Menorrhagia and primary dysmenorrhea: 100 mg PO three times per day for up to 6 days. RA/OA: 200 to 400 mg/day PO divided three to four times per day. [Generic only: Caps 50, 100 mg.] ▶L ♀B (D in 3rd trimester) ▶– $$$

MEFENAMIC ACID (*Ponstel, ✦ Ponstan*) Mild to moderate pain, primary dysmenorrhea: 500 mg PO initially, then 250 mg PO q 6 h prn for no more than 1 week. [Trade only: Caps 250 mg.] ▶L ♀D ▶– $$$$$ ■

NSAIDs—If one class fails, consider another. *Salicylic acid derivatives*: ASA, diflunisal, salsalate, Trilisate. *Propionic acids*: flurbiprofen, ibuprofen, ketoprofen, naproxen, oxaprozin. *Acetic acids*: diclofenac, etodolac, indomethacin, ketorolac, nabumetone, sulindac, tolmetin. *Fenamates*: meclofenamate. *Oxicams*: meloxicam, piroxicam. *COX-2 inhibitors*: celecoxib.

MELOXICAM (*Mobic*, ✦*Mobicox*) RA/OA: 7.5 mg PO daily. JRA age 2 yo or older: 0.125 mg/kg PO daily. [Generic/Trade: Tabs 7.5, 15 mg. Susp 7.5 mg/5 mL (1.5 mg/mL).] ▶L ♀C (D in 3rd trimester) ▶? $ ■

NABUMETONE (*Relafen*) RA/OA: Initial: Two 500 mg tabs (1000 mg) PO daily. May increase to 1500 to 2000 mg PO daily or divided two times per day. [Generic only: Tabs 500, 750 mL.] ▶L ♀C (D in 3rd trimester) ▶−$$$

NAPROXEN (*Naprosyn, Aleve, Anaprox, EC-Naprosyn, Naprelan, Prevacid, NapraPac*) Immediate-release: 250 to 500 mg PO two times per day. Delayed-release: 375 to 500 mg PO two times per day (do not crush or chew). Controlled-release: 750 to 1000 mg PO daily. JRA: give 2.5 mL PO two times per day for wt 13 kg or less, give 5 mL PO two times per day for 14 to 25 kg, give 7.5 mL PO two times per day for 26 to 38 kg. 500 mg naproxen equivalent to 550 mg naproxen sodium. [OTC Generic/Trade (Aleve): Tabs immediate-release 200 mg. OTC Trade only (Aleve): Caps, Gelcaps immediate-release 200 mg. Rx Generic/Trade: Tabs immediate-release (Naprosyn) 250, 375, 500 mg, (Anaprox) 275, 550 mg. Tabs delayed-release enteric-coated (EC-Naprosyn) 375, 500 mg. Tabs, controlled-release (Naprelan) 375, 500, 750 mg. Susp (Naprosyn) 125 mg/5 mL. Prevacid NapraPac: 7 lansoprazole 15 mg caps packaged with 14 naproxen tabs 375 mg or 500 mg.] ▶L ♀B (D in 3rd trimester) ▶+ $$$ ■

OXAPROZIN (*Daypro*) 1200 mg PO daily. [Generic/Trade: Tabs 600 mg, trade scored.] ▶L ♀C (D in 3rd trimester) ▶−$$$ ■

PIROXICAM (*Feldene, Fexicam*) 20 mg PO daily. [Generic/Trade: Caps 10, 20 mg.] ▶L ♀B (D in 3rd trimester) ▶+ $$$ ■

SULINDAC (*Clinoril*) 150 to 200 mg PO two times per day. [Generic/Trade: Tabs 200 mg. Generic only: Tabs 150 mg.] ▶L ♀B (D in 3rd trimester) ▶−$$$ ■

TOLMETIN (*Tolectin*) 200 to 600 mg PO three times per day. [Generic/Trade: Tabs 200 (trade scored), 600 mg. Caps 400 mg.] ▶L ♀C (D in 3rd trimester) ▶+ $$$$ ■

Opioid Agonist-Antagonists

BUPRENORPHINE (*Buprenex, Butrans, Subutex*) Analgesia: 0.3 to 0.6 mg IV/IM q 6 h prn. Treatment of opioid dependence (must undergo special training and be registered to prescribe for this indication): Induction 8 mg SL on day 1, 16 mg SL on day 2. Maintenance: 16 mg SL daily. Can individualize to range of 4 to 24 mg SL daily. Moderate to severe chronic pain: 5 to 20 mcg/h patch changed q 7 days. [Generic/Trade (Subutex): SL Tabs 2, 8 mg. Trade only (Butrans): transdermal patches 5, 10, 20 mcg/h.] ▶L ♀C ▶−©III $ IV, $$$$$ SL ■

BUTORPHANOL (*Stadol, Stadol NS*) 0.5 to 2 mg IV or 1 to 4 mg IM q 3 to 4 h prn. Nasal spray (Stadol NS): 1 spray (1 mg) in 1 nostril q 3 to 4 h. Abuse potential. [Generic only: Nasal spray 1 mg/spray, 2.5 mL bottle (14 to 15 doses/bottle).] ▶LK ♀C ▶+©IV $$$

NALBUPHINE (*Nubain*) 10 to 20 mg IV/IM/SC q 3 to 6 h prn. ▶LK ♀? ▶? $

PENTAZOCINE (*Talwin NX*) 30 mg IV/IM q 3 to 4 h prn (Talwin). 1 tab PO q 3 to 4 h. (Talwin NX = 50 mg pentazocine/0.5 mg naloxone). [Generic/Trade: Tabs 50 mg with 0.5 mg naloxone, trade scored.] ▶LK ♀C ▶?©IV $$$ ■

Opioid Agonists

CODEINE 0.5 to 1 mg/kg up to 15 to 60 mg PO/IM/IV/SC q 4 to 6 h. Do not use IV in children. [Generic only: Tabs 15, 30, 60 mg. Oral soln: 15 mg/5 mL.] ▶LK ♀C ▶–©II $$

FENTANYL (*Duragesic, Actiq, Fentora, Sublimaze, IONSYS*) Transdermal (Duragesic): 1 patch q 72 h (some with chronic pain may require q 48 h dosing). May wear more than 1 patch to achieve the correct analgesic effect. Transmucosal lozenge (Actiq) for breakthrough cancer pain: 200 to 1600 mcg, goal is 4 lozenges on a stick per day in conjunction with long-acting opioid. Buccal tab (Fentora) for breakthrough cancer pain: 100 to 800 mcg, titrated to pain relief. Buccal soluble film (Onsolis) for breakthrough cancer pain: 200 to 1200 mcg, titrated to pain relief. Adult analgesia/procedural sedation: 50 to 100 mcg slow IV over 1 to 2 min; carefully titrate to effect. Analgesia: 50 to 100 mcg IM q 1 to 2 h prn. [Generic/Trade: Transdermal patches 12.5, 25, 50, 75, 100 mcg/h. Actiq lozenges on a stick, berry flavored 200, 400, 600, 800, 1200, 1600 mcg. Trade only: IONSYS: Iontophoretic transdermal system: 40 mcg fentanyl per activation; max 6 doses/h. Max per system is eighty 40 mcg doses over 24 h Trade only: (Fentora) buccal tab 100, 200, 300, 400, 600, 800 mcg. Trade only: (Onsolis) buccal soluble film 200, 400, 600, 800, and 1200 mcg in child-resistant, protective foil.] ▶L ♀C ▶+©II $$$$$ ■

HYDROMORPHONE (*Dilaudid, Dilaudid-5, Exalgo, ✦ Hydromorph Contin*) Adults: 2 to 4 mg PO q 4 to 6 h. 0.5 to 2 mg IM/SC or slow IV q 4 to 6 h. 3 mg PR q 6 to 8 h. Titrate dose as high as necessary to relieve cancer or nonmalignant pain where chronic opioids are necessary. Peds age 12 yo or younger: 0.03 to 0.08 mg/kg PO q 4 to 6 h prn or give 0.015 mg/kg/dose IV q 4 to 6 h prn. Controlled-release tabs: 8 to 64 mg daily. [Generic/Trade: Tabs 2, 4, 8 mg (8 mg trade scored). Oral soln 5 mg/mL. Suppository 3 mg. Controlled-release tabs (Exalgo): 8, 12, 16 mg.] ▶L ♀C ▶?©II $$ ■

LEVORPHANOL (*Levo-Dromoran*) 2 mg PO q 6 to 8 h prn. [Generic only: Tabs 2 mg, scored.] ▶L ♀C ▶?©II $$$$

MEPERIDINE (*Demerol*, pethidine) 1 to 1.8 mg/kg up to 150 mg IM/SC/PO or slow IV q 3 to 4 h. 75 mg meperidine IV/IM/SC is equivalent to 300 mg meperidine PO. [Generic/Trade: Tabs 50 (trade scored), 100 mg. Syrup 50 mg/5 mL (trade banana flavored).] ▶LK ♀C but ▶ ▶+©II $$$

METHADONE (*Diskets, Dolophine, Methadose, ✦ Metadol*) Severe pain in opioid-tolerant patients: 2.5 to 10 mg IM/SC/PO q 3 to 4 h prn. Titrate dose as high as necessary to relieve cancer or nonmalignant pain where chronic opioids are necessary. Opioid dependence: 20 to 100 mg PO daily. Treatment

(cont.)

OPIOID EQUIVALENCY*

Opioid	PO	IV/SC/IM	Opioid	PO	IV/SC/IM
buprenorphine	n/a	0.3–0.4 mg	meperidine	300 mg	75 mg
butorphanol	n/a	2 mg	methadone	5–15 mg	2.5–10 mg
codeine	130 mg	75 mg	morphine	30 mg	10 mg
fentanyl	?	0.1 mg	nalbuphine	n/a	10 mg
hydrocodone	20 mg	n/a	oxycodone	20 mg	n/a
hydromorphone	7.5 mg	1.5 mg	oxymorphone	10 mg	1 mg
levorphanol	4 mg	2 mg	pentazocine	50 mg	30 mg

*Approximate equianalgesic doses as adapted from the 2003 American Pain Society (www.ampainsoc.org) guidelines and the 1992 AHCPR guidelines. Not available = "n/a." See drug entries themselves for starting doses. Many recommend initially using lower than equivalent doses when switching between different opioids. IV doses should be titrated slowly with appropriate monitoring. All PO dosing is with immediate-release preparations. Individualize all dosing, especially in the elderly, children, and in those with chronic pain, opioid naïve, or hepatic/renal insufficiency.

longer than 3 weeks is maintenance and only permitted in approved treatment programs. [Generic/Trade: Tabs 5, 10 mg. Dispersible tabs 40 mg (for opioid dependence only). Oral concentrate (Intensol): 10 mg/mL. Generic only: Oral soln 5, 10 mg/5 mL.] ▶L ♀C ▶?©II $ ■

MORPHINE (*MS Contin, Kadian, Avinza, Roxanol, Oramorph SR, MSIR, DepoDur, ◆ Statex, M.O.S.*) PO: start at 30 mg PO q 8 to 12 h. IM/IV: give 0.1 to 0.2 mg/kg up to 15 mg IM/SC or slow IV q 4 h. Controlled-release caps (Kadian): 20 mg PO q 12 to 24 h. Extended-release caps (Avinza): Start at 30 mg PO daily. Do not break, chew, or crush MS Contin or Oramorph SR. Kadian and Avinza caps may be opened and sprinkled in applesauce for easier administration; however, the pellets should not be crushed or chewed. Titrate dose as high as necessary to relieve cancer or nonmalignant pain where chronic opioids are necessary. [Generic/Trade: Tabs, immediate-release 15, 30 mg. Oral soln: 10 mg/5 mL, 20 mg/5 mL, 20 mg/mL (concentrate). Rectal supps 5, 10, 20, 30 mg. Controlled-release tabs (MS Contin) 15, 30, 60, 100, 200 mg. Trade only: Controlled-release caps (Kadian) 10, 20, 30, 50, 60, 80, 100, 200 mg. Controlled-release tabs (Oramorph SR) 15, 30, 60, 100 mg. Extended-release caps (Avinza) 30, 45, 60, 75, 90, 120 mg.] ▶LK ♀C ▶+©II $$$$ ■

OXYCODONE (*Roxicodone, OxyContin, Percolone, OxyIR, OxyFAST, ◆ Supeudol*) Immediate-release preparations: 5 mg PO q 4 to 6 h prn. Controlled-release (OxyContin): 10 to 40 mg PO q 12 h (no supporting data for shorter dosing intervals for controlled-release tabs). Titrate dose as high as necessary to relieve cancer or nonmalignant pain where chronic opioids are necessary. Do not break, chew, or crush controlled-release preparations. [Generic/Trade: Immediate-release: Tabs 5 mg, scored. Caps 5 mg. Tabs 15, 30 mg. Oral soln 5 mg/5 mL. Oral

(cont.)

FENTANYL TRANSDERMAL DOSE (Dosing based on ongoing morphine requirement.)

Morphine* (IV/IM)	Morphine* (PO)	Transdermal fentanyl*
10–22 mg/d	60–134 mg/d	25 mcg/h
23–37 mg/d	135–224 mg/d	50 mcg/h
38–52 mg/d	225–314 mg/d	75 mcg/h
53–67 mg/d	315–404 mg/d	100 mcg/h

*For higher morphine doses, see product insert for transdermal fentanyl equivalencies.

concentrate 20 mg/mL. Generic only: Immediate-release tabs 10, 20 mg. Trade only: Controlled-release tabs: 10, 15, 20, 30, 40, 60, 80 mg.] ▶L ♀B ▶–©II $$$$$ ■

OXYMORPHONE (*Opana*) 10 to 20 mg PO q 4 to 6 h (immediate-release) or 5 mg q 12 h (extended-release) in opioid-naive patients, 1 h before or 2 h after meals. 1 to 1.5 mg IM/SC q 4 to 6 h prn. 0.5 mg IV q 4 to 6 h prn, increase dose until pain adequately controlled. [Trade only: Extended-release tabs (Opana ER) 5, 7.5, 10, 15, 20, 30, 40 mg. Immediate-release tabs (Opana IR) 5, 10 mg.] ▶L ♀C ▶©II $$$$ ■

Opioid Analgesic Combinations

NOTE: *Refer to individual components for further information. May cause drowsiness and/or sedation, which may be enhanced by alcohol and other CNS depressants. Opioids, carisoprodol, and butalbital may be habit forming. Avoid exceeding 4 g/day of acetaminophen in combination products. Caution people who drink 3 or more alcoholic drinks/day to limit acetaminophen use to 2.5 g/day due to additive liver toxicity. Opioids commonly cause constipation; concurrent laxatives are recommended. All opioids are pregnancy class D if used for prolonged periods or in high doses at term.*

ANEXSIA (hydrocodone + acetaminophen) Multiple strengths; write specific product on Rx. 1 tab PO q 4 to 6 h prn. [Generic/Trade: Tabs 5/325, 5/500, 7.5/325, 7.5/650, 10/750 mg hydrocodone/mg acetaminophen, scored.] ▶LK ♀C ▶–©III $$

CAPITAL WITH CODEINE SUSPENSION (acetaminophen + codeine) 15 mL PO q 4 h prn. Peds: Give 5 mL q 4 to 6 h prn for age 3 to 6 yo, give 10 mL PO q 4 to 6 h prn for age 7 to 12 yo, use adult dose for age older than 12 yo. [Generic equivalent to oral soln. Trade equivalent to susp. Both codeine 12 mg and acetaminophen 120 mg per 5 mL (trade, fruit punch flavor).] ▶LK ♀C ▶?©V $

COMBUNOX (oxycodone + ibuprofen) 1 tab PO q 6 h prn for no more than 7 days. Max 4 tabs per day. [Generic/Trade: Tabs 5 mg oxycodone/ 400 mg ibuprofen.] ▶L ♀C (D in 3rd trimester) ▶?©II $$$

EMPIRIN WITH CODEINE (acetylsalicylic acid + codeine) Multiple strengths; write specific product on Rx. 1 to 2 tabs PO q 4 h prn. [Generic only: Tabs 325/30, 325/60 mg aspirin/mg codeine. Empirin brand no longer made.] ▶LK ♀D ▶–©III $

FIORICET WITH CODEINE (acetaminophen + butalbital + caffeine + codeine) 1 to 2 caps PO q 4 h prn. Max 6 caps per day. [Generic/Trade: Caps 325 mg acetaminophen/50 mg butalbital/40 mg caffeine/ 30 mg codeine.] ▶LK ♀C ▶–©III $$$

FIORINAL WITH CODEINE (acetylsalicylic acid + butalbital + caffeine + codeine, ✦ *Fiorinal C-1/4, Fiorinal C-1/2*) 1 to 2 caps PO q 4 h prn. Max 6 caps/24 h. [Generic/Trade: Caps 300 mg aspirin/50 mg butalbital/40 mg caffeine/30 mg codeine.] ▶LK ♀D ▶–©III $$$

IBUDONE (hydrocodone + ibuprofen) 1 tab PO q 4 h prn, max dose 5 tabs/day. [Generic/Trade: Tabs 5/200 mg and 10/200 mg hydrocodone/ ibuprofen.] ▶LK ♀– ▶?©III $$$

LORCET (hydrocodone + acetaminophen) 1 to 2 caps (5/500) PO q 4 to 6 h prn, max dose 8 caps/day. 1 tab PO q 4 to 6 h prn (7.5/650 and 10/650), max dose 6 tabs/day. [Generic/Trade: Caps 5/500 mg, Tabs 7.5/ 650, 10/650 mg hydrocodone/acetaminophen.] ▶LK ♀C ▶–©III $

LORTAB (hydrocodone + acetaminophen) 1 to 2 tabs (2.5/500 and 5/500) PO q 4 to 6 h prn, max dose 8 tabs/day. 1 tab (7.5/500 and 10/500 PO) q 4 to 6 h prn, max dose 5 tabs/day. Elixir 15 mL PO q 4 to 6 h prn, max 6 doses/day. [Generic/Trade: Lortab 5/500 (scored), Lortab 7.5/500 (trade scored), Lortab 10/500 mg hydrocodone/mg acetaminophen. Elixir: 7.5/500 mg hydrocodone/mg acetaminophen/15 mL. Trade only: Tabs 2.5/500 mg.] ▶LK ♀C ▶–©III $$

MAXIDONE (hydrocodone + acetaminophen) 1 tab PO q 4 to 6 h prn, max dose 5 tabs/day. [Trade only: Tabs 10/750 mg hydrocodone/mg acetaminophen.] ▶LK ♀C ▶–©III $$$

✦*MERSYNDOL WITH CODEINE* (acetaminophen + codeine + doxylamine) Canada only. 1 to 2 tabs PO q 4 to 6 h prn. Max 12 tabs per day. [Canada Trade only: OTC tab 325 mg acetaminophen/8 mg codeine phosphate/5 mg doxylamine.] ▶LK ♀C ▶? $

NORCO (hydrocodone + acetaminophen) 1 to 2 tabs PO q 4 to 6 h prn (5/325), max dose 12 tabs/day. 1 tab (7.5/325 and 10/325) PO q 4 to 6 h prn, max dose 8 and 6 tabs/day respectively. [Trade only: Tabs 5/325, 7.5/325, 10/325 mg hydrocodone/acetaminophen, scored.] ▶L ♀C ▶?©III $$$

PERCOCET (oxycodone + acetaminophen, ✦ *Percocet-demi, Oxycocet, Endocet*) Multiple strengths; write specific product on Rx. 1 to 2 tabs PO q 4 to 6 h prn (2.5/325 and 5/325). 1 tab PO q 4 to 6 h prn (7.5/500 and 10/650). [Trade only: Tabs 2.5/325 oxycodone/acetaminophen. Generic/Trade: Tabs 5/325, 7.5/325, 7.5/500, 10/325, 10/650 mg. Generic only: 2.5/300, 5/300, 7.5/300, 10/300, 2.5/400, 5/400, 7.5/400, 10/400, 10/500 mg.] ▶L ♀C ▶–©II $$

PERCODAN (oxycodone + acetylsalicylic acid, ✦ *Oxycodan, Endodan*) 1 tab PO q 6 h prn. [Generic/Trade: Tabs 4.88/325 mg oxycodone/aspirin (trade scored).] ▶LK ♀D ▶–©II $$

ROXICET (oxycodone + acetaminophen) Multiple strengths; write specific product on Rx. 1 tab PO q 6 h prn. Soln: 5 mL PO q 6 h prn. [Generic/Trade: Tabs 5/325 mg. Caps 5/500 mg. Soln 5/325 per 5 mL, mg oxycodone/acetaminophen.] ▶L ♀C ▶—©III $

SOMA COMPOUND WITH CODEINE (carisoprodol + acetylsalicylic acid + codeine) Moderate to severe musculoskeletal pain: 1 to 2 tabs PO four times per day prn. [Generic/Trade: Tabs 200 mg carisoprodol/ 325 mg aspirin/16 mg codeine.] ▶L ♀D ▶—©III $$$

SYNALGOS-DC (dihydrocodeine + acetylsalicylic acid + caffeine) 2 caps PO q 4 h prn. [Trade only: Caps 16 mg dihydrocodeine/ 356.4 mg aspirin/30 mg caffeine. "Painpack" = 12 caps.] ▶L ♀C ▶—©III $

TALACEN (pentazocine + acetaminophen) 1 tab PO q 4 h prn. [Generic/Trade: Tabs 25 mg pentazocine/ 650 mg acetaminophen, trade scored.] ▶L ♀C ▶?©IV $$$

TYLENOL WITH CODEINE (codeine + acetaminophen, ◆Atasol -8,-15,-30, Triatec) Multiple strengths; write specific product on Rx. Give 1 to 2 tabs PO q 4 h prn. Elixir: give 5 mL q 4 to 6 h prn for age 3 to 6 yo; give 10 mL q 4 to 6 h prn for age 7 to 12 yo. [Generic only: Tabs Tylenol #2 (15/300). Tylenol with Codeine Elixir 12/120 per 5 mL, mg codeine/mg acetaminophen. Generic/Trade: Tabs Tylenol #3 (30/300), Tylenol #4 (60/300).] ▶LK ♀C ▶?©III $

TYLOX (oxycodone + acetaminophen) 1 cap PO q 6 h prn. [Generic/Trade: Caps 5 mg oxycodone/500 mg acetaminophen.] ▶L ♀C ▶—©III $

VICODIN (hydrocodone + acetaminophen) 5/500 (max dose 8 tabs/day) and 7.5/750 (max dose of 5 tabs/day). 10/660: 1 tab PO q 4 to 6 h prn (max of 6 tabs/day). [Generic/Trade: Tabs Vicodin (5/500), Vicodin ES (7.5/750), Vicodin HP (10/660), scored, mg hydrocodone/mg acetaminophen.] ▶LK ♀C ▶?©III $

VICOPROFEN (hydrocodone + ibuprofen) 1 tab PO q 4 to 6 h prn, max dose 5 tabs/day. [Generic/Trade: Tabs 7.5/200 mg hydrocodone/ibuprofen. Generic only: Tabs 2.5/200, 5/200, 10/200 mg.] ▶LK ♀− ▶?©III $$$

WYGESIC (propoxyphene + acetaminophen) 1 tab PO q 4 h prn. [Generic only: Tabs 65 mg propoxyphene/ 650 mg acetaminophen.] ▶L ♀C ▶?©IV $

XODOL (hydrocodone + acetaminophen) 1 tab PO q 4 to 6 h prn, max 6 doses/day. [Trade only: Tabs 5/300, 7.5/300, 10/300 mg hydrocodone/acetaminophen.] ▶LK ♀C ▶—©III $$

ZYDONE (hydrocodone + acetaminophen) 1 to 2 tabs (5/400) PO q 4 to 6 h prn, max dose 8 tabs/day. 1 tab (7.5/400, 10/400) q 4 to 6 h prn, max dose 6 tabs/day. [Trade only: Tabs 5/400, 7.5/400, 10/400 mg hydrocodone/mg acetaminophen.] ▶LK ♀C ▶?©III $$

Opioid Antagonists

NALOXONE (Narcan) Adult opioid overdose: 0.4 to 2 mg IV/IM/SC q 2 to 3 min prn. Adult post-op reversal: 0.1 to 0.2 mg IV/IM/SC q 2 to 3 min prn. Peds opioid overdose: 0.01 mg/kg IV; may give 0.1 mg/kg if inadequate response. Peds post-op reversal: 0.005 to 0.01 mg q 2 to 3 min prn. May use IM/SC/ET if IV not available. ▶LK ♀B ▶? $

Other Analgesics

ACETAMINOPHEN (*Tylenol, Panadol, Tempra, Ofirmev,* paracetamol, *◆ Abenol, Atasol, Pediatrix*) 325 to 650 mg PO/PR q 4 to 6 h prn. Max dose 4 g/day. Adults and adolescents wt less than 50 kg, give 15 mg/kg IV q 6 h or 12.5 mg/kg IV q 4 h. Max dose 75 mg/kg/day. Adults and adolescents wt 50 kg or greater, give 1000 mg IV q 6 h or 650 mg IV q 4 h. Max dose 4 g/day. <u>OA</u>: 2 extended-release caps (ie, 1300 mg) PO q 8 h around the clock. Peds: 10 to 15 mg/kg/dose PO/PR q 4 to 6 h prn. Children age 2 to 12 yo, give 15 mg/kg IV q 6 h or 12.5 mg/kg q 4 h. Max dose 75 mg/kg/day. [OTC: Tabs 325, 500, 650 mg. Chewable Tabs 80 mg. Oral disintegrating Tabs 80, 160 mg. Caps/gelcaps 500 mg. Extended-release caps 650 mg. Liquid 160 mg/5 mL, 500 mg/15 mL. Infant gtts 80 mg/0.8 mL. Supps 80, 120, 325, 650 mg.] ▶LK ♀B ▶+ $
TAPENTADOL (*Nucynta*) <u>Moderate to severe acute pain</u>: 50 to 100 mg PO q 4 to 6 h prn, max 600 mg/day. Adjust dose in elderly, renal, and hepatic dysfunction. Avoid in opioid-dependent patients. Seizures may occur with concurrent antidepressants or seizure disorder. [Trade only: Tabs 50, 75, 100 mg.] ▶LK ♀C ▶–©II $$$$
TRAMADOL (*Ultram, Ultram ER, Ryzolt*) <u>Moderate to moderately severe pain</u>: 50 to 100 mg PO q 4 to 6 h prn, max 400 mg/day. <u>Chronic pain, extended-release</u>: 100 to 300 mg PO daily. Adjust dose in elderly, renal, and hepatic dysfunction. Avoid in opioid-dependent patients. Seizures may occur with concurrent serotonergic agents or seizure disorder. [Generic/Trade: Tabs, immediate-release 50 mg. Trade only (Ultram ER, Ryzolt): Extended-release tabs 100, 200, 300 mg.] ▶KL ♀C ▶– $$$
WOMEN'S TYLENOL MENSTRUAL RELIEF (acetaminophen + pamabrom) 2 caps PO q 4 to 6 h. [OTC: Caps 500 mg acetaminophen/ 25 mg pamabrom (diuretic).] ▶LK ♀B ▶+ $

ANESTHESIA

Anesthetics and Sedatives

DEXMEDETOMIDINE (*Precedex*) <u>ICU sedation less than 24 h</u>: Load 1 mcg/kg over 10 min followed by infusion 0.2 to 0.7 mcg/kg/h titrated to desired sedation endpoint. Beware of bradycardia and hypotension. ▶LK ♀C ▶? $$$$
ETOMIDATE (*Amidate*) <u>Induction</u>: 0.2 to 0.6 mg/kg IV. ▶L ♀C ▶? $
FOSPROPOFOL (*Lusedra*) Initial dose 6.5 mg/kg IV (not to exceed 16.5 mL), then give 1.6 mg/kg supplemental dose q 4 min (not to exceed 4 mL). ▶L ♀– ▶? $$$$
KETAMINE (*Ketalar*) 1 to 2 mg/kg IV over 1 to 2 min or 4 mg/kg IM induces 10 to 20 min dissociative state. Concurrent atropine minimizes hypersalivation. ▶L ♀? ▶?©III $
METHOHEXITAL (*Brevital*) <u>Induction</u>: give 1 to 1.5 mg/kg IV, duration 5 min. ▶L ♀B ▶?©IV $

MIDAZOLAM (***Versed***) Adult sedation/anxiolysis: 5 mg or 0.07 mg/kg IM; or 1 mg IV slowly q 2 to 3 min up to 5 mg. Peds: 0.25 to 1 mg/kg to max of 20 mg PO, or 0.1 to 0.15 mg/kg IM. IV route (6 mo to 5 yo): initial dose 0.05 to 0.1 mg/kg IV, then titrated to max 0.6 mg/kg. IV route (6 to 12 yo): initial dose 0.025 to 0.05 mg/kg IV, then titrated to max 0.4 mg/kg. Monitor for respiratory depression. [Generic only: Oral liquid 2 mg/mL.] ▶LK ♀D ▶─©IV $

PENTOBARBITAL (***Nembutal***) Pediatric sedation: 1 to 6 mg/kg IV, adjusted in increments of 1 to 2 mg/kg to desired effect, or 2 to 6 mg/kg IM, max 100 mg. ▶LK ♀D ▶?©II $$

PROPOFOL (***Diprivan***) Induction dose: 20 to 40 mg IV q 10 sec until induction (2 to 2.5 mg/kg). ICU ventilator sedation: Infusion 5 to 50 mcg/kg/min. Deep sedation: 1 mg/kg IV over 20 to 30 seconds. Repeat 0.5 mg/kg IV prn. ▶L ♀B ▶─ $$$

Local Anesthetics

ARTICAINE (***Septocaine, Zorcaine***) 4% injection (includes epinephrine). [4% (includes epinephrine 1:100,000).] ▶LK ♀C ▶? $

BUPIVACAINE (***Marcaine, Sensorcaine***) Local and regional anesthesia. [0.25%, 0.5%, 0.75%, all with or without epinephrine.] ▶LK ♀C ▶? $

CETACAINE (**benzocaine + tetracaine + butamben**) Topical anesthetic of mucous membranes: Spray: Apply for no more than 1 sec. Liquid or gel: Apply with cotton applicator directly to site. [Trade only: (14%/2%/2%) Spray 56 mL. Topical liquid 56 mL. Topical gel 5, 29 g.] ▶LK ♀C ▶? $$

DUOCAINE (**bupivacaine + lidocaine—local anesthetic**) Local anesthesia, nerve block for eye surgery. [Vials contain bupivacaine 0.375% + lidocaine 1%.] ▶LK ♀C ▶? $

LIDOCAINE—LOCAL ANESTHETIC (***Xylocaine***) 0.5 to 1% injection with and without epinephrine. [0.5, 1, 1.5, 2%. With epi: 0.5, 1, 1.5, 2%.] ▶LK ♀B ▶? $

MEPIVACAINE (***Carbocaine, Polocaine***) 1 to 2% injection. [1, 1.5, 2, 3%.] ▶LK ♀C ▶? $

Neuromuscular Blockers

CISATRACURIUM (***Nimbex***) Paralysis: 0.15 to 0.2 mg/kg IV. Peds: 0.1 mg/kg. Duration 30 to 60 min. ▶Plasma ♀B ▶? $$

ROCURONIUM (***Zemuron***) Paralysis: 0.6 mg/kg IV. Duration 30 min. ▶L ♀B ▶? $$

SUCCINYLCHOLINE (***Anectine, Quelicin***) Paralysis: 0.6 to 1.1 mg/kg IV. Peds. 2 mg/kg IV. ▶Plasma ♀C ▶? $

VECURONIUM (***Norcuron***) Paralysis: 0.08 to 0.1 mg/kg IV. Duration 15 to 30 min. ▶LK ♀C ▶? $

ANTIMICROBIALS

Aminoglycosides

NOTE: *See also dermatology and ophthalmology. Can cause nephrotoxicity, ototoxicity.*

AMIKACIN 15 mg/kg/day (up to 1500 mg/day) IM/IV divided q 8 to 12 h. Peak 20 to 35 mcg/mL, trough < 5 mcg/mL. Alternative 15 mg/kg IV q 24 h. ▶K ♀D ▶? $$$ ∎

GENTAMICIN   Adults: 3 to 5 mg/kg/day IM/IV divided q 8 h. Peak 5 to 10 mcg/mL, trough < 2 mcg/mL. Alternative 5 to 7 mg/kg IV q 24 h. Peds: 2 to 2.5 mg/kg q 8 h. ▶K ♀D ▶+ $ ■

STREPTOMYCIN   Combo therapy for TB: 15 mg/kg (up to 1 g) IM daily. 10 mg/kg (up to 750 mg) for age 60 yo or older. Peds: 20 to 40 mg/kg (up to 1 g) IM daily. ▶K ♀D ▶+ $$$$$ ■

TOBRAMYCIN   *(TOBI)*   Adults: 3 to 5 mg/kg/day IM/IV divided q 8 h. Peak 5 to 10 mcg/mL, trough < 2 mcg/mL. Alternative 5 to 7 mg/kg IV q 24 h. Peds: 2 to 2.5 mg/kg q 8 h. Cystic fibrosis (TOBI): 300 mg nebulized two times per day 28 days on, then 28 days off. [Trade only: TOBI 300 mg ampules for nebulizer.] ▶K ♀D ▶? $$ ■

Antifungal Agents—Azoles

CLOTRIMAZOLE   *(Mycelex)*   Oral troches 5 times per day for 14 days. [Generic/Trade: Oral troches 10 mg.] ▶L ♀C ▶? $$$$

FLUCONAZOLE   *(Diflucan)*   Vaginal candidiasis: 150 mg PO single dose ($). All other dosing regimens IV/PO. Oropharyngeal candidiasis: 100 to 200 mg daily for 7 to 14 days. Esophageal candidiasis: 200 to 400 mg daily for 14 to 21 days. Candidemia: 800 mg on first day, then 400 mg daily. Cryptococcal meningitis in AIDS: 400 mg daily for 8 weeks, then 200 mg daily until immune reconstitution. Peds: Oropharyngeal candidiasis: 6 mg/kg on first day, then 3 mg/kg daily for 7 to 14 days. Esophageal candidiasis: 12 mg/kg on first day, then 6 mg/kg daily for 14 to 21 days. Systemic candidiasis; cryptococcal meningitis in AIDS: 12 mg/kg on first day, then 6 to 12 mg/kg daily. [Generic/Trade: Tabs 50, 100, 150, 200 mg. 150 mg tab in single-dose blister pack. Susp 10, 40 mg/mL (35 mL).] ▶K ♀C ▶+ $$$$

ITRACONAZOLE   *(Onmel, Sporanox)*   Oral caps for onychomycosis "pulse dosing": 200 mg PO two times per day for 1st week of month for 2 months (fingernails) or 3 to 4 months (toenails). Standard regimen, toenail onychomycosis: 200 mg PO daily with full meal for 12 weeks. Fluconazole-refractory oropharyngeal or esophageal candidiasis: Oral soln 200 mg PO daily for 14 to 21 days. CYP3A4 inhibitor. Contraindicated with dofetilide, ergot alkaloids, lovastatin, PO midazolam, pimozide, quinidine, simvastatin, triazolam. Negative inotrope; do not use for onychomycosis if ventricular dysfunction. [Trade: Tabs 200 mg. Oral soln 10 mg/mL (150 mL). Generic/Trade: Caps 100 mg.] ▶L ♀C ▶– $$$$$ ■

KETOCONAZOLE   *(Nizoral)*   200 to 400 mg PO daily. Hepatotoxicity. CYP3A4 inhibitor. Contraindicated with midazolam, pimozide, triazolam. H2 blockers, proton pump inhibitors, antacids impair absorption. [Generic/Trade: Tabs 200 mg.] ▶L ♀C ▶?+ $$$ ■

MICONAZOLE—BUCCAL   *(Oravig)*   Oropharyngeal candidiasis: Apply 50 mg buccal tab to gums once daily for 14 days. Increased INR with warfarin. [Trade: Buccal tabs, 50 mg.] ▶L ♀C ▶? $$$$$

POSACONAZOLE   *(Noxafil)*   Prevention of invasive Aspergillus or Candida infection, age 13 yo or older: 200 mg (5 mL) PO three times per day.

(cont.)

Oropharyngeal candidiasis, age 13 yo or older: 100 mg (2.5 mL) PO two times on day 1, then 100 mg PO once daily for 13 days. Oropharyngeal candidiasis resistant to itraconazole/fluconazole, age 13 yo or older: 400 mg (10 mL) PO two times per day. Take with full meal or liquid nutritional supplement. CYP3A4 inhibitor. [Trade only: Oral susp 40 mg/mL, 105 mL bottle.] ▶Glucuronidation ♀C ▶– $$$$$

VORICONAZOLE (*Vfend*) Aspergillosis, systemic Candida infections: 6 mg/kg IV q 12 h for 2 doses, then 3 to 4 mg/kg IV q 12 h (use 4 mg/kg for aspergillosis). Esophageal candidiasis or maintenance therapy of aspergillosis/candidiasis: 200 mg PO two times per day. For wt less than 40 kg, reduce to 100 mg PO two times per day. Dosage adjustment for efavirenz: Voriconazole 400 mg PO two times per day with efavirenz 300 mg PO once daily (use caps). Peds younger than 12 yo: 7 mg/kg IV q 12 h. Infuse IV over 2 h. Take tabs and/or susp 1 h before or after meals. CYP3A4 inhibitor. Many drug interactions. [Trade only: Tabs 50, 200 mg (contains lactose). Susp 40 mg/mL (75 mL).] ▶L ♀D ▶? $$$$$

Antifungal Agents—Echinocandins

ANIDULAFUNGIN (*Eraxis*) Candidemia: 200 mg IV load on day 1, then 100 mg IV once daily. Esophageal candidiasis: 100 mg IV load on day 1, then 50 mg IV once daily. Max infusion rate of 1.1 mg/min to prevent histamine reactions. ▶Degraded chemically ♀C ▶? $$$$$

CASPOFUNGIN (*Cancidas*) Infuse over 1 h, give 70 mg IV loading dose on day 1, then 50 mg once daily. Peds: 70 mg/m² IV loading dose on day 1, then 50 mg/m² once daily (max of 70 mg/day). ▶KL ♀C ▶? $$$$$

MICAFUNGIN (*Mycamine*) Infuse IV over 1 h. Esophageal candidiasis: 150 mg once daily. Prevention of candidal infections in bone marrow transplant patients: 50 mg once daily. Candidemia, acute disseminated candidiasis, Candida peritonitis/abscess: 100 mg once daily. ▶L, feces ♀C ▶? $$$$$

Antifungal Agents—Polyenes

AMPHOTERICIN B DEOXYCHOLATE (*Fungizone*) Test dose 0.1 mg/kg up to 1 mg slow IV. Wait 2 to 4 h, and if tolerated then begin 0.25 mg/kg IV daily and advance to 0.5 to 1.5 mg/kg/day depending on fungal type. Maximum dose 1.5 mg/kg/day. ▶Tissues ♀B ▶? $$$$ ■

AMPHOTERICIN B LIPID FORMULATIONS (*Abelcet, AmBisome, Amphotec*) Abelcet: 5 mg/kg/day IV at 2.5 mg/kg/h. AmBisome: 3 to 5 mg/kg/day IV over 2 h. Amphotec: Test dose of 10 mL over 15 to 30 min, observe for 30 min, then 3 to 4 mg/kg/day IV at 1 mg/kg/h. ▶? ♀B ▶? $$$$$

Antifungal Agents—Other

FLUCYTOSINE (*Ancobon*) 50 to 150 mg/kg/day PO divided four times per day. Myelosuppression. [Trade only: Caps 250, 500 mg.] ▶K ♀C ▶– $$$$$ ■

GRISEOFULVIN (*Grifulvin V*) <u>Tinea capitis</u>: 500 mg PO daily in adults; 15 to 20 mg/kg (up to 1 g) PO daily in peds. Treat for 4 to 6 weeks, continuing for 2 weeks past symptom resolution. [Generic/Trade: Susp 125 mg/5 mL (120 mL). Trade only: Tabs 250, 500 mg.] ▶Skin ♀C ▶? $$$$

NYSTATIN (✦ *Nilstat*) <u>Thrush</u>: 4 to 6 mL PO, swish and swallow four times per day. Infants: 2 mL/dose with 1 mL in each cheek four times per day. [Generic only: Susp 100,000 units/mL (60, 480 mL). Troches 500,000 units/tab.] ▶Not absorbed ♀B ▶? $$

TERBINAFINE (*Lamisil*) <u>Onychomycosis</u>: 250 mg PO daily for 6 weeks to treat <u>fingernails</u>, for 12 weeks to treat <u>toenails</u>. <u>Tinea capitis</u>, age 4 yo or older: Give granules PO once daily with food for 6 weeks: 125 mg for wt less than 25 kg, 187.5 mg for wt 25 to 35 kg, 250 mg for wt more than 35 kg. [Generic/Trade: Tabs 250 mg. Trade only: Oral granules 125, 187.5 mg/packet.] ▶LK ♀B ▶–$

Antimalarials

NOTE: *For help treating malaria or getting antimalarials, see www.cdc.gov/ malaria or call the CDC "malaria hotline" (770) 488-7788 Monday-Friday 9 am to 5 pm EST; after hours/weekend (770) 488-7100. Pediatric doses of antimalarials should never exceed adult doses.*

CHLOROQUINE (*Aralen*) <u>Malaria prophylaxis, chloroquine-sensitive areas</u>: 8 mg/kg up to 500 mg PO q week starting 1 to 2 weeks before exposure to 4 weeks after exposure. Chloroquine resistance is widespread. Can prolong QT interval and cause torsades de pointes. [Generic only: Tabs 250 mg. Generic/Trade: Tabs 500 mg (500 mg phosphate equivalent to 300 mg base).] ▶KL ♀C but + ▶+ $ ■

COARTEM (artemether + lumefantrine, *coartemether*) <u>Uncomplicated malaria</u>: Take PO with food two times per day for 3 days. On day 1, give 2nd dose 8 h after 1st dose. Dose based on wt: 1 tab for 5 to 14 kg; 2 tabs for 15 to 24 kg; 3 tabs for 25 to 34 kg; 4 tabs for 35 kg or greater. Repeat dose if vomiting occurs within 1 to 2 h. Can prolong QT interval. [Trade only: Tabs, artemether 20 mg + lumefantrine 120 mg.] ▶L ♀C ▶? $$$

MALARONE (atovaquone + proguanil) <u>Prevention of malaria</u>: Give the following dose PO once daily from 1 to 2 days before exposure until 7 days after. Dose based on wt: ½ ped tab for wt 5 to 8 kg; ¾ ped tab for wt 9 to 10 kg; 1 ped tab for wt 11 to 20 kg; 2 ped tabs for 21 to 30 kg; 3 ped tabs for 31 to 40 kg; 1 adult tab for all patients wt greater than 40 kg. <u>Treatment of malaria</u>: Give the following dose PO once daily for 3 days. Dose based on wt: 2 ped tabs for 5 to 8 kg; 3 ped tabs for 9 to 10 kg; 1 adult tab for 11 to 20 kg; 2 adult tabs for 21 to 30 kg; 3 adult tabs for 31 to 40 kg; 4 adult tabs for all patients wt greater than 40 kg. Take with food or milky drink. [Generic/Trade: Adult tabs atovaquone 250 mg + proguanil 100 mg. Trade only: Pediatric tabs 62.5 mg + 25 mg.] ▶Fecal excretion; LK ♀C ▶? $$$$$

MEFLOQUINE <u>Malaria prophylaxis for chloroquine-resistant areas</u>: 250 mg PO once a week from 1 week before exposure to 4 weeks after. Treatment: 1250 mg PO single dose. <u>Peds malaria prophylaxis</u>: Give the following dose PO once a

(cont.)

week starting 1 week before exposure to 4 weeks after: Dose based on wt: 5 mg/kg (prepared by pharmacist) for wt 9 kg or less; ¼ tab for wt greater than 9 kg to 19 kg; ½ tab for wt greater than 19 kg to 30 kg; ¾ tab for wt greater than 30 to 45 kg; 1 tab for wt 45 kg or greater. Peds treatment: 20 to 25 mg/kg PO single dose or divided into 2 doses given 6 to 8 h apart. Take on full stomach. [Generic only: Tabs 250 mg.] ▶L ♀C ▶? $$

PRIMAQUINE Prevention of relapse, P. vivax/ovale malaria: 0.5 mg/kg (up to 30 mg) base PO daily for 14 days. Do not use unless normal G6PD level. [Generic only: Tabs 26.3 mg (equiv to 15 mg base).] ▶L ♀– ▶– $$ ■

QUININE (*Qualaquin*) Malaria: 648 mg PO three times per day. Peds: 25 to 30 mg/kg/day (up to 2 g/day) PO divided q 8 h. Treat for 3 days (Africa/South America) or 7 days (Southeast Asia). Also give 7-day course of doxycycline, tetracycline, or clindamycin. Nocturnal leg cramps: 325 mg PO at bedtime. FDA warns that risks exceed potential benefit for this indication. Can cause life-threatening adverse effects: Cinchonism with overdose; hemolysis with G6PD deficiency; hypersensitivity; thrombocytopenia; HUS/TTP; QT interval prolongation; many drug interactions. [Trade only: Caps 324 mg.] ▶L ♀C ▶+? $$$$ ■

Antimycobacterial Agents

NOTE: *Treat active mycobacterial infection with at least 2 drugs. See guidelines at www.thoracic.org/statements/index.php and www.aidsinfo.nih.gov.*

DAPSONE (*Aczone*) Pneumocystis prophylaxis, leprosy: 100 mg PO daily. Pneumocystis treatment: 100 mg PO daily with trimethoprim 5 mg/kg PO three times per day for 21 days. Acne (Aczone; $$$$): Apply two times per day. [Generic only: Tabs 25, 100 mg. Trade only (Aczone): Topical gel 5% 30 or 60 g.] ▶LK ♀C ▶– $

ETHAMBUTOL (*Myambutol*, ✦ *Etibi*) 15 to 20 mg/kg PO daily. Dose with whole tabs: Give 800 mg PO daily for wt 40 to 55 kg, 1200 mg for wt 56 to 75 kg, 1600 mg for wt 76 to 90 kg. Base dose on estimated lean body wt. Peds: 15 to 20 mg/kg (up to 1 g) PO daily. [Generic/Trade: Tabs 100, 400 mg.] ▶LK ♀C but ▶+ $$$$

ISONIAZID (*INH*) Adults: 5 mg/kg (up to 300 mg) PO daily. Peds: 10 to 15 mg/kg (up to 300 mg) PO daily. Hepatotoxicity. Consider supplemental pyridoxine up to 50 mg per day to prevent neuropathy. [Generic only: Tabs 100, 300 mg. Syrup 50 mg/5 mL.] ▶LK ♀C but ▶+ $ ■

PYRAZINAMIDE (*PZA*) 20 to 25 mg/kg (up to 2000 mg) PO daily. Dose with whole tabs: Give 1000 mg PO daily for wt 40 to 55 kg, 1500 mg for wt 56 to 75 kg, 2000 mg for wt 76 to 90 kg. Base dose on estimated lean body wt. Peds: 15 to 30 mg/kg (up to 2000 mg) PO daily. Hepatotoxicity. [Generic only: Tabs 500 mg.] ▶LK ♀C ▶? $$$$ ■

RIFABUTIN (*Mycobutin*) 300 mg PO daily or 150 mg PO two times per day. Dosage reduction required with protease inhibitors. [Trade only: Caps 150 mg.] ▶L ♀B ▶? $$$$$

RIFAMATE (isoniazid + rifampin) 2 caps PO daily on empty stomach. [Generic/Trade: Caps isoniazid 150 mg + rifampin 300 mg.] ▶LK ♀C but ▶+ $$$$ ■

RIFAMPIN (*Rifadin*, ✦ *Rofact*) <u>TB</u>: 10 mg/kg (up to 600 mg) PO/IV daily. Peds: 10 to 20 mg/kg (up to 600 mg) PO/IV daily. <u>Neisseria meningitidis carriers</u>: 600 mg PO two times per day for 2 days. Peds: Age 1 mo or older: 10 mg/kg (up to 600 mg) two times per day for 2 days. Age younger than 1 mo: 5 mg/kg PO two times per day for 2 days. IV and PO doses are the same. Take oral doses on empty stomach. [Generic/Trade: Caps 150, 300 mg. Pharmacists can make oral susp.] ▶L ♀C but +▶+ $$$ ■

RIFAPENTINE (*Priftin*) <u>TB</u>: 600 mg PO two times per week for 2 months, then once a week for 4 months. Use for continuation therapy only in selected HIV-negative patients. [Trade only: Tabs 150 mg.] ▶Esterases, fecal ♀C ▶? $$$$

RIFATER (**isoniazid + rifampin + pyrazinamide**) <u>TB</u>: 4 tabs daily for wt less than 45 kg, 5 tabs daily for wt 45 to 54 kg, 6 tabs daily for wt 55 kg or greater. [Trade only: Tabs isoniazid 50 mg + rifampin 120 mg + pyrazinamide 300 mg.] ▶LK ♀C ▶? $$$$$ ■

Antiparasitics

ALBENDAZOLE (*Albenza*) <u>Hydatid disease, neurocysticercosis</u>: 15 mg/kg/day (up to 800 mg/day) PO divided in two doses for wt less than 60 kg; 400 mg PO two times per day for wt 60 kg or greater. [Trade only: Tabs 200 mg.] ▶L ♀C ▶? $$$

ATOVAQUONE (*Mepron*) <u>Pneumocystis treatment</u>: 750 mg PO two times per day for 21 days. <u>Pneumocystis prevention</u>: 1500 mg PO daily. Take with meals. [Trade only: Susp 750 mg/5 mL (210 mL), foil pouch 750 mg/5 mL (5, 10 mL).] ▶Fecal ♀C ▶? $$$$$

IVERMECTIN (*Stromectol*) Single PO dose of 200 mcg/kg for <u>strongyloidiasis</u>, 200 mcg/kg for <u>scabies</u> (may need to repeat dose in 10 to 14 days), 150 mcg/kg for <u>onchocerciasis</u>. <u>Peds head lice</u>: 200 to 400 mcg/kg PO single dose; repeat in 7 days. Not for children less than 15 kg. Take on empty stomach with water. [Trade only: Tabs 3 mg.] ▶L ♀C ▶? $$

MEBENDAZOLE (*Vermox*) <u>Pinworm</u>: 100 mg PO once; repeat in 2 weeks. <u>Roundworm, whipworm, hookworm</u>: 100 mg PO two times per day for 3 days. [Generic only: Chewable tabs 100 mg.] ▶L ♀C ▶? $$$

NITAZOXANIDE (*Alinia*) <u>Cryptosporidial or Giardial diarrhea</u>: 100 mg two times per day for age 1 to 3 yo, 200 mg two times per day for 4 to 11 yo, 500 mg two times per day for adults and children 12 yo or older. Give PO with food for 3 days. Use susp if less than 12 yo. [Trade only: Oral susp 100 mg/5 mL, 60 mL bottle. Tabs 500 mg.] ▶L ♀B ▶? $$$$

PAROMOMYCIN 25 to 35 mg/kg/day PO divided three times per day with or after meals. [Generic only: Caps 250 mg.] ▶Not absorbed ♀C ▶– $$$$

PENTAMIDINE (*Pentam, NebuPent*) <u>Pneumocystis treatment</u>: 4 mg/kg IM/IV daily for 21 days. <u>Pneumocystis prevention</u>: 300 mg nebulized q 4 weeks. [Trade only: Aerosol 300 mg.] ▶K ♀C ▶– $$$

PRAZIQUANTEL (*Biltricide*) <u>Schistosomiasis</u>: 20 mg/kg PO q 4 to 6 h for 3 doses. [Trade only: Tabs 600 mg.] ▶LK ♀B ▶– $$$

PYRANTEL (*Pin-X, Pinworm*, ✦ *Combantrin*) <u>Pinworm, roundworm</u>: 11 mg/kg (up to 1 g) PO single dose. Repeat in 2 weeks for pinworm. [OTC Trade

(cont.)

only (Pin-X): Susp 144 mg/mL (equivalent to 50 mg/mL of pyrantel base) 30, 60 mL. Tabs 720.5 mg (equivalent to 250 mg of pyrantel base). OTC Generic only: Caps 180 mg (equivalent to 62.5 mg of pyrantel base).] ▶Not absorbed ♀–▶? $

PYRIMETHAMINE (*Daraprim*) <u>CNS toxoplasmosis in AIDS.</u> Acute therapy: First dose 200 mg PO, then 50 mg PO daily for wt less than 60 kg; use 75 mg PO once daily for 60 kg or greater. Treat for at least 6 weeks with pyrimethamine + sulfadiazine + leucovorin 10 to 25 mg PO once daily (can increase leucovorin to 50 mg/day). <u>Secondary prevention:</u> Pyrimethamine 25 to 50 mg PO once daily + sulfadiazine + leucovorin 10 to 25 mg PO once daily. [Trade only: Tabs 25 mg.] ▶L ♀C ▶+ $$

TINIDAZOLE (*Tindamax*) Adults: 2 g PO daily for 1 day for <u>trichomoniasis</u> or <u>giardiasis</u>, for 3 days for <u>amebiasis.</u> <u>Bacterial vaginosis:</u> 2 g PO once daily for 2 days or 1 g PO once daily for 5 days. Peds, age older than 3 yo: 50 mg/kg (up to 2 g) PO daily for 1 day for <u>giardiasis</u>, for 3 days for <u>amebiasis.</u> Take with food. [Trade only: Tabs 250, 500 mg. Pharmacists can compound oral susp.] ▶KL ♀C ▶?- $ ■

Antiviral Agents—Anti-CMV

CIDOFOVIR (*Vistide*) <u>CMV retinitis in AIDS:</u> 5 mg/kg IV once a week for 2 weeks, then 5 mg/kg every 2 weeks. Severe nephrotoxicity. ▶K ♀C ▶– $$$$$ ■

FOSCARNET <u>CMV retinitis:</u> 60 mg/kg IV (over 1 h) q 8 h or 90 mg/kg IV (over 1.5 to 2 h) q 12 h for 2 to 3 weeks, then 90 to 120 mg/kg IV daily over 2 h. HSV infection: 40 mg/kg (over 1 h) q 8 to 12 h. Nephrotoxicity, seizures. ▶K ♀C ▶? $$$$$ ■

GANCICLOVIR (*Cytovene*) <u>CMV retinitis:</u> Induction 5 mg/kg IV q 12 h for 14 to 21 days. Maintenance 6 mg/kg IV daily for 5 days per week. Myelosuppression. Potential carcinogen, teratogen. May impair fertility. [Generic only: Caps 250, 500 mg.] ▶K ♀C ▶– $$$$$ ■

VALGANCICLOVIR (*Valcyte*) <u>CMV retinitis.</u> 900 mg PO two times per day for 21 days, then 900 mg PO daily. <u>Prevention of CMV disease in high-risk transplant patients:</u> 900 mg PO daily given within 10 days post-transplant until 100 days post-transplant for heart or kidney and/or pancreas or 200 days for kidney transplant. See package insert for peds dose. Greater bioavailability than oral ganciclovir. Give with food. Impaired fertility, myelosuppression, potential carcinogen and teratogen. [Trade only: Tabs 450 mg. Oral soln 50 mg/mL.] ▶K ♀C ▶– $$$$$ ■

Antiviral Agents—Anti-Herpetic

ACYCLOVIR (*Zovirax*) <u>Genital herpes:</u> 400 mg PO three times per day for 7 to 10 days for first episode, or for 5 days for recurrent episodes. <u>Chronic suppression of genital herpes:</u> 400 mg PO two times per day; in HIV infection use 400 to 800 mg PO two to three times per day. <u>Zoster:</u> 800 mg PO five times

(cont.)

per day for 7 to 10 days. <u>Chickenpox:</u> 20 mg/kg (up to 800 mg) PO four times per day for 5 days. Adult IV: 5 to 10 mg/kg IV q 8 h, each dose over 1 h. <u>Herpes encephalitis:</u> 20 mg/kg IV q 8 h for 10 days for age 3 mo to 12 yo; 10 mg/kg IV q 8 h for 10 days for age 12 yo or older. <u>Neonatal herpes:</u> 20 mg/kg IV q 8 h for 21 days for disseminated/CNS disease, for 14 days for skin/mucous membrane infections. [Generic/Trade: Caps 200 mg. Tabs 400, 800 mg. Susp 200 mg/5 mL.] ▶K ♀B ▶+ $

FAMCICLOVIR (*Famvir*) <u>First episode genital herpes:</u> 250 mg PO three times per day for 7 to 10 days. <u>Recurrent genital herpes:</u> 1000 mg PO two times per day for 2 days; give 500 mg two times per day for 7 days if HIV infected. <u>Chronic suppression of genital herpes:</u> 250 mg PO two times per day; 500 mg PO two times per day if HIV infected. <u>Recurrent herpes labialis:</u> 1500 mg PO single dose; 500 mg two times per day for 7 days if HIV-infected. <u>Zoster:</u> 500 mg PO three times per day for 7 days. [Generic/Trade: Tabs 125, 250, 500 mg.] ▶K ♀B ▶? $$

VALACYCLOVIR (*Valtrex*) <u>First episode genital herpes:</u> 1 g PO two times per day for 10 days. <u>Recurrent genital herpes:</u> 500 mg PO two times per day for 3 days; if HIV infected give 1 g PO two times per day for 5 to 10 days. <u>Chronic suppression of genital herpes:</u> 500 to 1000 mg PO daily; if HIV infected give 500 mg PO two times per day. <u>Reduction of genital herpes transmission</u> in immunocompetent patients with no more than 9 recurrences per year: 500 mg PO daily for source partner, in conjunction with safer sex practices. <u>Herpes labialis,</u> age 12 yo or older: 2 g PO q 12 h for 2 doses. <u>Zoster:</u> 1000 mg PO three times per day for 7 days. <u>Chickenpox,</u> age 2 to 18 yo: 20 mg/kg (max of 1 g) PO three times per day for 5 days. [Generic/Trade: Tabs 500, 1000 mg.] ▶K ♀B ▶+ $$$$$

Antiviral Agents—Anti-HIV—CCR5 Antagonists

MARAVIROC (*Selzentry, MVC*) 150 mg PO two times per day with strong CYP3A4 inhibitors (most protease inhibitors, ketoconazole, itraconazole, clarithromycin); 300 mg PO two times per day with drugs that are not strong CYP3A4 inducers/inhibitors (NRTIs, tipranavir-ritonavir, nevirapine, raltegravir; rifabutin without a strong CYP3A4 inhibitor or inducer); 600 mg PO two times per day with strong CYP3A4 inducers (efavirenz, etravirine, rifampin, carbamazepine, phenobarbital, phenytoin). Tropism test before treatment; not for dual/mixed or CXCR4-tropic HIV infection. Hepatotoxicity with allergic features. [Trade only: Tabs 150, 300 mg.] ▶LK ♀B ▶− $$$$$ ■

Antiviral Agents—Anti-HIV—Combinations

ATRIPLA (*efavirenz + emtricitabine + tenofovir*) 1 tab PO once daily on empty stomach, preferably at bedtime. [Trade only: Tabs efavirenz 600 mg + emtricitabine 200 mg + tenofovir 300 mg.] ▶KL ♀D ▶− $$$$$ ■

COMBIVIR (*lamivudine + zidovudine*) 1 tab PO two times per day for wt 30 kg or greater. [Generic/Trade: Tabs lamivudine 150 mg + zidovudine 300 mg.] ▶LK ♀C ▶– $$$ ■

COMPLERA (*emtricitabine + rilpivirine + tenofovir*) 1 tab PO once daily with a meal. [Trade only: Tabs emtricitabine 200 mg + rilpivine 25 mg + tenofovir 300 mg.] ▶KL ♀B ▶– $$$$$ ■

EPZICOM (*abacavir + lamivudine*) 1 tab PO daily. [Trade only: Tabs abacavir 600 mg + lamivudine 300 mg.] ▶LK ♀C ▶– $$$$$ ■

TRIZIVIR (*abacavir + lamivudine + zidovudine*) 1 tab PO two times per day. [Trade only: Tabs abacavir 300 mg + lamivudine 150 mg + zidovudine 300 mg.] ▶LK ♀C ▶– $$$$$ ■

TRUVADA (*emtricitabine + tenofovir*) 1 tab PO daily. [Trade only: Tabs emtricitabine 200 mg + tenofovir 300 mg.] ▶K ♀B ▶– $$$$$ ■

Antiviral Agents—Anti-HIV—Integrase Strand Transfer Inhibitor

RALTEGRAVIR (*Isentress, RAL*) 400 mg PO two times per day. Increase to 800 mg PO two times per day if given with rifampin. [Trade only: Tabs 400 mg.] ▶Glucuronidation ♀C ▶– $$$$$

Antiviral Agents—Anti-HIV—Non-Nucleoside Reverse Transcriptase Inhibitors

EFAVIRENZ (*Sustiva, EFV*) Adults and children wt 40 kg or greater: 600 mg PO at bedtime. With voriconazole: Use voriconazole 400 mg PO two times per day and efavirenz 300 mg PO once daily. Peds, age 3 yo or older: Give PO at bedtime 200 mg for wt 10 kg to less than 15 kg, 250 mg for wt 15 kg to less than 20 kg, 300 mg for wt 20 kg to less than 25 kg, 350 mg for wt 25 kg to less than 32.5 kg, 400 mg for wt 32.5 kg to less than 40 kg. Do not give with high-fat meal. [Trade only: Caps 50, 100, 200 mg. Tabs 600 mg.] ▶L ♀D ▶– $$$$$

ETRAVIRINE (*Intelence, ETR*) Combination therapy for treatment-resistant HIV infection: 200 mg PO two times per day after meals. [Trade only: Tabs 100, 200 mg.] ▶L ♀B ▶– $$$$$

NEVIRAPINE (*Viramune, Viramune XR, NVP*) 200 mg PO daily for 14 days initially. If tolerated, increase to 200 mg PO two times per day or Viramune XR 400 mg PO once daily. Patients maintained on immediate-release tabs can switch directly to Viramune XR. Peds, age 15 days or older: 150 mg/m² PO once daily for 14 days, then 150 mg/m² two times per day (max dose 200 mg two times per day). Severe skin reactions and hepatotoxicity. [Trade only: Tabs 200 mg, susp 50 mg/5 mL (240 mL), extended-release tabs (Viramune XR) 400 mg.] ▶LK ♀C ▶– $$$$$ ■

RILPIVIRINE (*Edurant, RPV*) Combination therapy of treatment-naive HIV infection in adults: 25 mg PO once daily with a meal. [Trade only: Tabs 25 mg.] $$$$$ ▶L ♀B ▶–

Antiviral Agents—Anti-HIV—Nucleoside/Nucleotide Reverse Transcriptase Inhibitors

ABACAVIR (*Ziagen, ABC*) Adult: 300 mg PO two times per day or 600 mg PO daily. Peds. Oral soln, age 3 mo or older: 8 mg/kg (up to 300 mg) PO two times per day. Peds, tabs: 150 mg 75 mg two times per day for wt 14 to 21 kg, 150 mg PO q am and 300 mg PO q pm for wt 22 to 29 kg, 300 mg PO two times per day for wt 30 kg or greater. Potentially fatal hypersensitivity. HLA-B*5701 predisposes to hypersensitivity; screen before starting and avoid if positive test. Never rechallenge with abacavir after suspected reaction. [Trade only: Tabs 300 mg scored. Oral soln 20 mg/mL (240 mL).] ▶L ♀C ▶– $$$$$ ■

DIDANOSINE (*Videx, Videx EC, DDI*) Videx EC: Give 200 mg PO once daily for wt 20 to 24 kg, 250 mg PO once daily for wt 25 to 59 kg, 400 mg PO once daily for wt 60 kg or greater. Dosage reduction of Videx EC with tenofovir in adults: 200 mg for wt less than 60 kg, 250 mg for wt 60 kg or greater. Dosage reduction unclear with tenofovir if CrCl <60 mL/min. Buffered powder, peds: 100 mg/m² PO two times per day for age 2 weeks to 8 mo; 120 mg/m² PO two times per day for age older than 8 mo. All formulations usually taken on empty stomach. [Generic/Trade: Pediatric powder for oral soln 10 mg/mL (buffered with antacid). Delayed-release caps (Videx EC): 125, 200, 250, 400 mg.] ▶LK ♀B ▶– $$$$ ■

EMTRICITABINE (*Emtriva, FTC*) Adult: 200 mg cap or 240 mg oral soln PO once daily. Peds, oral soln: 3 mg/kg PO once daily for age 3 mo or younger; 6 mg/kg PO once daily (up to 240 mg) for age older than 3 mo. Can give 200 mg cap PO once daily if wt greater than 33 kg. [Trade only: Caps 200 mg. Oral soln 10 mg/mL (170 mL).] ▶K ♀B ▶– $$$$$ ■

LAMIVUDINE (*Epivir, Epivir-HBV, 3TC, ✦ Heptovir*) Epivir for HIV infection. Adults and teens older than 16 yo: 150 mg PO two times per day or 300 mg PO daily. Peds: 4 mg/kg (up to 150 mg) PO two times per day. Can use tabs if wt 14 kg or greater. Epivir-HBV for hepatitis B: Adults: 100 mg PO daily. Peds: 3 mg/kg (up to 100 mg) PO daily. [Trade only: Epivir, 3TC: Tabs 150 (scored), 300 mg, oral soln 10 mg/mL. Epivir-HBV, Heptovir: Tabs 100 mg, oral soln 5 mg/mL.] ▶K ♀C ▶– $$$$$ ■

TENOFOVIR (*Viread, TDF*) Adults and adolescents: 300 mg PO daily. [Trade only: Tabs 300 mg.] ▶K ♀B ▶– $$$$$ ■

ZIDOVUDINE (*Retrovir, AZT, ZDV*) 600 mg/day PO divided two or three times per day for wt 30 kg or greater. Peds dose based on wt: give 24 mg/kg/day PO divided two or three times per day for wt 4 to 8 kg, 18 mg/kg/day PO divided two or three times per day for wt 9 to 29 kg. [Generic/Trade: Caps 100 mg. Tabs 300 mg. Syrup 50 mg/5 mL (240 mL).] ▶LK ♀C ▶– $$$$$ ■

Antiviral Agents—Anti-HIV—Protease Inhibitors

NOTE: See www.aidsinfo.nih.gov for AIDS treatment guidelines and use of rifamycins with protease inhibitors. Many serious drug interactions: Always check before prescribing. Protease inhibitors inhibit CYP3A4. Contraindicated with most antiarrhythmics, alfuzosin, ergot alkaloids, lovastatin, pimozide,

(cont.)

rifampin, salmeterol, high-dose sildenafil for pulmonary hypertension, simvastatin, St. John's wort, triazolam. Midazolam contraindicated in labeling; but can use single dose IV cautiously with monitoring for procedural sedation. Monitor INR with warfarin. Avoid inhaled/nasal fluticasone with ritonavir if possible; increased fluticasone levels can cause Cushing's syndrome/adrenal suppression. Other protease inhibitors may increase fluticasone levels; find alternatives for long-term use. May need to reduce trazodone dose. Reduce colchicine dose; do not coadminister colchicine and protease inhibitors in patients with renal or hepatic dysfunction. Adjust dose of bosentan or tadalafil for pulmonary hypertension. Erectile dysfunction: Single dose of sildenafil 25 mg every 48 h, tadalafil 5 mg (not more than 10 mg) every 72 h, or vardenafil initially 2.5 mg every 72 h. Adverse effects include spontaneous bleeding in hemophiliacs, hyperglycemia, hyperlipidemia, immune reconstitution syndrome, and fat redistribution. Coinfection with hepatitis C or other liver disease increases the risk of hepatotoxicity with protease inhibitors; monitor LFTs at least twice in first month of therapy, then every 3 months.

ATAZANAVIR (*Reyataz, ATV*) Adults, therapy-naive: 400 mg PO once daily (without ritonavir) OR 300 mg + ritonavir 100 mg PO both once daily. With tenofovir, therapy naive: 300 mg + ritonavir 100 mg PO both once daily. With efavirenz, therapy-naive: 400 mg + ritonavir 100 mg PO both once daily. Do not give atazanavir with efavirenz in therapy-experienced patients. Therapy-experienced: 300 mg + ritonavir 100 mg PO both once daily. Peds, therapy-naive, age 6 yo or older: Give following dose PO once daily based on wt: atazanavir 8.5 mg/kg for wt 15 to 19 kg; 7 mg/kg (up to 300 mg) for wt 20 kg or greater. Give with ritonavir 4 mg/kg (up to 100 mg) PO once daily. Peds, therapy-experienced, age 6 yo or older and wt 25 kg or greater: atazanavir 7 mg/kg (up to 300 mg) with ritonavir 4 mg/kg (up to 100 mg) PO once daily. Therapy-naive, ritonavir-intolerant, age 13 yo or older and wt 39 kg or greater: 400 mg PO once daily. Give caps with food. Give atazanavir 2 h before or 1 h after buffered didanosine. [Trade only: Caps 100, 150, 200, 300 mg.] ▶L ♀B ▶– $$$$$

DARUNAVIR (*Prezista, DRV*) Therapy-naive or -experienced adults with no darunavir resistance substitutions: 800 mg + ritonavir 100 mg PO both once daily. Therapy-experienced adults with at least 1 darunavir resistance substitution: 600 mg + ritonavir 100 mg both PO two times per day. Peds, age 6 yo or older: 375 mg + ritonavir 50 mg PO both two times per day for wt 20 to 29 kg; 450 mg + ritonavir 60 mg PO both two times per day for wt 30 kg to 39 kg; 600 mg + ritonavir 100 mg PO both two times per day for wt 40 kg or greater. Take with food. [Trade only: Tabs 75, 150, 400, 600 mg.] ▶L ♀B ▶– $$$$$

FOSAMPRENAVIR (*Lexiva, FPV, ✦Telzir*) Therapy-naive adults: 1400 mg PO two times per day (without ritonavir) OR 1400 mg + ritonavir 100/200 mg PO both once daily OR 700 mg + ritonavir 100 mg PO both two times per day. Protease inhibitor-experienced adults: 700 mg + ritonavir 100 mg PO both two times per day. Peds, therapy-naive, 2 to 5 yo: Susp 30 mg/kg PO two times per day. Therapy-naive, 6 yo or older: Susp 30 mg/kg PO two times

(cont.)

per day OR susp 18 mg/kg + ritonavir 3 mg/kg PO both two times per day. Therapy-experienced, 6 yo or older: Susp 18 mg/kg + ritonavir 3 mg/kg PO both two times per day. Do not exceed adult dose in children. For unboosted fosamprenavir, can use tabs for peds patients wt 47 kg or greater. For ritonavir-boosted fosamprenavir, can use tabs for peds patients wt 39 kg or greater. Take tabs without regard to meals. Adults should take susp without food; children should take with food. [Trade only: Tabs 700 mg. Susp 50 mg/mL.] ▶L ♀C ▶– $$$$$

INDINAVIR (*Crixivan, IDV*) 800 mg PO q 8 h between meals with water (at least 48 oz/day to prevent kidney stones). [Trade only: Caps 100, 200, 400 mg.] ▶LK ♀C ▶– $$$$$

LOPINAVIR-RITONAVIR (*Kaletra, LPV/r*) Adults: 400/100 mg PO two times per day (tabs or oral soln). Can use 800/200 mg PO once daily in patients with less than 3 lopinavir resistance-associated substitutions. Coadministration with efavirenz, nevirapine, fosamprenavir, or nelfinavir: 500/125 mg tabs (use two 200/50 mg + one 100/25 mg tab) or 533/133 mg oral soln (6.5 mL) PO two times per day. Infants, age 14 days to 6 mo: Lopinavir 16 mg/kg PO two times per day. Peds, age 6 mo to 12 yo: Lopinavir 12 mg/kg PO two times per day for wt less than 15 kg, use 10 mg/kg PO two times per day for wt 15 to 40 kg. Coadministration with efavirenz, nevirapine, fosamprenavir, or nelfinavir: Lopinavir 13 mg/kg PO two times per day for wt less than 15 kg, 11 mg/kg PO two times per day for wt 15 to 45 kg. Do not exceed adult dose in children. No once-daily dosing for pediatric or pregnant patients; coadministration with carbamazepine, phenobarbital, phenytoin, efavirenz, nevirapine, fosamprenavir, or nelfinavir; or in patients with 3 or more lopinavir resistance-associated substitutions. Give tabs without regard to meals; give oral soln with food. [Trade only: Tabs 200/50 mg, 100/25 mg. Oral soln 80/20 mg/mL (160 mL).] ▶L ♀C ▶– $$$$$

NELFINAVIR (*Viracept, NFV*) 750 mg PO three times per day or 1250 mg PO two times per day. Peds: 45 to 55 mg/kg PO two times per day (up to 2500 mg/day). Take with meals. [Trade only: Tabs 250, 625 mg. Oral powder 50 mg/g (114 g).] ▶L ♀B ▶– $$$$$

RITONAVIR (*Norvir, RTV*) Adult doses of 100 mg PO daily to 400 mg PO two times per day used to boost levels of other protease inhibitors. Full-dose regimen (600 mg PO two times per day) is poorly tolerated. Peds, full-dose regimen: Start with 250 mg/m^2 two times per day and increase q 2 to 3 days by 50 mg/m^2 two times per day to achieve usual dose of 350 to 400 mg/m^2 (up to 600 mg) PO two times per day for age older than 1 mo. If 400 mg/m^2 two times per day not tolerated, consider other alternatives. See specific protease inhibitor entries (atazanavir, darunavir, fosamprenavir, tipranavir) for pediatric boosting doses of ritonavir. [Trade only: Caps 100 mg, tabs 100 mg. Oral soln 80 mg/mL (240 mL).] ▶L ♀B ▶– $$$$$ ■

SAQUINAVIR (*Invirase, SQV*) Regimens must contain ritonavir. Saquinavir 1000 mg + ritonavir 100 mg both PO two times per day within 2 h after meals. Saquinavir 1000 mg + Kaletra 400/100 mg PO both two times per day. [Trade only: Invirase (hard gel) Caps 200 mg. Tabs 500 mg.] ▶L ♀B ▶? $$$$$

TIPRANAVIR *(Aptivus, TPV)* 500 mg boosted by ritonavir 200 mg PO two times per day with food. Peds: 14 mg/kg with 6 mg/kg ritonavir PO two times per day; do not exceed adult dose. Hepatotoxicity. [Trade only: Caps 250 mg. Oral soln 100 mg/mL (95 mL in unit-of-use amber glass bottle).] ▶Feces ♀C ▶– $$$$$ ■

Antiviral Agents—Anti-Influenza

AMANTADINE *(Symmetrel, ◆ Endantadine)* Parkinsonism: 100 mg PO two times per day. Max 300 to 400 mg/day divided three to four times per day. Prevention/treatment of influenza A: 5 mg/kg/day up to 150 mg/day PO divided two times per day for age 1 to 9 yo and any child wt less than 40 kg. Give 100 mg PO two times per day for adults and children age 10 yo or older; reduce to 100 mg PO daily if age 65 yo or older. The CDC generally recommends against amantadine/rimantadine for treatment/prevention of influenza A in the United States due to high levels of resistance. [Generic only: Caps 100 mg. Tabs 100 mg. Syrup 50 mg/5 mL (480 mL).] ▶K ♀C ▶? $$

OSELTAMIVIR *(Tamiflu)* Influenza A/B: For treatment, give each dose two times per day for 5 days starting within 2 days of symptom onset. For prevention, give each dose once daily for 10 days starting within 2 days of exposure. For adults each dose is 75 mg. For peds, age 1 yo or older, each dose is 30 mg for wt 15 kg or less; 45 mg for wt 16 to 23 kg; 60 mg for wt 24 to 40 kg; and 75 mg for wt greater than 40 kg or age 13 yo or older. Influenza treatment in infants younger than 1 yo: 3 mg/kg/dose PO two times per day for 5 days. Influenza prophylaxis in infants 3 to 11 months old. 3 mg/kg/dose PO once daily. Due to limited data, prophylaxis is not recommended for infants younger than 3 mo unless the situation is critical. Can take with food to improve tolerability. [Trade only: Caps 30, 45, 75 mg. Susp 6 mg/mL (60 mL) with 10 mL dosing device. Pharmacist can also compound susp (6 mg/mL). Before July 2011, Tamiflu susp concentration was 12 mg/mL and pharmacists compounded 15 mg/mL susp. Both 6 mg/mL and 12 mg/mL strengths may be available during 2011-2012 flu season. Instructions for compounding new 6 mg/mL susp are in Tamiflu package insert.] ▶LK ♀C but + ▶? $$$

RIMANTADINE *(Flumadine)* Treatment or prevention of influenza A in adults: 100 mg PO two times per day. Reduce dose to 100 mg PO once daily for age older than 65 yo. Peds influenza A prophylaxis: 5 mg/kg (up to 150 mg/day) PO once daily for age 1 to 9 yo. Use adult dose for age 10 yo or older. Start treatment within 2 days of symptom onset and continue for 7 days. The CDC generally recommends against amantadine/rimantadine for treatment/prevention of influenza A in the United States due to high levels of resistance. [Generic/Trade: Tabs 100 mg. Pharmacist can compound suspension.] ▶LK ♀C ▶– $$

ZANAMIVIR *(Relenza)* Influenza A/B treatment: 2 puffs two times per day for 5 days for adults and children 7 yo or older. Influenza A/B prevention: 2 puffs once daily for 10 days for adults and children 5 yo or older starting within 2 days of exposure. Do not use if chronic airway disease. [Trade only: Rotadisk inhaler 5 mg/puff (20 puffs).] ▶K ♀C ▶? $$$

OVERVIEW OF BACTERIAL PATHOGENS (Selected)

By bacterial class

Gram-Positive Aerobic Cocci: *Staph epidermidis* (coagulase negative), *Staph aureus* (coagulase positive), Streptococci: *S pneumoniae* (pneumococcus), *S pyogenes* (Group A), *S agalactiae* (Group B), enterococcus

Gram-Positive Aerobic/Facultatively Anaerobic Bacilli: *Bacillus, Corynebacterium diphtheriae, Erysipelothrix rhusiopathiae, Listeria monocytogenes, Nocardia*

Gram-Negative Aerobic Diplococci: *Moraxella catarrhalis, Neisseria gonorrhoeae, Neisseria meningitidis*

Gram-Negative Aerobic Coccobacilli: *Haemophilus ducreyi, Influenzae*

Gram-Negative Aerobic Bacilli: *Acinetobacter, Bartonella* species, *Bordetella pertussis, Brucella, Burkholderia cepacia, Campylobacter, Francisella tularensis, Helicobacter pylori, Legionella pneumophila, Pseudomonas aeruginosa, Stenotrophomonas maltophilia, Vibrio cholerae, Yersinia*

Gram-Negative Facultatively Anaerobic Bacilli: *Aeromonas hydrophila, Eikenella corrodens, Pasteurella multocida,* Enterobacteriaceae: *E coli, Citrobacter, Shigella, Salmonella, Klebsiella, Enterobacter, Hafnia, Serratia, Proteus, Providencia*

Anaerobes: *Actinomyces, Bacteroides fragilis, Clostridium botulinum, Clostridium difficile, Clostridium perfringens, Clostridium tetani, Fusobacterium, Lactobacillus, Peptostreptococcus*

Defective Cell Wall Bacteria: *Chlamydia pneumoniae, Chlamydia psittaci, Chlamydia trachomatis, Coxiella burnetii, Mycoplasma pneumoniae, Rickettsia prowazekii, Rickettsia rickettsii, Rickettsia typhi, Ureaplasma urealyticum*

Spirochetes: *Borrelia burgdorferi, Leptospira, Treponema pallidum*

Mycobacteria: *M avium complex, M kansasii, M leprae, M TB*

By bacterial name

Acinetobacter **Gram-Negative Aerobic Bacilli**
Actinomyces **Anaerobes**
Aeromonas hydrophila **Gram-Negative Facultatively Anaerobic Bacilli**
Bacillus **Gram-Positive Aerobic/Facultatively Anaerobic Bacilli**
Bacteroides fragilis **Anaerobes**
Bartonella species **Gram-Negative Aerobic Bacilli**
Bordetella pertussis **Gram-Negative Aerobic Bacilli**
Borrelia burgdorferi **Spirochetes**
Brucella **Gram-Negative Aerobic Bacilli**
Burkholderia cepacia **Gram-Negative Aerobic Bacilli**
Campylobacter **Gram-Negative Aerobic Bacilli**
Chlamydia pneumoniae **Defective Cell Wall Bacteria**
Chlamydia psittaci **Defective Cell Wall Bacteria**
Chlamydia trachomatis **Defective Cell Wall Bacteria**
Citrobacter **Gram-Negative Facultatively Anaerobic Bacilli**
Clostridium botulinum **Anaerobes**
Clostridium difficile **Anaerobes**
Clostridium perfringens **Anaerobes**
Clostridium tetani **Anaerobes**
Corynebacterium diphtheriae **Gram-Positive Aerobic/Facultatively Anaerobic Bacilli**
Coxiella burnetii **Defective Cell Wall Bacteria**
E coli **Gram-Negative Facultatively Anaerobic Bacilli**
Eikenella corrodens **Gram-Negative Facultatively Anaerobic Bacilli**
Enterobacter **Gram-Negative Facultatively Anaerobic Bacilli**
Enterobacteriaceae **Gram-Negative Facultatively Anaerobic Bacilli**
Enterococcus **Gram-Positive Aerobic Cocci**
Erysipelothrix rhusiopathiae **Gram-Positive Aerobic/Facultatively Anaerobic Bacilli**

Francisella tularensis Gram-Negative Aerobic Bacilli
Fusobacterium Anaerobes
Haemophilus ducreyi Gram-Negative Aerobic Coccobacilli
Haemophilus influenzae Gram-Negative Aerobic Coccobacilli
Hafnia Gram-Negative Facultatively Anaerobic Bacilli
Helicobacter pylori Gram-Negative Aerobic Bacilli
Klebsiella Gram-Negative Facultatively Anaerobic Bacilli
Lactobacillus Anaerobes
Legionella pneumophila Gram-Negative Aerobic Bacilli
Leptospira Spirochetes
Listeria monocytogenes Gram-Positive Aerobic/Facultatively Anaerobic Bacilli
M avium complex Mycobacteria
M kansasii Mycobacteria
M leprae Mycobacteria
M tuberculosis Mycobacteria
Moraxella catarrhalis Gram-Negative Aerobic Diplococci
Mycoplasma pneumoniae Defective Cell Wall Bacteria
Neisseria gonorrhoeae Gram-Negative Aerobic Diplococci
Neisseria meningitidis Gram-Negative Aerobic Diplococci
Nocardia Gram-Positive Aerobic/Facultatively Anaerobic Bacilli
Pasteurella multocida Gram-Negative Facultatively Anaerobic Bacilli
Peptostreptococcus Anaerobes
Pneumococcus Gram-Positive Aerobic Cocci
Proteus Gram-Negative Facultatively Anaerobic Bacilli
Providencia Gram-Negative Facultatively Anaerobic Bacilli
Pseudomonas aeruginosa Gram-Negative Aerobic Bacilli
Rickettsia prowazekii Defective Cell Wall Bacteria
Rickettsia rickettsii Defective Cell Wall Bacteria
Rickettsia typhi Defective Cell Wall Bacteria
Salmonella Gram-Negative Facultatively Anaerobic Bacilli
Serratia Gram-Negative Facultatively Anaerobic Bacilli
Shigella Gram-Negative Facultatively Anaerobic Bacilli
Staph aureus (coagulase positive) Gram-Positive Aerobic Cocci
Staph epidermidis (coagulase negative) Gram-Positive Aerobic Cocci
Stenotrophomonas maltophilia Gram-Negative Aerobic Bacilli
Strep agalactiae (Group B) Gram-Positive Aerobic Cocci
Strep pneumoniae (pneumococcus) Gram-Positive Aerobic Cocci
Strep pyogenes (Group A) Gram-Positive Aerobic Cocci
Streptococci Gram-Positive Aerobic Cocci
Treponema pallidum Spirochetes
Ureaplasma urealyticum Defective Cell Wall Bacteria
Vibrio cholerae Gram-Negative Aerobic Bacilli
Yersinia Gram-Negative Aerobic Bacilli

Antiviral Agents—Other

ADEFOVIR (*Hepsera*) <u>Chronic hepatitis B</u>: 10 mg PO daily. Nephrotoxic; lactic acidosis and hepatic steatosis; discontinuation may exacerbate hepatitis B; may result in HIV resistance in untreated HIV infection. [Trade only: Tabs 10 mg.] ▶K ♀C ▶– $$$$$ ■

BOCEPREVIR (*Victrelis*) <u>Chronic hepatitis C, genotype 1</u>: 800 mg PO three times per day (q 7 to 9 h) in combo with peginterferon and ribavirin. Take with

(cont.)

food. Start boceprevir after 4 weeks of peginterferon plus ribavirin. Treatment duration is based on response at weeks 8, 12, and 24. Stop boceprevir if HCV-RNA is 100 IU/mL or greater at week 12 or confirmed detectable at week 24. Neutropenia, anemia. Many drug interactions. [Trade only: Caps 200 mg.] ▶L ♀B ▶– $$$$$

ENTECAVIR (*Baraclude*) <u>Chronic hepatitis B</u>: 0.5 mg PO once daily if treatment-naive; give 1 mg if lamivudine-resistant, history of viremia despite lamivudine treatment, or HIV coinfected. Give on empty stomach. [Trade only: Tabs 0.5, 1 mg.] ▶K ♀C ▶– $$$$$ ■

INTERFERON ALFA-2B (*Intron A*) <u>Chronic hepatitis B</u>: 5 million units/day or 10 million units 3 times per week SC/IM for 16 weeks if HBeAg+, for 48 weeks if HBeAg–. [Trade only: Powder/soln for injection 10, 18, 50 million units/vial. Soln for injection 18, 25 million units/multidose vial. Multidose injection pens 3, 5, 10 million units/0.2 mL (1.5 mL), 6 doses/pen.] ▶K ♀C ▶?+ $$$$$ ■

PALIVIZUMAB (*Synagis*) <u>Prevention of respiratory syncytial virus pulmonary disease in high-risk infants</u>: 15 mg/kg IM once monthly during RSV season. ▶L ♀C ▶? $$$$$

PEGINTERFERON ALFA-2A (*Pegasys*) <u>Chronic hepatitis C</u>: 180 mcg SC in abdomen or thigh once a week for 48 weeks with or without PO ribavirin. <u>Hepatitis B</u>: 180 mcg SC in abdomen or thigh once a week for 48 weeks. May cause or worsen severe autoimmune, neuropsychiatric, ischemic, and infectious diseases. Frequent clinical and lab monitoring. [Trade only: 180 mcg/1 mL soln in single-use vial, 180 mcg/0.5 mL prefilled syringe.] ▶LK ♀C ▶– $$$$$ ■

PEGINTERFERON ALFA-2B (*PEG-Intron*) <u>Chronic hepatitis C</u>: Give SC once a week on same day each week. Monotherapy 1 mcg/kg/week. In combo with oral ribavirin: 1.5 mcg/kg/week with ribavirin 800 to 1400 mg/day PO divided two times per day. Peds, age older than 3 yo: 60 mcg/m^2 SC once a week with ribavirin 15 mg/kg/day PO divided two times per day. May cause or worsen severe autoimmune, neuropsychiatric, ischemic, and infectious diseases. Frequent clinical and lab monitoring. [Trade only: 50, 80, 120, 150 mcg/ 0.5 mL single-use vials with diluent, 2 syringes, and alcohol swabs. Disposable single-dose Redipen 50, 80, 120, 150 mcg.] ▶K? ♀C ▶– $$$$$ ■

RIBAVIRIN—INHALED (*Virazole*) <u>Severe respiratory syncytial virus infection in children</u>: Aerosol 12 to 18 h/day for 3 to 7 days. Beware of sudden pulmonary deterioration; drug precipitation can cause ventilator dysfunction. ▶Lung ♀X ▶– $$$$$ ■

RIBAVIRIN—ORAL (*Rebetol, Copegus, Ribasphere*) In combination with ribavirin for chronic hepatitis C, peginterferon is preferred over interferon alfa because of substantially higher response rate. Regimen and duration of treatment is based on genotype. Divide daily dose of ribavirin two times per day and give with food. <u>Chronic hepatitis C, genotypes 1 and 4</u>: Treat for 48 weeks, evaluating response after 12 weeks. Ribavirin in combo with peginterferon alfa-2b (PegIntron): 800 mg/day PO for wt 65 kg or less, 1000 mg/day for wt 66 kg to 85 kg, 1200 mg/day for wt 86 kg to 105 kg, 1400 mg/day for wt greater than 105 kg. Ribavirin in combo with peginterferon alfa-2a (Pegasys): 1000 mg/day PO for wt less than 75 kg, 1200 mg/day for wt 75 kg or greater.

(cont.)

Chronic hepatitis C, genotypes 2 and 3: Treat for 24 weeks with ribavirin 800 mg/day in combo with peginterferon. Chronic hepatitis C, children age 2 yo and older: Treat for 48 weeks with peginterferon alfa-2b in combo with ribavirin 15 mg/kg/day PO divided two times per day. Can cause hemolytic anemia; dosage adjustments required based on hemoglobin. [Generic/Trade: Caps 200 mg, Tabs 200, 500 mg. Generic only: Tabs 400, 600 mg. Trade only (Rebetol): Oral soln 40 mg/mL (100 mL).] ▶Cellular, K ♀X ▶– $$$$$ ■

TELAPREVIR (*Incivek*) Chronic hepatitis C, genotype 1: 750 mg PO three times per day (q 7 to 9 h) taken with food (not low-fat). Give with peginterferon and ribavirin for 12 weeks. Give peginterferon and ribavirin for additional 12 to 36 weeks based on HCV RNA levels at weeks 4 and 12, and whether patient was partial/null responder to prior therapy. Stop telaprevir if HCV RNA is greater than 1000 international units per/mL at week 4 or 12, or detectable at week 24. Many drug interactions. Can cause serious skin reactions and anemia. [Trade only: 375 mg tabs in 28-day blister pack or bottle of 168 tabs.] ▶L ♀B ▶– $$$$$

TELBIVUDINE (*Tyzeka*) Chronic hepatitis B: 600 mg PO once daily. [Trade only: Tabs 600 mg. Oral soln 100 mg/5 mL (300 mL).] ▶K ♀B ▶– $$$$$ ■

Carbapenems

DORIPENEM (*Doribax*) 500 mg IV q 8 h. ▶K ♀B ▶? $$$$$

ERTAPENEM (*Invanz*) 1 g IV/IM q 24 h. Prophylaxis, colorectal surgery: 1 g IV 1 h before incision. Peds, younger than 13 yo: 15 mg/kg IV/IM q 12 h (up to 1 g/day). Infuse IV over 30 min. ▶K ♀B ▶? $$$$$

IMIPENEM-CILASTATIN (*Primaxin*) 250 to 1000 mg IV q 6 to 8 h. Peds, age older than 3 mo: 15 to 25 mg/kg IV q 6 h. Seizures (especially if given with ganciclovir, elderly with renal dysfunction, or cerebrovascular or seizure disorder). ▶K ♀C ▶? $$$$$

MEROPENEM (*Merrem IV*) Complicated skin infections: 10 mg/kg up to 500 mg IV q 8 h. Intra-abdominal infections: 20 mg/kg up to 1 g IV q 8 h. Peds meningitis: 40 mg/kg IV q 8 h for age 3 mo or older; 2 g IV q 8 h for wt greater than 50 kg. ▶K ♀B ▶? $$$$$

Cephalosporins—1st Generation

CEFADROXIL 1 to 2 g/day PO once daily or divided two times per day. Peds: 30 mg/kg/day divided two times per day. [Generic only: Tabs 1 g. Caps 500 mg. Susp 125, 250, 500 mg/5 mL.] ▶K ♀B ▶+ $$$

CEFAZOLIN 0.5 to 1.5 g IM/IV q 6 to 8 h. Peds: 25 to 50 mg/kg/day divided q 6 to 8 h (up to 100 mg/kg/day for severe infections). ▶K ♀B ▶+ $$

CEPHALEXIN (*Keflex, Panixine DisperDose*) 250 to 500 mg PO four times per day. Peds: 25 to 50 mg/kg/day. Not for otitis media, sinusitis. [Generic/Trade: Caps 250, 500 mg. Generic only: Tabs 250, 500 mg. Susp 125, 250 mg/5 mL. Panixine DisperDose 125, 250 mg scored tabs for oral susp. Trade only: Caps 333, 750 mg.] ▶K ♀B ▶? $$$

Cephalosporins—2nd Generation

CEFACLOR (*Raniclor*) 250 to 500 mg PO three times per day. Peds: 20 to 40 mg/kg/day PO divided three times per day. <u>Otitis media:</u> 40 mg/kg/day PO divided two times per day. <u>Group A streptococcal pharyngitis:</u> 20 mg/kg/day PO divided two times per day. Serum sickness-like reactions with repeated use. [Generic only: Caps 250, 500 mg, Susp, Chewable tabs 125, 187, 250, 375 mg per 5 mL or tab.] ▸K ♀B ▸? $$$$

CEFOXITIN 1 to 2 g IM/IV q 6 to 8 h. Peds: 80 to 160 mg/kg/day IV divided q 4 to 8 h. ▸K ♀B ▸+ $$$$$

CEFPROZIL (*Cefzil*) 250 to 500 mg PO two times per day. Peds otitis media: 15 mg/kg/dose PO two times per day. <u>Peds group A streptococcal pharyngitis (2nd line to penicillin):</u> 7.5 mg/kg/dose PO two times per day for 10 days. [Generic only: Tabs 250, 500 mg. Susp 125, 250 mg/5 mL.] ▸K ♀B ▸+ $$$$

CEFUROXIME (*Zinacef, Ceftin*) Adult: 750 to 1500 mg IM/IV q 8 h. 250 to 500 mg PO two times per day. Peds: 50 to 100 mg/kg/day IV divided q 6 to 8 h; not for meningitis; 20 to 30 mg/kg/day susp PO divided two times per day. [Generic only: Tabs 125, 250, 500 mg. Susp 125, 250 mg/5 mL.] ▸K ♀B ▸? $$$

Cephalosporins—3rd Generation

CEFDINIR 14 mg/kg/day up to 600 mg/day PO once daily or divided two times per day. [Generic only: Caps 300 mg. Susp 125, 250 mg/5 mL.] ▸K ♀B ▸? $$$$

CEFDITOREN (*Spectracef*) 200 to 400 mg PO two times per day with food. [Trade only: Tabs 200, 400 mg.] ▸K ♀B ▸? $$$$$

CEFIXIME (*Suprax*) 400 mg PO once daily. <u>Gonorrhea:</u> 400 mg PO single dose. Peds: 8 mg/kg/day once daily or divided two times per day. [Trade only: Susp 100, 200 mg/5 mL. Chewable tabs 100, 150, 200 mg. Tabs 400 mg.] ▸K/Bile ♀B ▸? $$

CEFOTAXIME (*Claforan*) Usual dose: 1 to 2 g IM/IV q 6 to 8 h. Peds: 50 to 180 mg/kg/day IM/IV divided q 4 to 6 h. <u>AAP dose for pneumococcal meningitis:</u> 225 to 300 mg/kg/day IV divided q 6 to 8 h. ▸KL ♀B ▸+ $$$$$

CEFPODOXIME (*Vantin*) 100 to 400 mg PO two times per day. Peds: 10 mg/kg/day divided two times per day. [Generic/Trade: Tabs 100, 200 mg. Susp 50, 100 mg/5 mL.] ▸K ♀B ▸? $$$$

CEFTAZIDIME (*Fortaz, Tazicef*) 1 g IM/IV or 2 g IV q 8 to 12 h. 30 to 50 mg/kg IV q 8 h. ▸K ♀B ▸+ $$$$$

CEFTIBUTEN (*Cedax*) 400 mg PO once daily. Peds: 9 mg/kg (up to 400 mg) PO once daily. [Trade only: Caps 400 mg. Susp 90 mg/5 mL.] ▸K ♀B ▸? $$$$$

CEFTIZOXIME 1 to 2 g IV q 8 to 12 h. Peds: 50 mg/kg/dose IV q 6 to 8 h. ▸K ♀B ▸? $$$$$

CEFTRIAXONE (*Rocephin*) 1 to 2 g IM/IV q 24 h. <u>Meningitis:</u> 2 g IV q 12 h. <u>Gonorrhea:</u> 250 mg IM plus azithromycin 1 g PO both single dose. Peds: 50 to

(cont.)

CEPHALOSPORINS – GENERAL ANTIMICROBIAL SPECTRUM

1st **generation**: gram-positive (including Staphylococcus aureus); basic gram-negative coverage

2nd **generation** diminished Staph aureus, improved gram-negative coverage compared to 1st generation; some with anaerobic coverage

3rd **generation** further diminished Staph aureus, further improved gram negative coverage compared to 1st and 2nd generation; some with Pseudomonal coverage & diminished gram-positive coverage

4th **generation**: same as 3rd generation plus coverage against Pseudomonas

5th **generation**: gram-negative coverage similar to 3rd generation; also active against *S aureus* (including MRSA) and *S pneumoniae*.

75 mg/kg/day (up to 2 g/day) divided q 12 to 24 h. <u>Peds meningitis</u>: 100 mg/kg/day (up to 4 g/day) IV divided q 12 to 24 h. <u>Otitis media</u>: 50 mg/kg up to 1 g IM single dose. May dilute in 1% lidocaine for IM. Contraindicated in neonates who require (or are expected to require) IV calcium (including calcium in TPN); fatal lung/kidney precipitation of calcium ceftriaxone has been reported in neonates. In other patients, do not give ceftriaxone and calcium-containing solns simultaneously, but sequential administration is acceptable if lines are flushed with a compatible fluid between infusions. ▶K/Bile ♀B ▶+ $$$

Cephalosporins—4th Generation

CEFEPIME (*Maxipime*) 0.5 to 2 g IM/IV q 12 h. Peds: 50 mg/kg IV q 8 to 12 h. ▶K ♀B ▶? $$$$$

Cephalosporins—5th Generation

CEFTAROLINE (*Teflaro*) <u>Community-acquired bacterial pneumonia, acute bacterial skin and skin structure infections</u>: 600 mg IV q 12 h infused over 1 h. ▶K ♀B ▶? $$$$$

Macrolides

AZITHROMYCIN (*Zithromax, Zmax*) 500 mg IV daily 10 mg/kg (up to 500 mg) PO on day 1, then 5 mg/kg (up to 250 mg) daily for 4 days. <u>Otitis media</u>: 30 mg/kg PO single dose or 10 mg/kg PO daily for 3 days. <u>Peds sinusitis</u>: 10 mg/kg PO daily for 3 days. <u>Group A streptococcal pharyngitis</u> (second-line to penicillin): 12 mg/kg PO daily for 5 days. <u>Adult acute sinusitis or exacerbation of chronic bronchitis</u>: 500 mg PO daily for 3 days. <u>Zmax for community-acquired pneumonia, acute sinusitis</u>: 60 mg/kg (up to 2 g) PO single dose on empty stomach; give adult dose of 2 g for wt 34 kg or greater. <u>Chlamydia (including pregnancy), chancroid</u>: 1 g PO single dose. <u>Prevention of disseminated Mycobacterium avium complex disease</u>: 1200 mg PO once a week. <u>Pertussis treatment/post-exposure prophylaxis</u>:

(cont.)

SEXUALLY TRANSMITTED DISEASES & VAGINITIS*

Bacterial vaginosis: (1) metronidazole 5 g of 0.75% gel intravaginally daily for 5 days OR 500 mg PO two times per day for 7 days; (2) clindamycin 5 g of 2% cream intravaginally at bedtime for 7 days. In pregnancy: (1) metronidazole 500 mg PO two times per day for 7 days OR 250 mg PO three times per day for 7 days; (2) clindamycin 300 mg PO two times per day for 7 days.

Candidal vaginitis: (1) intravaginal clotrimazole, miconazole, terconazole, nystatin, tioconazole, or butoconazole; (2) fluconazole 150 mg PO single dose.

Chancroid: (1) azithromycin 1 g PO single dose; (2) ceftriaxone 250 mg IM single dose; (3) ciprofloxacin 500 mg PO two times per day for 3 days.

Chlamydia: First line either azithromycin 1 g PO single dose or doxycycline 100 mg PO two times per day for 7 days. Second line fluoroquinolones or erythromycin. In pregnancy: (1) azithromycin 1 g PO single dose; (2) amoxicillin 500 mg PO three times per day for 7 days. Repeat NAAT[c] 3 weeks after treatment in pregnant women.

Epididymitis: (1) ceftriaxone 250 mg IM single dose + doxycycline 100 mg PO two times per day for 10 days; (2) ofloxacin 300 mg PO two times per day or levofloxacin 500 mg PO daily for 10 days if enteric organisms suspected, or negative gonococcal culture or NAAT.[†]

Gonorrhea: Single dose of: (1) ceftriaxone 250 mg IM + azithromycin 1 g PO single dose (preferred) or doxycycline 100 mg PO two times per day for 7 days; (2) cefixime 400 mg PO (not for pharyngeal) + azithromycin/doxycycline if ceftriaxone is not an option.[†] Consult infectious disease expert if severe cephalosporin allergy.

Gonorrhea, disseminated: Initially treat with ceftriaxone 1 g IM/IV q 24 h until 24 to 48 h after improvement. Second-line alternatives: (1) cefotaxime 1 g IV q 8 h; (2) ceftizoxime 1 g IV q 8 h. Complete at least 1 week of treatment with cefixime tabs 400 mg PO two times per day.[†]

Gonorrhea, meningitis: ceftriaxone 1 to 2 g IV q 12 h for 10 to 14 days.

Gonorrhea, endocarditis: ceftriaxone 1 to 2 g IV q 12 h for at least 4 weeks.

Granuloma inguinale: doxycycline 100 mg PO two times per day for at least 3 weeks and until lesions completely healed. Alternative azithromycin 1 g PO once weekly for at least 3 weeks and until lesions completely healed.

Herpes simplex (genital, first episode): (1) acyclovir 400 mg PO three times per day for 7 to 10 days; (2) famciclovir 250 mg PO three times per day for 7 to 10 days; (3) valacyclovir 1 g PO two times per day for 7 to 10 days.

Herpes simplex (genital, recurrent): (1) acyclovir 400 mg PO three times per day for 5 days; (2) acyclovir 800 mg PO three times per day for 2 days or two times per day for 5 days; (3) famciclovir 125 mg PO two times per day for 5 days; (4) famciclovir 1 g PO two times per day for 1 day; (5) famciclovir 500 mg PO first dose, then 250 mg PO two to three times per day for 2 days; (6) valacyclovir 500 mg PO two times per day for 3 days; (7) valacyclovir 1 g PO daily for 5 days.

Herpes simplex (suppressive therapy): (1) acyclovir 400 mg PO two times per day; (2) famciclovir 250 mg PO two times per day; (3) valacyclovir 500 to 1000 mg PO daily. Valacyclovir 500 mg PO daily may be less effective than other valacyclovir/acyclovir regimens in patients who have 10 or more recurrences per year.

Herpes simplex (genital, recurrent in HIV infection): (1) acyclovir 400 mg PO three times per day for 5 to 10 days; (2) famciclovir 500 mg PO two times per day for 5 to 10 days; (3) valacyclovir 1 g PO two times per day for 5 to 10 days.

Herpes simplex (suppressive therapy in HIV infection): (1) acyclovir 400 to 800 mg PO two to three times per day; (2) famciclovir 500 mg PO two times per day; (3) valacyclovir 500 mg PO two times per day.

Herpes simplex (prevention of transmission in immunocompetent patients with not more than 9 recurrences/year): Valacyclovir 500 mg PO daily by source partner, in conjunction with safer sex practices.

(cont.)

SEXUALLY TRANSMITTED DISEASES & VAGINITIS* (continued)

Lymphogranuloma venereum: (1) doxycycline 100 mg PO two times per day for 21 days. Alternative: erythromycin base 500 mg PO four times per day for 21 days.

Pelvic inflammatory disease (PID), inpatient regimens: (1) cefoxitin 2 g IV q 6 h + doxycycline 100 mg IV/PO q 12 h; (2) clindamycin 900 mg IV q 8 h + gentamicin 2 mg/kg IM/IV loading dose, then 1.5 mg/kg IM/IV q 8 h (Can substitute 3 to 5 mg/kg once-daily dosing). Can switch to PO therapy within 24 h of improvement.

Pelvic inflammatory disease (PID), outpatient treatment: (1) ceftriaxone 250 mg IM single dose + doxycycline 100 mg PO two times per day +/– metronidazole 500 mg PO two times per day for 14 days.

Proctitis, proctocolitis, enteritis: ceftriaxone 250 mg IM single dose + doxycycline 100 mg PO two times per day for 7 days.

Sexual assault prophylaxis: ceftriaxone 250 mg IM or cefixime 400 mg PO single dose + metronidazole 2 g PO single dose + azithromycin 1 g PO single dose/doxycycline 100 mg PO two times per day for 7 days.

Syphilis (primary and secondary): (1) benzathine penicillin 2.4 million units IM single dose. (2) doxycycline 100 mg PO two times per day for 2 weeks if penicillin-allergic.

Syphilis (early latent, i.e. duration less than 1 year): (1) benzathine penicillin 2.4 million units IM single dose; (2) doxycycline 100 mg PO two times per day for 2 weeks if penicillin-allergic.

Syphilis (late latent or unknown duration): (1) benzathine penicillin 2.4 million units IM q week for 3 doses; (2) doxycycline 100 mg PO two times per day for 4 weeks if penicillin-allergic.

Syphilis (tertiary): benzathine penicillin 2.4 million units IM q week for 3 doses. Consult infectious disease specialist for management of penicillin-allergic patients.

Syphilis (neuro): (1) penicillin G 18 to 24 million units/day continuous IV infusion or 3 to 4 million units IV q 4 h for 10 to 14 days; (2) if compliance can be ensured, consider procaine penicillin 2.4 million units IM daily + probenecid 500 mg PO four times per day, both for 10 to 14 days.

Syphilis in pregnancy: Treat only with penicillin regimen for stage of syphilis as noted above. Use penicillin desensitization protocol if penicillin-allergic.

Trichomoniasis: metronidazole (can use in pregnancy) or tinidazole, each 2 g PO single dose.

Urethritis, Cervicitis: Test for chlamydia and gonorrhea with NAAL.† Treat based on test results or treat presumptively if high-risk of infection (Chlamydia: age 25 yo or younger, new/multiple sex partners, or unprotected sex. Gonorrhea: population prevalence greater than 5%), esp. if NAAI† unavailable or patient unlikely to return for follow-up.

Urethritis (persistent/recurrent): metronidazole/ tinidazole 2 g PO single dose + azithromycin 1 g PO single dose (if not used in first episode).

---

*MMWR 2010;59:RR-12 or http://www.cdc.gov/STD/treatment/. Treat sexual partners for all except herpes, candida, and bacterial vaginosis.

† There is a growing threat of multi-drug resistant gonorrhea, with high level azithromycin resistance and reduced cephalosporin susceptibility reported in the US in 2011. Ceftriaxone is the most effective cephalosporin for treatment of gonorrhea. If cefixime treatment failure occurs, retreat with ceftriaxone 250 mg IM plus azithromycin 2 g PO both single dose and perform culture (preferred) or NAAT in 1 week. If ceftriaxone treatment failure occurs, consult infectious disease expert and CDC. Do not use azithromycin monotherapy for routine treatment of gonorrhea. If azithromycin is used in patients with cephalosporin allergy, use azithromycin 2 g PO single dose and perform culture (preferred) or NAAT in 1 week. Report treatment failure to state/local health department within 24 hours. As of April 2007, the CDC no longer recommends fluoroquinolones for gonorrhea or PID because of high resistance rates. Do not consider fluoroquinolone unless antimicrobial susceptibility can be documented by culture. If parenteral cephalosporin not feasible for PID (and NAAT is negative or culture documents fluoroquinolone susceptibility), can consider levofloxacin 500 mg PO once daily or ofloxacin 400 mg PO two times per day +/– metronidazole 500 mg PO two times per day for 14 days.

‡ NAAT = nucleic acid amplification test.

10 mg/kg PO once daily for 5 days for infants age younger than 6 mo; 10 mg/ kg (max 500 mg) PO on day 1, then 5 mg/kg (max 250 mg) PO once daily for 4 days for children 6 mo and older; 500 mg PO on day 1, then 250 mg PO daily for 4 days for adolescents and adults. [Generic/Trade: Tabs 250, 500, 600 mg. Susp 100, 200 mg/5 mL. Packet only: Z-Pak: #6: 250 mg tab. Tri-Pak: #3: 500 mg tab. Zmax extended-release oral susp: 2 g in 60 mL single-dose bottle.] ▶L ♀B ▶? $$

CLARITHROMYCIN (*Biaxin, Biaxin XL*) 250 to 500 mg PO two times per day. Peds: 7.5 mg/kg PO two times per day. *H pylori:* See table in GI section. See table for prophylaxis of bacterial endocarditis. Mycobacterium avium complex disease prevention: 7.5 mg/kg up to 500 mg PO two times per day. Biaxin XL: 1000 mg PO daily with food. [Generic/Trade: Tabs 250, 500 mg. Extended-release tab 500 mg. Susp 125, 250 mg/ 5 mL. Trade only: Biaxin XL-Pak: #14, 500 mg tabs. Generic only: Extended-release tab 1000 mg.] ▶KL ♀C ▶? $$$

ERYTHROMYCIN BASE (*Eryc, Ery-Tab*) Adult: 250 to 500 mg PO four times per day, 333 mg PO three times per day, or 500 mg PO two times per day. Peds: 30 to 50 mg/kg/day PO divided four times per day. [Generic/Trade: Tabs 250, 333, 500 mg, delayed-release cap 250 mg.] ▶L ♀B ▶+ $

ERYTHROMYCIN ETHYL SUCCINATE (*EryPed*) 400 mg PO four times per day. Peds: 30 to 50 mg/kg/day PO divided four times per day. [Generic/Trade: Tabs 400. Susp 200, 400 mg/5 mL. Trade only (EryPed): Susp 100 mg/2.5 mL (50 mL).] ▶L ♀B ▶+ $

ERYTHROMYCIN LACTOBIONATE (♦ *Erythrocin IV*) 15 to 20 mg/kg/day (max 4 g) IV divided q 6 h. Peds: 15 to 50 mg/kg/day IV divided q 6 h. ▶L ♀B ▶+ $$$$$

FIDAXOMICIN (*Dificid*) C difficile-associated diarrhea: 200 mg PO two times per day for 10 days. [Trade only: 200 mg tabs.] ▶minimal absorption ♀B ▶? $$$$$

ERYTHROMYCIN ETHYL SUCCINATE + SULFISOXAZOLE Otitis media: 50 mg/ kg/day (based on EES dose) PO divided three to four times per day. [Generic only: Susp, erythromycin ethyl succinate 200 mg + sulfisoxazole 600 mg/5 mL.] ▶KL ♀C ▶– $$

Penicillins—1st generation—Natural

BENZATHINE PENICILLIN (*Bicillin L-A*, ♦ *Megacillin*) Adults and peds wt greater than 27 kg: 1.2 million units IM. Peds wt 27 kg or less: 600,000 units IM. Doses last 2 to 4 weeks. Give IM q month for secondary prevention of rheumatic fever (q 3 weeks for high-risk patients). [Trade only: For IM use, 600,000 units/mL; 1, 2, 4 mL syringes.] ▶K ♀B ▶? $$ ■

BICILLIN C-R (procaine penicillin + benzathine penicillin) For IM use. Not for treatment of syphilis. [Trade only: For IM use 300/300 thousand units/mL procaine/benzathine penicillin; 1, 2, 4 mL syringes.] ▶K ♀B ▶? $$$ ■

PENICILLIN G Pneumococcal pneumonia and severe infections: 250,000 to 400,000 units/kg/day (8 to 12 million units/day in adult) IV divided q 4 to 6 h. Pneumococcal meningitis: 250,000 to 400,000 units/kg/day (24 million units/ day in adult) in 4 to 6 divided doses. ▶K ♀B ▶? $$$$

PENICILLIN V (✦ *PVF-K*) Adults: 250 to 500 mg PO four times per day. Peds: 25 to 50 mg/kg/day divided two to four times per day. <u>AHA doses for pharyngitis</u>: 250 mg (peds 27 kg or less) or 500 mg (adults and peds greater than 27 kg) PO two to three times per day for 10 days. [Generic only: Tabs 250, 500 mg, oral soln 125, 250 mg/5 mL.] ▸K ♀B ▸? $

PROCAINE PENICILLIN 0.6 to 1 million units IM daily (peak 4 h, lasts 24 h). [Generic: For IM use, 600,000 units/mL; 1, 2 mL syringes.] ▸K ♀B ▸? $$$$$ ■

Penicillins—2nd generation—Penicillinase-Resistant

DICLOXACILLIN 250 to 500 mg PO four times per day. Peds: 12.5 to 25 mg/kg/day PO divided four times per day. [Generic only: Caps 250, 500 mg.] ▸KL ♀B ▸? $$

NAFCILLIN 1 to 2 g IM/IV q 4 h. Peds: 50 to 200 mg/kg/day IM/IV divided q 4 to 6 h. ▸L ♀B ▸? $$$$$

OXACILLIN 1 to 2 g IM/IV q 4 to 6 h. Peds: 150 to 200 mg/kg/day IM/IV divided q 4 to 6 h. ▸KL ♀B ▸? $$$$$

Penicillins—3rd generation—Aminopenicillins

AMOXICILLIN (*DisperMox, Moxatag*) 250 to 500 mg PO three times per day, or 500 to 875 mg PO two times per day. <u>High-dose for community-acquired pneumonia, acute sinusitis</u>: 1 g PO three times per day. <u>Lyme disease</u>: 500 mg PO three times per day for 14 days for early disease, for 28 days for Lyme arthritis. <u>Chlamydia in pregnancy</u>: 500 mg PO three times per day for 7 days. AHA dosing for <u>group A streptococcal pharyngitis</u>: 50 mg/kg (max 1 g) PO once daily for 10 days. <u>Group A streptococcal pharyngitis/ tonsillitis</u>: 775 mg ER tab (Moxatag) PO for 10 days for age 12 yo or older. Peds AAP <u>otitis media</u>: 90 mg/kg/day divided two times per day. AAP recommends 5 to 7 days of therapy for age 6 yo or older with non-severe otitis media, and 10 days for younger children and those with severe disease. Peds infections other than otitis media: 40 mg/kg/day PO divided three times per day or 45 mg/kg/day divided two times per day. [Generic only: Caps 250, 500 mg, Tabs 500, 875 mg, Chewable tabs 125, 200, 250, 400 mg. Susp 125, 250 mg/5 mL. Susp 200, 400 mg/5 mL. Infant gtts 50 mg/mL. DisperMox 200, 400, 600 mg tabs for oral susp, Moxatag 775 mg extended-release tab.] ▸K ♀B ▸+ $

AMOXICILLIN-CLAVULANATE (*Augmentin, Augmentin ES-600, Augmentin XR*, ✦ *Clavulin*) 500 to 875 mg PO two times per day or 250 to 500 mg three times per day. Augmentin XR: 2 tabs PO q 12 h with meals. Peds AAP <u>otitis media</u>: Augmentin ES 90 mg/kg/day divided two times per day. AAP recommends 5 to 7 days of therapy for age 6 yo or older <u>non-severe otitis media</u>, and 10 days for younger children and those with severe disease. Peds: 45 mg/kg/day PO divided two times per day or 40 mg/kg/day divided three times per day for <u>sinusitis, pneumonia, otitis media</u>; 25 mg/kg/day

(cont.)

divided two times per day or 20 mg/kg/day divided three times per day for less severe infections. [Generic/Trade: (amoxicillin-clavulanate) Tabs 250/125, 500/125, 875/125 mg. Chewables, Susp 200/28.5, 400/57 mg per tab or 5 mL, 250/62.5 mg per 5 mL. (ES) Susp 600/42.9 mg per 5 mL. Trade only: Chewables, Susp 125/31.25 per tab or 5 mL, 250/62.5 mg per tab. Extended-release tabs (Augmentin XR) 1000/62.5 mg.] ▶K ♀B ▶? $$$$

AMPICILLIN Usual dose: 1 to 2 g IV q 4 to 6 h. <u>Sepsis, meningitis:</u> 150 to 200 mg/kg/day IV divided q 3 to 4 h. Peds: 100 to 400 mg/kg/day IM/IV divided q 4 to 6 h. [Generic only: Caps 250, 500 mg. Susp 125, 250 mg/5 mL.] ▶K ♀B ▶? $ for PO $$$$$ for IV

AMPICILLIN-SULBACTAM (*Unasyn*) 1.5 to 3 g IM/IV q 6 h. Peds: 100 to 400 mg/kg/day of ampicillin divided q 6 h. ▶K ♀B ▶? $$$$$

Penicillins—4th generation—Extended Spectrum

PIPERACILLIN-TAZOBACTAM (*Zosyn*, ✦*Tazocin*) 3.375 to 4.5 g IV q 6 h. <u>Peds appendicitis or peritonitis:</u> 80 mg/kg IV q 8 h for age 2 to 9 mo, 100 mg/kg piperacillin IV q 8 h for age older than 9 mo, use adult dose for wt greater than 40 kg. ▶K ♀B ▶? $$$$$

TICARCILLIN-CLAVULANATE (*Timentin*) 3.1 g IV q 4 to 6 h. Peds: 50 mg/kg up to 3.1 g IV q 4 to 6 h. ▶K ♀B ▶? $$$$$

PROPHYLAXIS FOR BACTERIAL ENDOCARDITIS*

Limited to dental or respiratory tract procedures in patients at highest risk. All regimens are single doses administered 30-60 minutes prior to procedure.	
Standard regimen	amoxicillin 2 g PO
Unable to take oral meds	ampicillin 2 g IM/IV; or cefazolin† or ceftriaxone† 1 g IM/IV
Allergic to penicillin	clindamycin 600 mg PO; or cephalexin† 2 g PO; or azithromycin or clarithromycin 500 mg PO
Allergic to penicillin and unable to take oral meds	clindamycin 600 mg IM/IV; or cefazolin† or ceftriaxone† 1 g IM/IV
Pediatric drug doses	Pediatric dose should not exceed adult dose. Amoxicillin 50 mg/kg, ampicillin 50 mg/kg, azithromycin 15 mg/kg, cephalexin† 50 mg/kg, cefazolin† 50 mg/kg, ceftriaxone† 50 mg/kg, clarithromycin 15 mg/kg, clindamycin 20 mg/kg.

*For additional details of the 2007 AHA guidelines, see http://www.americanheart.org.
†Avoid cephalosporins if prior penicillin-associated anaphylaxis, angioedema, or urticaria.

PENICILLINS — GENERAL ANTIMICROBIAL SPECTRUM

1st generation: Most streptococci; oral anaerobic coverage
2nd generation: Most streptococci; *Staph aureus* (but not MRSA)
3rd generation: Most streptococci; basic Gram-negative coverage
4th generation: *Pseudomonas*

QUINOLONES—GENERAL ANTIMICROBIAL SPECTRUM

1st **generation:** Gram-negative (excluding *Pseudomonas*), urinary tract only, no atypicals

2nd **generation:** Gram-negative (including *Pseudomonas*); Staph aureus (but not MRSA or *pneumococcus*); some atypicals

3rd **generation:** Gram-negative (including *Pseudomonas*); Gram-positive, including *pneumococcus* and *Staph aureus* (but not MRSA); expanded atypical coverage

4th **generation:** same as 3rd generation plus enhanced coverage of *pneumococcus*, decreased activity vs. *Pseudomonas*

Quinolones—2nd Generation

CIPROFLOXACIN *(Cipro, Cipro XR, ProQuin XR)* 200 to 400 mg IV q 8 to 12 h. 250 to 750 mg PO two times per day. <u>Simple UTI</u>: 250 mg two times per day for 3 days or Cipro XR/ProQuin XR 500 mg PO daily for 3 days. Give ProQuin XR with main meal of day. Cipro XR for <u>pyelonephritis or complicated UTI</u>: 1000 mg PO daily for 7 to 14 days. [Generic/Trade: Tabs 100, 250, 500, 750 mg. Extended-release tabs 500, 1000 mg. Trade only (ProQuin XR): Extended-release tabs 500 mg, blister pack 500 mg (#3 tabs).] ▶LK ♀C but teratogenicity unlikely ▶?+ $ ■

NORFLOXACIN *(Noroxin)* <u>Simple UTI</u>: 400 mg PO two times per day for 3 days. [Trade only: Tabs 400 mg.] ▶LK ♀C ▶? $ ■

OFLOXACIN *(Floxin)* 200 to 400 mg PO two times per day. [Generic/Trade: Tabs 200, 300, 400 mg.] ▶LK ♀C ▶?+ $$$ ■

Quinolones—3rd Generation

LEVOFLOXACIN *(Levaquin)* 250 to 750 mg PO/IV daily. [Generic/Trade: Tabs 250, 500, 750 mg. Oral soln 25 mg/mL. Trade only: Leva-Pak: #5, 750 mg tabs.] ▶KL ♀C ▶? $$$$ ■

Quinolones—4th Generation

GEMIFLOXACIN *(Factive)* 320 mg PO daily for 5 to 7 days. [Trade only: Tabs 320 mg.] ▶Feces, K ♀C ▶− $$$$ ■

MOXIFLOXACIN *(Avelox)* 400 mg PO/IV daily for 5 days (<u>chronic bronchitis exacerbation</u>), 5 to 14 days (<u>complicated intra-abdominal infection</u>), 7 days (<u>uncomplicated skin infections</u>), 10 days (<u>acute sinusitis</u>), 7 to 14 days (<u>community-acquired pneumonia</u>), 7 to 21 days (<u>complicated skin infections</u>). [Trade only: Tabs 400 mg.] ▶LK ♀C ▶− $$$ ■

Sulfonamides

SULFADIAZINE <u>CNS toxoplasmosis in AIDS.</u> Acute treatment: 1000 mg PO four times per day for wt less than 60 kg; 1500 mg PO four times per day for wt 60 kg or greater. Secondary prevention: 2000 to 4000 mg/day PO divided two to four times per day. Give with pyrimethamine + leucovorin. [Generic only: Tabs 500 mg.] ▶K ♀C ▶+ $$$$

TRIMETHOPRIM-SULFAMETHOXAZOLE (*Bactrim,   Septra,   Sulfatrim, cotrimoxazole*) 1 tab PO two times per day, double-strength (DS, 160 mg/800 mg) or single-strength (SS, 80 mg/400 mg). Pneumocystis treatment: 15 to 20 mg/kg/day (based on TMP) IV divided q 6 to 8 h or PO divided three times per day for 21 days total. Pneumocystis prophylaxis: 1 DS tab PO daily. Peds usual dose: 1 mL/kg/day susp PO divided two times per day (up to 20 mL PO two times per day). Use adult dose for wt greater than 40 kg. Community-acquired MRSA skin infections. Adults: 1 to 2 DS tabs PO two times per day for 7 to 10 days. Peds: 1 to 1.5 mL/kg/day PO divided two times per day. [Generic/Trade: Tabs 80 mg TMP/400 mg SMX (single strength), 160 mg TMP/800 mg SMX (double strength; DS), susp 40 mg TMP/200 mg SMX per 5 mL. 20 mL susp = 2 SS tabs = 1 DS tab.] ▶K ♀C ▶+ $

Tetracyclines

DEMECLOCYCLINE (*Declomycin*) Usual dose: 150 mg PO four times per day or 300 mg PO two times per day on empty stomach. Syndrome of inappropriate antidiuretic hormone hypersecretion (SIADH): 600 to 1200 mg/day PO given in 3 to 4 divided doses. [Generic/Trade: Tabs 150, 300 mg.] ▶K, feces ♀D ▶?+ $$$$

DOXYCYCLINE (*Doryx, Monodox, Oracea, Periostat, Vibramycin, Vibra-Tabs, ◆Doxycin*) 100 mg PO two times per day on 1st day, then 50 mg two times per day or 100 mg daily. Severe infections: 100 mg PO/IV two times per day. Community-acquired MRSA skin infections: 100 mg PO two times per day. Lyme disease: 100 mg PO two times per day for 14 days for early disease, for 28 days for Lyme arthritis. Acne: Up to 100 mg PO two times per day. Periostat for periodontitis: 20 mg PO two times per day. Oracea ($$$$$) for inflammatory rosacea: 40 mg PO once every morning on empty stomach. Malaria prophylaxis: 2 mg/kg/day up to 100 mg PO daily starting 1 to 2 days before exposure until 4 weeks after. Avoid in children age younger than 8 yo due to teeth staining. [Generic/Trade: Tabs 20, 75, 100 mg, Caps 50, 100 mg. Generic only: Caps 75, 150 mg, Tabs 50, 150 mg. Susp 25 mg/5 mL (60 mL). Trade only: (Vibramycin) Syrup 50 mg/5 mL (480 mL). Delayed-release tabs (Doryx $$$$$): Generic/Trade: 75, 100 mg. Trade only: 150 mg. Delayed-release caps (Oracea $$$$$): Generic/Trade: 40 mg.] ▶LK ♀D ▶?+ $

MINOCYCLINE (*Minocin, Dynacin, Solodyn*) 200 mg IV/PO initially, then 100 mg q 12 h. Community-acquired MRSA skin infections: 200 mg PO first dose, then 100 mg PO two times per day for 5 to 10 days. Acne (traditional dosing, not Solodyn): 50 mg PO two times per day. Solodyn ($$$$$) for inflammatory acne in adults and children 12 yo and older: Give PO once daily at dose of 45 mg for wt 45 to 54 kg, 65 mg for wt 55 to 77 kg, 90 mg for wt 78 to 102 kg, 115 mg for wt 103 to 125 kg, 135 mg for wt 126 to 136 kg. [Generic/Trade: Caps, Tabs 50, 75, 100 mg. Tabs, extended-release (Solodyn) 45, 90, 135 mg. Trade only: Tabs, extended-release (Solodyn) 65, 115 mg.] ▶LK ♀D ▶?+ $$

TETRACYCLINE 250 to 500 mg PO four times per day. [Generic only: Caps 250, 500 mg.] ▶LK ♀D ▶?+ $

Other Antimicrobials

AZTREONAM (*Azactam, Cayston*) 0.5 to 2 g IM/IV q 6 to 12 h. Peds: 30 mg/kg IV q 6 to 8 h. [Trade only: 75 mg/vial with diluent for inhalation (Cayston).] ▶K ♀B ▶+ $$$$$

CHLORAMPHENICOL (*Chloromycetin*) 50 to 100 mg/kg/day IV divided q 6 h. Aplastic anemia. ▶LK ♀C ▶– $$$$$ ■

CLINDAMYCIN (*Cleocin*, ◆ *Dalacin C*) 150 to 450 mg PO four times per day. 600 to 900 mg IV q 8 h. Community-acquired MRSA skin infections: 300 to 450 mg PO three times per day for 5 to 10 days for adults; 10 to 13 mg/kg/dose PO q 6 to 8 h (max 40 mg/kg/day) for peds. Peds usual dose: 20 to 40 mg/kg/day IV divided q 6 to 8 h or give 8 to 25 mg/kg/day susp PO divided q 6 to 8 h. [Generic only: Caps 75, 150, 300 mg. Generic/Trade: Oral soln 75 mg/5 mL (100 mL).] ▶L ♀B ▶?+ $$$ ■

DAPTOMYCIN (*Cubicin, Cidecin*) Complicated skin infections (including MRSA): 4 mg/kg IV daily for 7 to 14 days. S. aureus bacteremia (including MRSA): 6 mg/kg IV daily for at least 2 to 6 weeks. Infuse over 30 min. Not for pneumonia (inactived by surfactant). Not approved in children. ▶K ♀B ▶? $$$$$

FOSFOMYCIN (*Monurol*) Simple UTI: One 3 g packet PO single dose. [Trade only: 3 g packet of granules.] ▶K ♀B ▶? $$

LINEZOLID (*Zyvox*, ◆ *Zyvoxam*) Pneumonia, complicated skin infections (including MRSA), vancomycin-resistant E. faecium infections: 10 mg/kg (up to 600 mg) IV/PO q 8 h for age younger than 12 yo, 600 mg IV/PO q 12 h for adults and age 12 yo or older. Myelosuppression, drug interactions due to MAO inhibition. Limit tyramine foods to less than 100 mg/meal. [Trade only: Tabs 600 mg. Susp 100 mg/5 mL.] ▶Oxidation/K ♀C ▶? $$$$$

METRONIDAZOLE (*Flagyl, Flagyl ER*, ◆ *Florazole ER*) Bacterial vaginosis: 500 mg PO two times per day or Flagyl ER 750 mg PO daily for 7 days. H. pylori: See table in GI section. Anaerobic bacterial infections: Load 1 g or 15 mg/kg IV, then 500 mg or 7.5 mg/kg (up to 4 g/day) IV/PO q 6 to 8 h, each IV dose over 1 h. Peds: 7.5 mg/kg IV q 6 h. C. difficile associated diarrhea: Adults: 500 mg three times per day for 10 to 14 days. Peds: 30 mg/kg/day PO divided four times per day for 10 to 14 days. See table for management of C. difficile infection. Trichomoniasis: 2 g PO single dose for patient and sex partners (may be used in pregnancy per CDC). Giardia: 250 mg (5 mg/kg/dose for peds) PO three times per day for 5 to 7 days. [Generic/Trade: Tabs 250, 500 mg, Caps 375 mg. Trade only: Tabs, extended-release 750 mg.] ▶KL ♀B ▶?– $ ■

NITROFURANTOIN (*Furadantin, Macrodantin, Macrobid*) 50 to 100 mg PO four times per day. Peds: 5 to 7 mg/kg/day divided four times per day. Macrobid: 100 mg PO two times per day. [Generic/Trade (Macrodantin): Caps 25, 50, 100 mg. Generic/Trade (Macrobid): Caps 100 mg. Generic/Trade (Furadantin): Susp 25 mg/5 mL.] ▶KL ♀B ▶+ $

C. DIFFICILE INFECTION IN ADULTS: IDSA/SHEA TREATMENT RECOMMENDATIONS

Severity	Clinical signs	Treatment
Initial episode		
Mild to moderate	Leukocytosis with WBC count 15,000 or lower AND Serum creatinine less than 1.5 times premorbid level	Metronidazole 500 mg PO q 8 h for 10 to 14 days
Severe	Leukocytosis with WBC count 15,000 or higher OR Serum creatinine at least 1.5 times greater than premorbid level	Vancomycin 125 mg PO q 6 h for 10 to 14 days
Severe complicated	Hypotension or shock, ileus, megacolon	Vancomycin 500 mg PO/NG q 6 h plus metronidazole 500 mg IV q 8 h. Consider vancomycin 500 mg/100 mL normal saline retention enema q 6 h if complete ileus.
Recurrent episodes		
First recurrence	—	Same as initial episode, stratified by severity. Use vancomycin if WBC count 15,000 or higher, or serum creatinine is increasing.
Second recurrence	—	Vancomycin taper* and/or pulsed regimen

Adapted from Infect Control Hosp Epidemiol 2010; 31(5). Available online at: http://www.idsociety.org.
* Example: Vancomycin 125 mg PO four times per day for 10 to 14 days, then 125 mg two times per day for 7 days, then 125 mg once daily for 7 days, then 125 mg every 2 or 3 days for 2 to 8 weeks.

RIFAXIMIN (*Xifaxan*) Traveler's diarrhea: 200 mg PO three times per day for 3 days. Prevention of recurrent hepatic encephalopathy ($$$$$): 550 mg PO two times per day. [Trade only: Tabs 200, 550 mg.] ▶Feces, no GI absorption ♀C ▶? $$$

SYNERCID (quinupristin + dalfopristin) 7.5 mg/kg IV q 12 h, each dose over 1 h. MRSA bacteremia (2nd line): 7.5 mg/kg IV q 8 h. Not active against E. faecalis. ▶Bile ♀B ▶? $$$$$

TELAVANCIN (*Vibativ*) Complicated skin infections including MRSA: 10 mg/kg IV once daily for 7 to 14 days. Infuse over 1 h. Teratogenic; get serum pregnancy test before use in women of childbearing potential. Nephrotoxicity. Not approved in children. ▶K ♀C ▶? $$$$$ ∎

TELITHROMYCIN (*Ketek*) 800 mg PO daily for 7 to 10 days for community-acquired pneumonia. No longer indicated for acute sinusitis or acute exacerbation of chronic bronchitis (risks exceed potential benefit). Contraindicated in myasthenia gravis. [Trade only: Tabs 300, 400 mg. Ketek Pak: #10, 400 mg tabs.] ▶LK ♀C ▶? $$$ ∎

TIGECYCLINE (*Tygacil*) <u>Complicated skin infections, complicated intra-abdominal infections, community-acquired pneumonia</u>: 100 mg IV first dose, then 50 mg IV q 12 h. Infuse over 30 to 60 min. Consider other antibiotics for severe infection because mortality is higher with tigecycline, especially in ventilator-associated pneumonia. ▶Bile, K ♀D ▶?+ $$$$$

TRIMETHOPRIM (*Primsol*, ✦*Proloprim*) 100 mg PO two times per day or 200 mg PO daily. [Generic only: Tabs 100 mg. Trade only (Primsol): Oral soln 50 mg/5 mL.] ▶K ♀C ▶– $

VANCOMYCIN (*Vancocin*) Usual dose: 15 to 20 mg/kg IV q 8 to 12 h; consider loading dose of 25 to 30 mg/kg for severe infection. Infuse over 1 h; infuse over 1.5 to 2 h if dose greater than 1 g. Peds: 10 to 15 mg/kg IV q 6 h. <u>C. difficile diarrhea</u>: 40 to 50 mg/kg/day PO up to 500 mg/day divided four times per day for 10 to 14 days. IV administration ineffective for this indication. Dose depends on severity and complications, see table for management of C. difficile infection. [Trade only: Caps 125, 250 mg.] ▶K ♀C ▶? $$$$$

CARDIOVASCULAR

ACE Inhibitors

NOTE: *See also antihypertensive combinations. Hyperkalemia possible, especially if used concomitantly with other drugs that increase K+ (including K+ containing salt substitutes) and in patients with heart failure, diabetes mellitus, or renal impairment. An increase in serum creatinine up to 35% above baseline is acceptable and is not reason to withhold therapy unless hyperkalemia occurs. Coadministration with NSAIDS, including selective COX-2 inhibitors, may further deteriorate renal function (usually reversible) and decrease antihypertensive effects. ACE inhibitors are contraindicated during pregnancy. Contraindicated with a history of angioedema. Renoprotection and decreased cardiovascular morbidity/mortality seen with some ACE inhibitors are most likely a class effect.*

BENAZEPRIL (*Lotensin*) <u>HTN</u>: Start 10 mg PO daily, usual maintenance dose 20 to 40 mg PO daily or divided two times per day, max 80 mg/day. [Generic/Trade: Tabs unscored 5, 10, 20, 40 mg.] ▶LK ♀– ▶? $$

CAPTOPRIL (*Capoten*) <u>HTN</u>: Start 25 mg PO two to three times per day, usual maintenance dose 25 to 150 mg two to three times per day, max 450 mg/day. <u>Heart failure</u>: Start 6.25 to 12.5 mg PO three times per day, usual dose 50 to 100 mg PO three times per day, max 450 mg/day. <u>Diabetic nephropathy</u>: 25 mg PO three times per day. [Generic/Trade: Tabs scored 12.5, 25, 50, 100 mg.] ▶LK ♀– ▶+ $

CILAZAPRIL (✦*Inhibace*) Canada only. <u>HTN</u>: 1.25 to 10 mg PO daily. [Generic/Trade: Tabs, scored 1, 2.5, 5 mg.] ▶LK ♀– ▶? $

ENALAPRIL (*enalaprilat, Vasotec*) <u>HTN</u>: Start 5 mg PO daily, usual maintenance dose 10 to 40 mg PO daily or divided two times per day, max

(cont.)

ACE INHIBITOR DOSING	HTN		Heart Failure	
	Initial	Max/day	Initial	Max/day
benazepril (*Lotensin*)	10 mg daily*	80 mg	-	-
captopril (*Capoten*)	25 mg bid/tid	450 mg	6.25 mg tid	450 mg
enalapril (*Vasotec*)	5 mg daily*	40 mg	2.5 mg bid	40 mg
fosinopril (*Monopril*)	10 mg daily*	80 mg	5–10 mg daily	40 mg
lisinopril (*Zestril/ Prinivil*)	10 mg daily	80 mg	2.5–5 mg daily	40 mg
moexipril (*Univasc*)	7.5 mg daily*	30 mg	-	-
perindopril (*Aceon*)	4 mg daily*	16 mg	2 mg daily	16 mg
quinapril (*Accupril*)	10–20 mg daily*	80 mg	5 mg bid	40 mg
ramipril (*Altace*)	2.5 mg daily*	20 mg	1.25–2.5 mg bid	10 mg
trandolapril (*Mavik*)	1–2 mg daily*	8 mg	1 mg daily	4 mg

bid=two times per day; tid=three times per day.

Data taken from prescribing information and *Circulation* 2009;119:e391–e479.

*May require bid dosing for 24-h BP control.

40 mg/day. If oral therapy not possible, can use enalaprilat 1.25 mg IV q 6 h over 5 min, and increase up to 5 mg IV q 6 h if needed. <u>Renal impairment or concomitant diuretic therapy</u>: Start 2.5 mg PO daily. <u>Heart failure</u>: Start 2.5 mg PO two times per day, usual 10 to 20 mg PO two times per day, max 40 mg/day. [Generic/Trade: Tabs, scored 2.5, 5 mg, unscored 10, 20 mg.] ▶LK ♀− ▶+ $$

FOSINOPRIL (*Monopril*) <u>HTN</u>: Start 10 mg PO daily, usual maintenance dose 20 to 40 mg PO daily or divided two times per day, max 80 mg/day. <u>Heart failure</u>: Start 5 to 10 mg PO daily, usual dose 20 to 40 mg PO daily, max 40 mg/day. [Generic/Trade: Tabs scored 10, unscored 20, 40 mg.] ▶LK ♀− ▶? $

LISINOPRIL (*Prinivil, Zestril*) <u>HTN</u>: Start 10 mg PO daily, usual maintenance dose 20 to 40 mg PO daily, max 80 mg/day. <u>Heart failure, acute MI</u>: Start 2.5 to 5 mg PO daily, usual dose 5 to 20 mg PO daily, max dose 40 mg. [Generic/Trade: Tabs unscored (Zestril) 2.5, 5, 10, 20, 30, 40 mg. Tabs scored (Prinivil) 10, 20, 40 mg.] ▶K ♀− ▶? $

MOEXIPRIL (*Univasc*) <u>HTN</u>: Start 7.5 mg PO daily, usual maintenance dose 7.5 to 30 mg PO daily or divided two times per day, max 30 mg/day. [Generic/Trade: Tabs scored 7.5, 15 mg.] ▶LK ♀− ▶? $$

PERINDOPRIL (*Aceon*, ✦ *Coversyl*) <u>HTN</u>: Start 4 mg PO daily, usual maintenance dose 4 to 8 mg PO daily or divided two times per day, max 16 mg/day. Reduction of cardiovascular events in stable CAD: Start 4 mg PO daily for 2 weeks, max 8 mg/day. Elderly (age older than 65 yo): 4 mg PO daily, max 8 mg/day. [Generic/Trade: Tabs scored 2, 4, 8 mg.] ▶K ♀− ▶? $$

QUINAPRIL (*Accupril*) <u>HTN</u>: Start 10 to 20 mg PO daily (start 10 mg/day if elderly), usual maintenance dose 20 to 80 mg PO daily or divided two times per day, max 80 mg/day. <u>Heart failure</u>: Start 5 mg PO two times per day, usual maintenance dose 10 to 20 mg two times per day. [Generic/Trade: Tabs scored 5, unscored 10, 20, 40 mg.] ▶LK ♀− ▶? $$

RAMIPRIL (*Altace*) HTN: 2.5 mg PO daily, usual maintenance dose 2.5 to 20 mg PO daily or divided two times per day, max 20 mg/day. Heart failure post MI: Start 2.5 mg PO two times per day, usual maintenance dose 5 mg PO two times per day. Reduce risk of MI, CVA, death from cardiovascular causes: 2.5 mg PO daily for 1 week, then 5 mg daily for 3 weeks, increase as tolerated to max 10 mg/day. [Generic/Trade: Caps 1.25, 2.5, 5, 10 mg.] ▶LK ♀– ▶? $$$

TRANDOLAPRIL (*Mavik*) HTN: Start 1 mg PO daily, usual maintenance dose 2 to 4 mg PO daily or divided two times per day, max 8 mg/day. Heart failure/post MI: Start 0.5 to 1 mg PO daily, usual maintenance dose 4 mg PO daily. [Generic/Trade: Tabs scored 1, unscored 2, 4 mg.] ▶LK ♀– ▶? $$

Aldosterone Antagonists

EPLERENONE (*Inspra*) HTN: Start 50 mg PO daily; max 50 mg two times per day. Improve survival of stable patients with LV systolic dysfunction (LVEF 40% or less) and heart failure post MI: Start 25 mg PO daily; titrate to target dose 50 mg daily within 4 weeks, if tolerated. [Generic/trade: Tabs unscored 25, 50 mg.] ▶L ♀B ▶? $$$

SPIRONOLACTONE (*Aldactone*) HTN: 50 to 100 mg PO daily or divided two times per day. Edema: 25 to 200 mg/day. Hypokalemia: 25 to 100 mg PO daily. Primary hyperaldosteronism, maintenance: 100 to 400 mg/day PO. Heart failure, NYHA III or IV: 25 to 50 mg PO daily. [Generic/Trade: Tabs unscored 25 mg scored 50, 100 mg.] ▶LK ♀D ▶+ $

Angiotensin Receptor Blockers (ARBs)

NOTE: *See also antihypertensive combinations. An increase in serum creatinine up to 35% above baseline is acceptable and is not reason to withhold therapy unless hyperkalemia occurs. Do not use during pregnancy. Coadministration with NSAIDs, including selective COX-2 inhibitors, may further deteriorate renal function (usually reversible) and decrease antihypertensive effects.*

AZILSARTAN (*Edarbi*) HTN: 80 mg daily. [Trade only: Tabs unscored 40, 80 mg.] ▶L – ♀– ▶? $$$

CANDESARTAN (*Atacand*) HTN: Start 16 mg PO daily, maximum 32 mg/day. Heart failure (NYHA II–IV and LVEF 40% or less): Start 4 mg PO daily, maximum 32 mg/day; has added effect when used with ACE inhibitor. [Trade only: Tabs unscored 4, 8, 16, 32 mg.] ▶K ♀– ▶? $$$

EPROSARTAN (*Teveten*) HTN: Start 600 mg PO daily, maximum 800 mg/day given daily or divided two times per day. [Trade only: Tabs unscored 400, 600 mg.] ▶Fecal excretion ♀– ▶? $$$

IRBESARTAN (*Avapro*) HTN: Start 150 mg PO daily, maximum 300 mg/day. Type 2 diabetic nephropathy: Start 150 mg PO daily, target dose 300 mg daily. [Trade only: Tabs unscored 75, 150, 300 mg.] ▶L ♀– ▶? $$$

HTN Therapy[1]

Area of Concern	BP Target	Preferred Therapy[2]	Comments
General CAD prevention	<140/90 mm Hg	ACEI, ARB, CCB, thiazide, or combination	Start 2 drugs if systolic BP ≥ 160 or diastolic BP ≥ 100
High CAD risk[3]	<130/80 mm Hg		
Stable angina, un-stable angina, MI	<130/80 mm Hg	Beta-blocker[4] + (ACEI or ARB)[5]	May add dihydropyridine CCB or thiazide
Left heart failure[6,7]	<120/80 mm Hg	Beta-blocker + (ACEI or ARB) + diuretic[8] + aldosterone antagonist[9]	

1. ACEI = angiotensin converting enzyme inhibitor; ARB = angiotensin-receptor blocker; CCB = calcium-channel blocker; MI = myocardial infarction. Adapted from *Circulation* 2007;115:2761–2788. 2. All patients should attempt lifestyle modifications: optimize wt, healthy diet, sodium restriction, exercise, smoking cessation, alcohol moderation. 3. Diabetes mellitus, chronic kidney disease, known CAD or risk equivalent (eg, peripheral artery disease, abdominal aortic aneurysm, carotid artery disease, and prior ischemic CVA/TIA), 10-year Framingham risk score ≥ 10%. 4. Use only if hemodynamically stable. If beta-blocker contraindications or intolerable side effects (and no bradycardia or heart failure), may substitute verapamil or diltiazem. 5. Preferred if anterior wall MI, persistent HTN, heart failure, or diabetes mellitus. 6. Avoid verapamil, diltiazem, clonidine, beta-blockers. 7. For blacks with NYHA class III or IV HF, consider adding hydralazine/isosorbide dinitrate. 8. Loop or thiazide. 9. Use if NYHA class III or IV, or if clinical heart failure + LVEF < 40%.

LOSARTAN (*Cozaar*) HTN: Start 50 mg PO daily, max 100 mg/day given daily or divided two times per day. <u>Volume-depleted patients or history of hepatic impairment</u>: Start 25 mg PO daily. <u>CVA risk reduction in patients with HTN and LV hypertrophy</u> (may not be effective in black patients): Start 50 mg PO daily. If need more BP reduction add HCTZ 12.5 mg PO daily, then increase losartan to 100 mg/day, then increase HCTZ to 25 mg/day. <u>Type 2 diabetic nephropathy</u>: Start 50 mg PO daily, target dose 100 mg daily. [Generic/Trade: Tabs unscored 25, 50, 100 mg.] ▶L ♀− ▶? $$$
OLMESARTAN (*Benicar*) HTN: Start 20 mg PO daily, max 40 mg/day. [Trade only: Tabs unscored 5, 20, 40 mg.] ▶K ♀− ▶? $$$
TELMISARTAN (*Micardis*) HTN: Start 40 mg PO daily, max 80 mg/day. <u>Cardiovascular risk reduction</u>: Start 80 mg PO daily, max 80 mg/day. [Trade only: Tabs unscored 20, 40, 80 mg.] ▶L ♀− ▶? $$$
VALSARTAN (*Diovan*) HTN: Start 80 to 160 mg PO daily, max 320 mg/day. <u>Heart failure</u>: Start 40 mg PO two times per day, target dose 160 mg two times per day; there is no evidence of added benefit when used with adequate dose of ACE inhibitor. <u>Reduce mortality/morbidity post MI with LV systolic dysfunction/failure</u>: Start 20 mg PO two times per day, target dose 160 mg two times per day. [Trade only: Tabs scored 40, unscored 80, 160, 320 mg.] ▶L ♀− ▶? $$$

Antiadrenergic Agents

CLONIDINE (*Catapres, Catapres-TTS, Jenloga, Kapvay, ✦Dixarit*) <u>Immediate-release, HTN</u>: Start 0.1 mg PO two times per day, usual maintenance dose 0.2 to 0.6 mg/day in 2 to 3 divided doses, max 2.4 mg

(cont.)

daily. <u>Extended-release (Jenloga)</u>, HTN: Start 0.1 mg daily at bedtime, max 0.6 mg daily. Rebound HTN with abrupt discontinuation, taper dose slowly. <u>Transdermal (Catapres-TTS)</u>, HTN: Start 0.1 mg/24 h patch once a week, titrate to desired effect, max effective dose 0.6 mg/24 h (two 0.3 mg/24 h patches). Transdermal Therapeutic System (TTS) is designed for 7-day use so that a TTS-1 delivers 0.1 mg/day for 7 days. May supplement 1st dose of TTS with oral for 2 to 3 days while therapeutic level is achieved. <u>Extended-release (Kapvay)</u>, ADHD (6 to 17 yo): Start 0.1 mg PO at bedtime; may increase by 0.1 mg/day each week; give two times per day with equal or higher dose at bedtime, max 0.4 mg daily. <u>Immediate-release</u>, ADHD (unapproved peds): Start 0.05 mg PO at bedtime, titrate based on response over 8 weeks to max 0.2 mg/day (for wt less than 45 kg) or to max 0.4 mg/day (for wt 45 kg or greater) in 2 to 4 divided doses. <u>Tourette syndrome</u> (unapproved peds and adult): 3 to 5 mcg/kg/day PO divided two to four times per day. Opioid withdrawal, adjunct: 0.1 to 0.3 mg PO three to four times per day or 0.1 to 0.2 mg PO q 4 h for 3 days tapering off over 4 to 10 days. <u>Alcohol withdrawal, adjunct</u>: 0.1 to 0.2 mg PO q 4 h prn. <u>Smoking cessation</u>: Start 0.1 mg PO two times per day, increase 0.1 mg/day at weekly intervals to 0.75 mg/day as tolerated, transdermal (Catapres TTS): 0.1 to 0.2 mg/24 h patch once a week for 2 to 3 weeks after cessation. <u>Menopausal flushing</u>: 0.1 to 0.4 mg/day PO divided two to three times per day. Transdermal system applied weekly: 0.1 mg/day. Monitor for bradycardia when taking concomitant digitalis, nondihydropyridine calcium channel blockers, or beta-blockers. [Generic/Trade: Tabs Immediate-release unscored (Catapres) 0.1, 0.2, 0.3 mg. Transdermal weekly patch 0.1 mg/day (TTS-1), 0.2 mg/day (TTS-2), 0.3 mg/day (TTS-3). Generic only: Oral Susp, Extended-release, 0.09 mg/mL (118 mL). Tabs extended-release unscored (Jenloga, Kapvay) 0.1, 0.2 mg.] ▶LK ♀C ▶? $$

DOXAZOSIN (**Cardura, Cardura XL**) <u>BPH</u>: Immediate-release: Start 1 mg PO at bedtime, max 8 mg/day. Extended-release (not approved for HTN): 4 mg PO q am with breakfast, max 8 mg/day. <u>HTN</u>: Start 1 mg PO at bedtime, max 16 mg/day. Take first dose at bedtime to minimize orthostatic hypotension. [Generic/Trade: Tabs scored 1, 2, 4, 8 mg. Trade only (Cardura XL): Tabs extended-release 4, 8 mg.] ▶L ♀C ▶? $$

GUANFACINE (**Tenex**) <u>HTN</u>: Start 1 mg PO at bedtime, increase to 2 to 3 mg at bedtime if needed after 3 to 4 weeks, max 3 mg/day. <u>ADHD in children</u>: Start 0.5 mg PO daily, titrate by 0.5 mg q 3 to 4 days as tolerated to 0.5 mg PO three times per day. [Generic/Trade: Tabs unscored 1, 2 mg.] ▶K ♀B ▶? $

METHYLDOPA (**Aldomet**) <u>HTN</u>: Start 250 mg PO 2 to 3 times daily, maximum 3000 mg/day. May cause hemolytic anemia. May be used to manage BP during pregnancy. [Generic only: Tabs unscored 125, 250, 500 mg.] ▶LK ♀B ▶+ $

PRAZOSIN (**Minipress**) <u>HTN</u>: Start 1 mg PO two to three times per day, max 40 mg/day. Take 1st dose at bedtime to minimize orthostatic hypotension. [Generic/Trade: Caps 1, 2, 5 mg.] ▶L ♀C ▶? $$

TERAZOSIN (*Hytrin*) <u>HTN</u>: Start 1 mg PO at bedtime, usual effective dose 1 to 5 mg PO daily or divided two times per day, max 20 mg/day. Take first dose at bedtime to minimize orthostatic hypotension. BPH: Start 1 mg PO at bedtime, usual effective dose 10 mg/day, max 20 mg/day. [Generic/Trade: Tabs/caps 1, 2, 5, 10 mg.] ▶LK ♀C ▶? $$

Anti-Dysrhythmics/Cardiac Arrest

ADENOSINE (*Adenocard*) <u>PSVT conversion (not A-fib)</u>: Adult and peds wt 50 kg or greater: 6 mg rapid IV and flush, preferably through a central line. If no response after 1 to 2 min, then 12 mg. A 3rd dose of 12 mg may be given prn. Peds wt less than 50 kg: Initial dose 50 to 100 mcg/kg, subsequent doses 100 to 200 mcg/kg q 1 to 2 min prn up to a max single dose of 300 mcg/kg or 12 mg, whichever is less. Half-life is less than 10 sec. Give doses by rapid IV push followed by NS flush. Need higher dose if on theophylline or caffeine, lower dose if on dipyridamole or carbamazepine ▶Plasma ♀C ▶? $$$

AMIODARONE (*Cordarone, Pacerone*) Proarrhythmic. <u>Life-threatening ventricular arrhythmia without cardiac arrest</u>: Load 150 mg IV over 10 min, then 1 mg/min for 6 h, then 0.5 mg/min for 18 h. Mix in D5W. Oral loading dose 800 to 1600 mg PO daily for 1 to 3 weeks, reduce to 400 to 800 mg PO daily for 1 month when arrhythmia is controlled, reduce to lowest effective dose thereafter, usually 200 to 400 mg PO daily. Photosensitivity with oral therapy. Pulmonary and hepatic toxicity. Hypo- or hyperthyroidism possible. Coadministration of fluoroquinolones, macrolides, loratadine, trazodone, azoles, or Class IA and III antiarrhythmic drugs may prolong QTc. May increase digoxin levels; discontinue digoxin or decrease dose by 50%. May increase INR with warfarin by up to 100%; decrease warfarin dose by 33 to 50%. Do not use with grapefruit juice. Do not use with simvastatin dose greater than 10 mg/day, lovastatin dose greater than 40 mg/day; caution with atorvastatin; increases risk of myopathy and rhabdomyolysis. Caution with beta-blockers and calcium channel blockers. IV therapy may cause hypotension. Contraindicated with marked sinus bradycardia and 2nd or 3rd degree heart block in the absence of a functioning pacemaker. [Trade only (Pacerone): tabs unscored 100 mg. Generic/Trade: Tabs scored 200, 400 mg.] ▶L ♀D ▶– $$$$

ATROPINE (*AtroPen*) <u>Bradyarrhythmia/CPR</u>: 0.5 to 1 mg IV q 3 to 5 min to max 0.04 mg/kg (3 mg). <u>Peds</u>: 0.02 mg/kg IV, minimum single dose, 0.1 mg; max cumulative dose, 1 mg. <u>AtroPen</u>: Injector pens for insecticide or nerve agent poisoning. [Trade only: Prefilled auto-injector pen: 0.25 mg (yellow), 0.5 mg (blue), 1 mg (dark red), 2 mg (green).] ▶K ♀C ▶– $

BICARBONATE <u>Severe acidosis</u>: 1 mEq/kg IV up to 50 to 100 mEq/dose. ▶K ♀C ▶? $

DIGOXIN (*Lanoxin, Lanoxicaps, Digitek*) Proarrhythmic. <u>Systolic heart failure/rate control of chronic A-fib</u>: 0.125 to 0.25 mg PO daily; impaired renal function: 0.0625 to 0.125 mg PO daily. <u>Rapid A-fib</u>: Load 0.5 mg IV, then 0.25 mg IV q 6 h for 2 doses, maintenance 0.125 to 0.375 mg IV/PO daily. [Generic/Trade: Tabs, scored (Lanoxin, Digitek) 0.125, 0.25 mg; elixir 0.05 mg/mL. Trade only: Caps (Lanoxicaps), 0.1, 0.2 mg.] ▶KL ♀C ▶+ $

SELECTED DRUGS THAT MAY PROLONG THE QT INTERVAL

alfuzosin	epirubicin	methadone*†	ranolazine
amantadine	erythromycin*†	moexipril/HCTZ	risperidone‡
amiodarone*†	escitalopram	moxifloxacin	salmeterol
apomorphine	famotidine	nicardipine	sertindole
arsenic trioxide*	felbamate	nilotinib	sertraline
atazanavir	flecainide†	octreotide	sotalol*†
azithromycin*	foscarnet	ofloxacin	sunitinib
chloroquine*†	fosphenytoin	ondansetron	tacrolimus
chlorpromazine	gatifloxacin	oxytocin	tamoxifen
cisapride*†	gemifloxacin	paliperidone	telithromycin*
citalopram*	granisetron	pentamidine*†	thioridazine*
clarithromycin*	halofantrine*┃	phenothiazines‡	tizanidine
clozapine	haloperidol*‡	pimozide*†	tolterodine
cocaine*	ibutilide*†	polyethylene	vandetanib*
dasatinib	indapamide*	glycol (PEG-salt	vardenafil
disopyramide*†	isradipine	soln)§	venlafaxine
dofetilide*	lapatinib	procainamide*†	visicol§
dolasetron	levofloxacin*	quetiapine‡	voriconazole*
dronedarone	lithium	quinidine*†	vorinostat
droperidol*	mefloquine	quinine	ziprasidone‡

Note: This table may not include all drugs that prolong the QT interval or cause torsades. Risk of drug-induced QT prolongation may be increased in women, elderly, hypokalemia, hypomagnesemia, bradycardia, starvation, CHF, and CNS injuries. Hepatorenal dysfunction and drug interactions can increase the concentration of QT interval-prolonging drugs. Coadministration of QT interval-prolonging drugs can have additive effects. Avoid these (and other) drugs in congenital prolonged QT syndrome (www.qtdrugs.org). *Torsades reported in product labeling/case reports. †Increased risk in women. ‡QT prolongation: thioridazine > ziprasidone > risperidone, quetiapine, haloperidol. §May be due to electrolyte imbalance.

DIGOXIN IMMUNE FAB (*Digibind, DigiFab*) Digoxin toxicity: Dose varies. Acute ingestion of known amount: 1 vial binds approximately 0.5 mg digoxin. Acute ingestion of unknown amount: 10 vials IV, may repeat once. Toxicity during chronic therapy: 6 vials usually adequate; one formula is: Number vials is equivalent to (serum dig level in ng/mL) × (kg)/100. ▶K ♀C ▶? $$$$$

DISOPYRAMIDE (*Norpace, Norpace CR,* ✦ *Rythmodan, Rythmodan-LA*) Proarrhythmic. Rarely indicated, consult cardiologist. Ventricular arrhythmia: 400 to 800 mg PO daily in divided doses (immediate-release is divided q 6 h; extended-release is divided q 12 h). [Generic/Trade: Caps immediate-release 100, 150 mg; extended-release 150 mg. Trade only: Caps, extended-release 100 mg.] ▶KL ♀C ▶+ $$$$

DOFETILIDE (*Tikosyn*) Proarrhythmic. Conversion of A-fib/flutter: Specialized dosing based on CrCl and QTc interval. Available only to hospitals and prescribers who have received appropriate dosing and treatment-initiation education. [Trade only: Caps, 0.125, 0.25, 0.5 mg.] ▶KL ♀C ▶— $$$$

DRONEDARONE (*Multaq*) Reduce risk of CV hospitalization with paroxysmal or persistent atrial fib/flutter, with recent episode of atrial fib/flutter and CV risk factors (ie, age older than 70 yo, HTN, diabetes, prior CVA, left atrial diameter 50 mm or greater, or LVEF less than 40%), who are in sinus rhythm or will be converted: 400 mg PO two times per day with morning and evening

(cont.)

meals. Do not use with any of the following: 2nd or 3rd degree AV block or sick sinus syndrome without functioning pacemaker; bradycardia < 50 bpm; QTc Bazett interval > 500 ms; or severe hepatic impairment. Do not use with grapefruit juice; other antiarrhythmic agents; potent inhibitors of CYP3A4 enzyme system (clarithromycin, erythromycin, itraconazole, ketoconazole, nefazodone, ritonavir, voriconazole); or inducers of CYP3A4 enzyme system (carbamazepine, phenytoin, phenobarbital, rifampin, St. John's Wort). May increase INR when added to warfarin therapy. May increase digoxin levels; discontinue digoxin or decrease dose by 50%. Caution with beta-blockers and calcium channel blockers. May increase levels of sirolimus, tacrolimus, and CYP3A4 substrates with narrow therapeutic index. May initiate or worsen HF symptoms. Do not use with NYHA Class IV heart failure or NYHA Class II–III heart failure with recent decompensation requiring hospitalization or referral to heart failure clinic. [Trade: Tabs unscored 400 mg.] ▶L ♀X ▶– $$$$

FLECAINIDE *(Tambocor)* Proarrhythmic. Prevention of paroxysmal atrial fib/flutter or PSVT, with symptoms and no structural heart disease: Start 50 mg PO q 12 h, may increase by 50 mg two times per day q 4 days, max 300 mg/day. Use with AV nodal slowing agent (beta-blocker, verapamil, diltiazem) to minimize risk of 1:1 atrial flutter. Life-threatening ventricular arrhythmias without structural heart disease: Start 100 mg PO q 12 h, may increase by 50 mg two times per day q 4 days, max 400 mg/day. With severe renal impairment (CrCl less than 35 mL/min): Start 50 mg PO two times per day. [Generic/Trade: Tabs unscored 50, scored 100, 150 mg.] ▶K ♀C ▶– $$$$

IBUTILIDE *(Corvert)* Proarrhythmic. Recent onset A-fib/flutter: 0.01 mg/kg up to 1 mg IV over 10 min, may repeat once if no response after 10 additional min. Keep on cardiac monitor at least 4 h. ▶LK ♀C ▶? $$$$$

ISOPROTERENOL *(Isuprel)* Refractory bradycardia or 3rd degree AV block: bolus method: 0.02 to 0.06 mg IV: infusion method, dilute 2 mg in 250 mL D5W (8 mcg/mL), a rate of 37.5 mL/h delivers 5 mcg/min. Peds infusion method: 0.05 to 2 mcg/kg/min. Using the same concentration as adult for a 10 kg child, a rate of 8 mL/h delivers 0.1 mcg/kg/min. ▶LK ♀C ▶? $$$

LIDOCAINE *(Xylocaine, Xylocard)* Ventricular arrhythmia: Load 1 mg/kg IV, then 0.5 mg/kg q 8 to 10 min prn to max 3 mg/kg. IV infusion: 4 g in 500 mL D5W (8 mg/mL) run at rate of 7.5 to 30 mL/h to deliver 1 to 4 mg/min. Peds: 20 to 50 mcg/kg/min. ▶LK ♀B ▶? $

MEXILETINE *(Mexitil)* Proarrhythmic. Rarely indicated, consult cardiologist. Ventricular arrhythmia: Start 200 mg PO q 8 h with food or antacid, max dose 1200 mg/day. [Generic only: Caps 150, 200, 250 mg.] ▶L ♀C ▶– $$$

PROCAINAMIDE *(Pronestyl)* Proarrhythmic. Ventricular arrhythmia: Loading dose: 100 mg IV q 10 min or 20 mg/min (150 mL/h) until QRS widens more than 50%, dysrhythmia suppressed, hypotension, or total of 17 mg/kg or 1000 mg delivered. Infusion: Dilute 2 g in 250 mL D5W (8 mg/mL) rate of 15 to 45 mL/h to deliver 2 to 6 mg/min. ▶LK ♀C ▶? $

PROPAFENONE *(Rythmol, Rythmol SR)* Proarrhythmic. Prevention of paroxysmal atrial fib/flutter or PSVT, with symptoms and no structural heart disease; or life-threatening ventricular arrhythmias: Start (immediate-

(cont.)

release) 150 mg PO q 8 h; may increase after 3 to 4 days to 225 mg PO q 8 h; max 900 mg/day. <u>Prolong time to recurrence of symptomatic atrial fib without structural heart disease:</u> 225 mg SR PO q 12 h, may increase after 5 days to 325 mg SR PO q 12 h, max 425 mg SR PO q 12 h. Consider using with AV nodal blocking agent (beta-blocker, verapamil, diltiazem) to minimize risk of 1:1 atrial flutter. [Generic/Trade: Tabs immediate-release scored 150, 225, 300 mg. Trade only: SR, Caps 225, 325, 425 mg.] ▶L ♀C ▶? $$$$

QUINIDINE Proarrhythmic. <u>Arrhythmia:</u> Gluconate, extended-release: 324 to 648 mg PO q 8 to 12 h; sulfate, immediate-release: 200 to 400 mg PO q 6 to 8 h; sulfate, extended-release: 300 to 600 mg PO q 8 to 12 h. [Generic gluconate: Tabs, extended-release unscored 324 mg. Generic sulfate: Tabs, scored immediate-release 200, 300 mg, Tabs, extended-release 300 mg.] ▶LK ♀C ▶+ $$$- gluconate, $-sulfate

SOTALOL (*Betapace, Betapace AF*) Proarrhythmic. <u>Ventricular arrhythmia (Betapace), A-fib/A-flutter (Betapace AF):</u> Start 80 mg PO two times per day, max 640 mg/day. [Generic/Trade: Tabs, scored 80, 120, 160, 240 mg, Tabs, scored (Betapace AF) 80, 120, 160 mg.] ▶K ♀B ▶– $$$$

Anti-Hyperlipidemic Agents—Bile Acid Sequestrants

CHOLESTYRAMINE (*Questran, Questran Light, Prevalite, LoCHOLEST, LoCHOLEST Light*) <u>Elevated LDL-C:</u> Powder: Start 4 g PO daily to two times per day before meals, increase up to max 24 g/day. [Generic/Trade: Powder for oral susp, 4 g cholestyramine resin/9 g powder (Questran, LoCHOLEST), 4 g cholestyramine resin/5 g powder (Questran Light), 4 g cholestyramine resin/5.5 g powder (Prevalite, LoCHOLEST Light). Each available in bulk powder and single-dose packets.] ▶Not absorbed ♀C ▶+ $$$

COLESEVELAM (*Welchol*) <u>Glycemic control of type 2 diabetes or LDL-C reduction:</u> 3.75 g once daily or 1.875 g PO two times per day, max 3.75 g/day. Give with meal and 4 to 8 ounces of water, fruit juice, or diet soft drink. 3.75 g is equivalent to 6 tabs; 1.875 g is equivalent to 3 tabs. [Trade only: Tabs unscored 625 mg. Powder single-dose packets 1.875, 3.75 g.] ▶Not absorbed ♀B ▶– $$$$$

COLESTIPOL (*Colestid, Colestid Flavored*) <u>Elevated LDL-C:</u> Tabs: Start 2 g PO daily to two times per day, max 16 g/day. Granules: Start 5 g PO daily to two times per day, max 30 g/day. [Generic/Trade: Tabs 1 g. Granules for oral susp, 5 g/7.5 g powder.] ▶Not absorbed ♀B ▶+ $$$$

Anti-Hyperlipidemic Agents—HMG-CoA Reductase Inhibitors ("Statins") and Combinations

NOTE: *Atorvastatin, lovastatin, pitavastatin, rosuvastatin, and simvastatin have restricted maximum doses that are lower than typical maximum doses when used with certain interacting medications. Evaluate muscle symptoms before starting therapy, 6 to 12 weeks after starting/increasing therapy, and at each follow-up visit. Evaluate for low Vitamin D and hypothyroidism and obtain creatine kinase when patient complains of muscle soreness, tenderness, weakness, or pain. These factors increase the risk for myopathy: Advanced age (especially*

(cont.)

LIPID REDUCTION BY CLASS/AGENT[1]

Drug class/agent	LDL	HDL	TG
Bile acid sequestrants[2]	↓ 15–30%	↑ 3–5%	No change or ↑
Cholesterol absorption inhibitor[3]	↓ 18%	↑ 1%	↓8%
Fibrates[4]	↓ 5–20%	↑ 10–20%	↓ 20–50%
Lovastatin+ext'd release niacin[5]*	↓ 30–42%	↑ 20–30%	↓ 32–44%
Niacin[6]*	↓ 5–25%	↑ 15–35%	↓ 20–50%
Omega 3 fatty acids[7]	No change or ↑	↑ 9%	↓ 45%
Statins[8]	↓18–63%	↑ 5–15%	↓ 7–35%
Simvastatin+ezetimibe[9]	↓ 45–59%	↑ 6–10%	↓ 23–31%

1. LDL = low density lipoprotein. HDL = high density lipoprotein. TG = triglycerides. Adapted from NCEP: *JAMA* 2001; 285:2486 and prescribing information. 2. Cholestyramine (4–16 g), colestipol (5–20 g), colesevelam (2.6–3.8 g). 3. Ezetimibe (10 mg). When added to statin therapy, will ↓ LDL 25%, ↑ HDL 3%, ↓ TG 14% in addition to statin effects. 4. Fenofibrate (145–200 mg), gemfibrozil (600 mg two times per day). 5. Advicor® (20/1000–40/2000 mg). 6. Extended release nicotinic acid (Niaspan® 1–2 g), immediate release (crystalline) nicotinic acid (1.5–3 g), sustained release nicotinic acid (Slo-Niacin® 1–2 g). 7. Lovaza (4 g) 8. Atorvastatin (10–80 mg), fluvastatin (20–80 mg), lovastatin (20–80 mg), pravastatin (20–80 mg), rosuvastatin (5–40 mg), simvastatin (20–40 mg). 9. Vytorin® (10/10–10/40 mg). *Lowers lipoprotein a.

age older than 80 yo, women > men); multisystem disease (eg, chronic renal insufficiency, especially due to diabetes); multiple medications; perioperative periods; alcohol abuse; grapefruit juice (more than 1 quart/day); specific concomitant medications: fibrates (especially gemfibrozil), nicotinic acid (rare), amiodarone, clarithromycin, cyclosporine, daptomycin, diltiazem, erythromycin, itraconazole, ketoconazole, nefazodone, protease inhibitors, or verapamil. Weigh potential risk of combination therapy against potential benefit. Hepatotoxicity: Monitor LFTs initially, then when clinically indicated.

ADVICOR (lovastatin + niacin) Hyperlipidemia: 1 tab PO at bedtime with a low-fat snack. Establish dose using extended-release niacin first, or if already on lovastatin, substitute combo product with lowest niacin dose. Immediate-release aspirin or ibuprofen 30 min prior may decrease niacin flushing reaction. Do not use with potent inhibitors of CYP3A4 enzyme system (clarithromycin, erythromycin, grapefruit juice > 1 quart/day, HIV protease inhibitors, itraconazole, ketoconazole, nefazodone, telithromycin); increases risk of myopathy. Do not exceed 20 mg/day of lovastatin component when used with cyclosporine, danazol, fibrates, or niacin at doses 1 g/day or greater; do not exceed 40 mg/day of lovastatin component when used with amiodarone or verapamil. With concomitant cyclosporine or danazol, start with 10 mg daily of lovastatin component. [Trade only: Tabs, unscored extended- release lovastatin/niacin 20/500, 20/750, 20/1000, 40/1000 mg.] ▶LK ♀X ▶– $$$$

ATORVASTATIN (*Lipitor*) Hyperlipidemia/prevention of cardiovascular events, including type 2 DM: Start 10 to 40 mg PO daily, max 80 mg/day. Do not exceed 10 mg/day when used with cyclosporine. Use > 20 mg/day cautiously when used with clarithromycin, itraconazole, or combinations of HIV protease inhibitors that include ritonavir. [Trade only: Tabs unscored 10, 20, 40, 80 mg.] ▶L ♀X ▶– $$$$

CADUET (amlodipine + atorvastatin) <u>Simultaneous treatment of HTN and hypercholesterolemia</u>: Establish dose using component drugs first. Dosing interval: Daily. [Trade only: Tabs, 2.5/10, 2.5/20, 2.5/40, 5/10, 5/20, 5/40, 5/80, 10/10, 10/20, 10/40, 10/80 mg.] ▶L ♀X ▶− $$$$

FLUVASTATIN (*Lescol, Lescol XL*) <u>Hyperlipidemia</u>: Start 20 to 80 mg PO at bedtime, max 80 mg daily (XL) or divided two times per day. <u>Post percutaneous coronary intervention</u>: 80 mg of extended-release PO daily, max 80 mg daily. [Trade only: Caps 20, 40 mg. Tabs extended-release unscored 80 mg.] ▶L ♀X ▶− $$$

LOVASTATIN (*Mevacor, Altoprev*) <u>Hyperlipidemia/prevention of cardiovascular events</u>: Start 20 mg PO q pm, max 80 mg/day daily or divided two times per day. See package insert for dosing restrictions when used with amiodarone, cyclosporine, danazol, fibrates, niacin, or verapamil. [Generic/Trade: Tabs unscored 20, 40 mg. Trade only: Tabs extended-release (Altoprev) 20, 40, 60 mg.] ▶L ♀X ▶− $

PITAVASTATIN (*Livalo*) <u>Hyperlipidemia</u>: Start 2 mg PO at bedtime, max 4 mg daily. <u>Renal impairment</u> (GFR 15-59 mL/min) or <u>end stage renal disease receiving hemodialysis</u>: Max start 1 mg PO daily, max 2 mg daily. See package insert for dosing restrictions when used for patients taking erythromycin or rifampin. Do not use with cyclosporine. [Trade only: Tabs 1, 2, 4 mg.] ▶L − ♀X ▶− $$$$

PRAVASTATIN (*Pravachol*) <u>Hyperlipidemia/prevention of cardiovascular events</u>: Start 40 mg PO daily, max 80 mg/day. [Generic/Trade: Tabs unscored 10, 20, 40, 80 mg.] ▶L ♀X ▶− $$$

ROSUVASTATIN (*Crestor*) <u>Hyperlipidemia/slow progression of atherosclerosis/ primary prevention of cardiovascular disease</u>: Start 10 to 20 mg PO daily, max 40 mg/day. See package insert for dosing restrictions when used for Asians, patients with renal impairment, and patients taking cyclosporine, gemfibrozil, or protease inhibitor combinations that include ritonavir. [Trade only: Tabs unscored 5, 10, 20, 40 mg.] ▶L ♀X ▶− $$$$

SIMCOR (simvastatin + niacin) <u>Hyperlipidemia</u>: 1 tab PO at bedtime with a low-fat snack. If niacin-naive or switching from immediate-release niacin, start: 20/500 mg PO q pm. If receiving extended-release niacin, do not start with more than 40/2000 mg PO q pm. Max 40/2000 mg/day. Immediate-release aspirin or ibuprofen 30 min prior may decrease niacin flushing reaction. Contraindicated with strong CYP3A4 inhibitors, amiodarone, clarithromycin, cyclosporine, danazol, diltiazem, erythromycin, fenofibrate, gemfibrozil, grapefruit juice more than 1 quart/day, HIV protease inhibitors, itraconazole, ketoconazole, nefazodone, posaconazole, telithromycin, verapamil. Do not exceed 20/1000 with amlodipine, ranolazine, or Chinese patients. [Trade only: Tabs, unscored extended-release simvastatin/niacin 20/500, 20/750, 20/1000 mg.] ▶LK ♀X ▶− $$$

SIMVASTATIN (*Zocor*) Do not initiate therapy with or titrate to 80 mg/day; only use 80 mg/day in patients who have taken this dose for longer than 12 months without evidence of muscle toxicity. <u>Hyperlipidemia</u>: Start 10 to

(cont.)

Risk Category	LDL Goal	Lifestyle Changes[2]	Also Consider Meds at LDL (mg/dL)[3]
LDL CHOLESTEROL GOALS[1]			
High risk: CHD or equivalent risk,[4,5,6] 10-year risk >20%	<100 (optional <70)[7]	LDL ≥ 100[8]	≥100 (<100: consider Rx options)[9]
Moderately high risk: 2+ risk factors,[10] 10-year risk 10–20%	<130 (optional <100)	LDL ≥ 130[8]	≥130 (100–129: consider Rx options)[11]
Moderate risk: 2+ risk factors,[10] 10-year risk <10%	<130 mg/dL	LDL ≥ 130	≥160
Lower risk: 0 to 1 risk factor[5]	<160 mg/dL	LDL ≥ 160	≥190 (160–189: Rx optional)

1. CHD=coronary heart disease. LDL= low density lipoprotein. Adapted from NCEP: *JAMA* 2001; 285:2486; NCEP Report: *Circulation* 2004;110:227–239. All 10-year risks based upon Framingham stratification; calculator available at: http://hin.nhlbi.nih.gov/atpiii/calculator.asp?usertype=prof. 2. Dietary modification, wt reduction, exercise. 3. When using LDL lowering therapy, achieve at least 30-40% LDL reduction. 4. Equivalent risk defined as diabetes, other atherosclerotic disease (peripheral artery disease, abdominal aortic aneurysm, symptomatic carotid artery disease, CKD or prior ischemic CVA/TIA), or ≥ 2 risk factors such that 10-year risk >20%. 5. History of ischemic CVA or transient ischemic attack = CHD risk equivalents (*Stroke* 2006;37:577-617). 6. Chronic kidney disease = CHD risk equivalent (*Am J Kidney Dis* 2003 Apr;41 (4 suppl 3):I-IV,S1-91). 7. For any patient with atherosclerotic disease, may treat to LDL < 70 mg/dL (*Circulation* 2006;113:2363-72). 8. Regardless of LDL, lifestyle changes are indicated when lifestyle-related risk factors (obesity, physical inactivity, ↑TG, ↓HDL, or metabolic syndrome) are present. 9. If baseline LDL < 100, starting LDL lowering therapy is an option based on clinical trials. With ↑TG or ↓HDL, consider combining fibrate or nicotinic acid with LDL lowering drug. 10. Risk factors: Cigarette smoking, HTN (BP ≥140/90 mmHg or on antihypertensive meds), low HDL (< 40 mg/dL), family hx of CHD (1° relative: ♂ < 55 yo, ♀ < 65 yo), age (♂ ≥ 45 yo, ♀ ≥ 55 yo). 11. At baseline or after lifestyle changes - initiating therapy to achieve LDL < 100 is an option based on clinical trials.

20 mg PO q pm, max 40 mg/day. Reduce cardiovascular mortality/events in high risk for coronary heart disease event: Start 40 mg PO q pm, max 40 mg/day. Severe renal impairment: Start 5 mg/day, closely monitor. Do not use with clarithromycin, cyclosporine, danazol, erythromycin, gemfibrozil, grapefruit juice more than 1 quart/day, HIV protease inhibitors, itraconazole, ketoconazole, nefazodone, posaconazole, telithromycin. Do not exceed 10 mg/day when used with amiodarone, diltiazem, or verapamil; or 20 mg/day when used with amlodipine or ranolazine. For Chinese patients, do not exceed 20 mg/day with niacin 1 g or more daily. [Generic/Trade: Tabs unscored 5, 10, 20, 40, 80 mg.] ▶L ♀X ▶– $$$$

VYTORIN (ezetimibe + simvastatin) Hyperlipidemia: Start 10/10 or 10/20 mg PO q pm, max 10/40 mg/day. Restrict the use of the 10/80 mg dose to patients who have taken it at least 12 months without muscle toxicity. Do not use with clarithromycin, cyclosporine, danazol, erythromycin, gemfibrozil, grapefruit juice more than 1 quart/day, HIV protease inhibitors, itraconazole, ketoconazole, nefazodone, posaconazole, telithromycin. Max dose 10/10 mg/day when used with amiodarone, diltiazem, or verapamil. Max dose 20/10 mg/day when used with amlodipine or ranolazine. For Chinese patients, max dose 10/20 mg/day with niacin 1 g/day or more. [Trade only: Tabs, unscored ezetimibe/simvastatin 10/10, 10/20, 10/40, 10/80 mg.] ▶L ♀X ▶– $$$$

Anti-Hyperlipidemic Agents—Other

BEZAFIBRATE (✦ *Bezalip*) Canada only. Hyperlipidemia/hypertriglyceridemia: 200 mg immediate-release PO two to three times per day, or 400 mg of sustained-release PO daily. [Canada Trade only: Sustained-release tab 400 mg.] ▶K ♀D ▶– $$$

EZETIMIBE (*Zetia*, ✦ *Ezetrol*) Hyperlipidemia: 10 mg PO daily. [Trade only: Tabs, unscored 10 mg.] ▶L ♀C ▶? $$$$

FENOFIBRATE (*TriCor, Antara, Fenoglide Lipofen, Triglide*, ✦ *Lipidil Micro, Lipidil Supra, Lipidil EZ*) Hypertriglyceridemia: TriCor tabs: 48 to 145 mg PO daily, max 145 mg daily. Antara: 43 to 130 mg PO daily; max 130 mg daily. Fenoglide: 40 to 120 mg PO daily; max 120 mg daily. Lipofen: 50 to 150 mg PO daily, max 150 mg daily. Triglide: 50 to 160 mg PO daily, max 160 mg daily. Generic tabs: 54 to 160 mg, max 160 mg daily. Generic caps: 67 to 200 mg PO daily; max 200 mg daily. Hypercholesterolemia/mixed dyslipidemia: TriCor tabs: 145 mg PO daily. Antara: 130 mg PO daily. Fenoglide: 120 mg daily. Lipofen: 150 mg daily. Triglide: 160 mg daily. Generic tabs: 160 mg daily. Generic caps 200 mg PO daily. All formulations, except Antara, TriCor, and Triglide, should be taken with food. [Generic only: Tabs unscored 54, 160 mg. Generic caps 67, 134, 200 mg. Trade only: Tabs (TriCor) unscored 48, 145 mg. Caps (Antara) 43, 130 mg. Caps (Fenoglide) unscored 40, 120 mg. Tabs (Lipofen) unscored 50, 100, 150 mg. Tabs (Triglide) unscored 50, 160 mg.] ▶LK ♀C ▶– $$$

FENOFIBRIC ACID (*Fibricor, TriLipix*) In combination with statin for mixed dyslipidemia and CHD or CHD risk equivalent: TriLipix: 135 mg PO daily. Hypertriglyceridemia: Fibricor: 35 to 105 mg PO daily, max 105 mg daily. TriLipix: 45 to 135 mg PO daily, max 135 mg daily. Hypercholesterolemia/mixed dyslipidemia: Fibricor: 105 mg PO daily. TriLipix: 135 mg PO daily. [Trade only: Caps (TriLipix) delayed-release 45, 135 mg. Tabs (Fibricor) 35, 105 mg.] ▶LK ♀C ▶– $$$

STATINS

Minimum Dose for 30-40% LDL Reduction	LDL *
atorvastatin 10 mg	-39%
fluvastatin 40 mg two times per day	-36%
fluvastatin XL 80 mg	-35%
lovastatin 40 mg	-31%
pitavastatin 2 mg	-36%
pravastatin 40mg	-34%
rosuvastatin 5 mg	-45%
simvastatin 20 mg	-38%

LDL=low-density lipoprotein. Will get ~6% decrease in LDL with every doubling of dose.
*Adapted from *Circulation* 2004;110:227-239.

GEMFIBROZIL (*Lopid*) <u>Hypertriglyceridemia/primary prevention of CAD</u>: 600 mg PO two times per day 30 min before meals. [Generic/Trade: Tabs scored 600 mg.] ▶LK ♀C ▶? $$$

Antihypertensive Combinations

NOTE: *Dosage should first be adjusted by using each drug separately. See component drugs for further details.*

BY TYPE: ACE Inhibitor/Diuretic: ACE Inhibitor/Diuretic: *Accuretic, Capozide, ✦Inhibace Plus, Lotensin HCT, Monopril HCT, Prinzide, Uniretic, Vaseretic, Zestoretic.* **ACE Inhibitor/Calcium Channel Blocker:** *Lexxel, Lotrel, Tarka.* **Angiotensin Receptor Blocker/Diuretic:** *Atacand HCT, Avalide, Benicar HCT, Diovan HCT, Hyzaar, Micardis HCT, Teveten HCT.* **Angiotensin Receptor Blocker/Calcium Channel Blocker:** *Azor, Exforge, Twynsta.* **Angiotensin Receptor Blocker/Calcium Channel Blocker/Diuretic:** *Exforge HCT, Tribenzor.* **Angiotensin Receptor Blocker/Direct renin inhibitor:** *Valturna.* **Beta-blocker/Diuretic:** *Corzide, Inderide, Lopressor HCT, Tenoretic, Ziac.* **Direct renin inhibitor/Calcium Channel Blocker:** *Tekamlo.* **Direct renin inhibitor/Calcium Channel Blocker/Diuretic:** *Amturnide.* **Direct renin inhibitor/Diuretic:** *Tekturna HCT.* **Diuretic combinations:** *Aldactazide, Dyazide, Maxzide, Moduretic.* **Diuretic/miscellaneous antihypertensive:** *Aldoril, Apresazide, Clorpres, Minizide.*

BY NAME: *Accuretic* (quinapril + HCTZ): Generic/Trade: Tabs, scored 10/12.5, 20/12.5, unscored 20/25 mg. *Aldactazide* (spironolactone + HCTZ): Generic/Trade: Tabs, unscored 25/25, scored 50/50 mg. *Aldoril* (methyldopa + HCTZ): Generic: Tabs, unscored 250/15, 250/25 mg. *Amturnide* (aliskiren + amlodipine + HCTZ): Trade only: Tabs, unscored 150/5/12.5, 300/5/12.5, 300/5/25, 300/10/12.5, 300/10/25 mg. *Apresazide* (hydralazine + HCTZ): Generic only: Caps 25/25, 50/50 mg. *Atacand HCT* (candesartan + HCTZ, ✦Atacand Plus): Trade only: Tab, unscored 16/12.5, 32/12.5, 32/25 mg. *Avalide* (irbesartan + HCTZ): Trade only: Tabs, unscored 150/12.5, 300/12.5, 300/25 mg. *Azor* (amlodipine + olmesartan): Trade only: Tabs, unscored 5/20, 5/40, 10/20, 10/40 mg. *Benicar HCT* (olmesartan + HCTZ): Trade only: Tabs, unscored 20/12.5, 40/12.5, 40/25 mg. *Capozide* (captopril + HCTZ): Generic/ Trade: Tabs, scored 25/15, 25/25, 50/15, 50/25 mg. *Clorpres* (clonidine + chlorthalidone): Trade only: Tabs, scored 0.1/15, 0.2/15, 0.3/15 mg. *Corzide* (nadolol + bendroflumethiazide): Generic/Trade: Tabs 40/5, 80/5 mg. *Diovan HCT* (valsartan + HCTZ): Trade only: Tabs, unscored 80/12.5, 160/12.5, 160/25, 320/12.5, 320/25 mg. *Dyazide* (triamterene + HCTZ): Generic/Trade: Caps, (Dyazide) 37.5/25, (generic only) 50/25 mg. *Exforge* (amlodipine + valsartan): Trade only: Tabs, unscored 5/160, 5/320, 10/160, 10/320 mg. *Exforge HCT* (amlodipine + valsartan + HCTZ): Trade only: Tabs, unscored 5/160/12.5, 5/160/25, 10/160/12.5, 10/160/25, 10/320/25 mg. *Hyzaar* (losartan + HCTZ): Generic/Trade: Tabs, unscored 50/12.5, 100/12.5, 100/25 mg. *Inderide* (propranolol + HCTZ): Generic/Trade: Tabs, scored 40/25, 80/25 mg. ✦*Inhibace Plus* (cilazapril + HCTZ): Trade only:

(cont.)

Tabs, scored 5/12.5 mg. **Lexxel (enalapril + felodipine):** Trade only: Tabs, unscored 5/2.5, 5/5 mg. **Lopressor HCT (metoprolol + HCTZ):** Generic/ Trade: Tabs, scored 50/25, 100/25, 100/50 mg. **Lotensin HCT (benazepril + HCTZ):** Generic/ Trade: Tabs, scored 5/6.25, 10/12.5, 20/12.5, 20/25 mg. **Lotrel (amlodipine + benazepril):** Generic/Trade: Cap, 2.5/10, 5/10, 5/20, 10/20 mg. Trade only: Cap, 5/40, 10/40 mg. **Maxzide (triamterene + HCTZ, ◆Triazide):** Generic/ Trade: Tabs, scored (Maxzide-25) 37.5/25 (Maxzide) 75/50 mg. **Micardis HCT (telmisartan + HCTZ, ◆Micardis Plus):** Trade only: Tabs, unscored 40/12.5, 80/12.5, 80/25 mg. **Minizide (prazosin + polythiazide):** Trade only: cap, 1/0.5, 2/0.5, 5/0.5 mg. **Moduretic (amiloride + HCTZ, ◆Moduret):** Generic/Trade: Tabs, scored 5/50 mg. **Monopril HCT (fosinopril + HCTZ):** Generic/Trade: Tabs, unscored 10/12.5, scored 20/12.5 mg. **Prinzide (lisinopril + HCTZ):** Generic/Trade: Tabs, unscored 10/12.5, 20/12.5, 20/25 mg. **Tarka (trandolapril + verapamil):** Trade only: Tabs, unscored 2/180, 1/240, 2/240, 4/240 mg. **Tekamlo (aliskiren + amlodipine):** Trade only: Tabs, unscored 150/5, 150/10, 300/5, 300/10 mg. **Tekturna HCT (aliskirin + HCTZ):** Trade only: Tabs, unscored 150/12.5, 150/25, 300/12.5, 300/25 mg. **Tenoretic (atenolol + chlorthalidone):** Generic/Trade: Tabs, scored 50/25, unscored 100/25 mg. **Teveten HCT (eprosartan + HCTZ):** Trade only: Tabs, unscored 600/12.5, 600/25 mg. **Tribenzor (amlodipine + olmesartan + HCTZ):** Trade only: Tabs, unscored 5/20/12.5, 5/40/12.5, 5/40/25,10/40/12.5,10/40/25 mg. **Twynsta (amlodipine + telmisartan):** Trade only: Tabs, unscored 5/40, 5/80, 10/40, 10/80 mg. **Uniretic (moexipril + HCTZ):** Generic/ Trade: Tabs, scored 7.5/12.5, 15/12.5, 15/25 mg. **Valturna (aliskiren + valsartan):** Tabs, unscored 150/160, 300/320 mg. **Vaseretic (enalapril + HCTZ):** Generic/Trade: Tabs, unscored 5/12.5, 10/25 mg. **Zestoretic (lisinopril HCTZ):** Generic/Trade: Tabs, unscored 10/12.5, 20/12.5, 20/25 mg. **Ziac (bisoprolol + HCTZ):** Generic/Trade: Tabs, unscored 2.5/6.25, 5/6.25, 10/6.25 mg.

Antihypertensives—Other

ALISKIREN *(Tekturna)* <u>HTN:</u> 150 mg PO daily, max 300 mg/day. Do not use with cyclosporine or itraconazole. [Trade only: Tabs unscored 150, 300 mg.] ▶LK ♀− ▶−? $$$

FENOLDOPAM *(Corlopam)* <u>Severe HTN:</u> 10 mg in 250 mL D5W (40 mcg/mL), start at 0.1 mcg/kg/min titrate q 15 min, usual effective dose 0.1 to 1.6 mcg/kg/min. ▶LK ♀B ▶? $$$

HYDRALAZINE *(Apresoline)* <u>Hypertensive emergency:</u> 10 to 50 mg IM or 10 to 20 mg IV, repeat prn. <u>HTN:</u> Start 10 mg PO two to four times per day, max 300 mg/day. Headaches, peripheral edema, SLE syndrome. [Generic only: Tabs unscored 10, 25, 50, 100 mg.] ▶LK ♀C ▶+ $

NITROPRUSSIDE *(Nitropress)* <u>Hypertensive emergency:</u> Dilute 50 mg in 250 mL D5W (200 mcg/mL), rate of 6 mL/h for 70 kg adult delivers starting dose of 0.3 mcg/kg/min. Max 10 mcg/kg/min. Protect from light. Cyanide toxicity with high doses (10 mcg/kg/min), hepatic/renal impairment, and prolonged infusions (longer than 3 to 7 days); check thiocyanate levels. ▶RBCs ♀C ▶− $

PHENTOLAMINE (*Regitine, Rogitine*) <u>Diagnosis of pheochromocytoma</u>: 5 mg increments IV/IM. Peds: 0.05 to 0.1 mg/kg IV/IM up to 5 mg per dose. Extravasation: 5 to 10 mg in 10 mL NS inject 1 to 5 mL SC (in divided doses) around extravasation site. ▶Plasma ♀C ▶? $$$

Antiplatelet Drugs

ABCIXIMAB (*ReoPro*) <u>Platelet aggregation inhibition, percutaneous coronary intervention</u>: 0.25 mg/kg IV bolus via separate infusion line before procedure, then 0.125 mcg/kg/min (max 10 mcg/min) IV infusion for 12 h. ▶Plasma ♀C ▶? $$$$$

AGGRENOX (**acetylsalicylic acid + dipyridamole**) <u>Prevention of CVA after TIA/CVA</u>: 1 cap PO two times per day. Headaches are common adverse effect. [Trade only: Caps, 25 mg aspirin/200 mg extended-release dipyridamole.] ▶LK ♀D ▶? $$$$

CLOPIDOGREL (*Plavix*) <u>Reduction of thrombotic events, recent acute MI/CVA, established peripheral arterial disease</u>: 75 mg PO daily; <u>non-ST segment elevation acute coronary syndrome</u>: 300 to 600 mg loading dose, then 75 mg PO daily in combination with aspirin. <u>ST segment elevation MI</u>: Start with/without 300 mg loading dose, then 75 mg PO daily in combination with aspirin, with/without thrombolytic. Avoid drugs that are strong or moderate CYP2C19 inhibors (eg, omeprazole, esomeprazole, cimetidine, etravirine, felbamate, fluconazole, fluoxetine, fluvoxamine, ketoconazole, voriconazole). [Trade: Tabs unscored 75, 300 mg.] ▶LK ♀B ▶? $$$$

DIPYRIDAMOLE (*Persantine*) <u>Antithrombotic</u>: 75 to 100 mg PO four times per day. [Generic/Trade: Tabs unscored 25, 50, 75 mg.] ▶L ♀B ▶? $$$

EPTIFIBATIDE (*Integrilin*) <u>Acute coronary syndrome</u>: Load 180 mcg/kg IV bolus, then infusion 2 mcg/kg/min for up to 72 h. Discontinue infusion prior to CABG. <u>Percutaneous coronary intervention</u>: Load 180 mcg/kg IV bolus just before procedure, followed by infusion 2 mcg/kg/min and a 2nd 180 mcg/kg IV bolus 10 min after the first bolus. Continue infusion for up to 18 to 24 h (minimum 12 h) after procedure. Reduce infusion dose to 1 mcg/kg/min with CrCl < 50 mL/min; contraindicated in dialysis patients. Thrombocytopenia possible; monitor platelets. ▶K ♀B ▶? $$$$$

PRASUGREL (*Effient*) <u>Reduction of thrombotic events after acute coronary syndrome managed with percutaneous coronary intervention (PCI)</u>: 60 mg loading dose, then 10 mg PO daily in combination with aspirin. For wt less than 60 kg consider lowering maintenance dose to 5 mg PO daily. [Trade: Tabs unscored 5, 10 mg.] ▶LK ♀B ▶? $$$$

TICAGRELOR (*Brilinta*) <u>Reduction of thrombotic events in patients with acute coronary syndrome (MI or unstable angina)</u>: 180 mg loading dose, then 90 mg PO two times daily in combination with aspirin (aspirin maintenance dose: 75-100 mg daily. After the initial dose of aspirin, do not use more than 100 mg of aspirin daily with ticagrelor.) Do not use with history of intracranial hemorrhage, active bleeding, severe hepatic

(cont.)

impairment, strong CYP3A inhibitors, or CYP3A inducers. Monitor digoxin levels when initiating or changing ticagrelor therapy. [Trade only: Tabs, unscored 90 mg.] ▶L - ♀C ▶? $$$$$ ■

TICLOPIDINE (*Ticlid*) Due to high incidence of neutropenia and thrombotic thrombocytopenia purpura, other antiplatelet agents preferred. Platelet aggregation inhibition/reduction of thrombotic CVA: 250 mg PO twice daily with food. [Generic/Trade: Tabs unscored 250 mg.] ▶L ♀B ▶? $$$$

TIROFIBAN (*Aggrastat*) Acute coronary syndromes: Start 0.4 mcg/kg/min IV infusion for 30 min, then decrease to 0.1 mcg/kg/min for 48 to 108 h or until 12 to 24 h after coronary intervention. Half dose with CrCl less than 30 mL/min. Use concurrent heparin to keep PTT 2× normal. ▶K ♀B ▶? $$$$$

Beta-Blockers

NOTE: *See also antihypertensive combinations. Not first line for HTN (unless to treat angina, post MI, LV dysfunction, or heart failure). Abrupt discontinuation may precipitate angina, MI, arrhythmias, or rebound HTN; discontinue by tapering over 1 to 2 weeks. Discontinue beta-blocker several days before discontinuing concomitant clonidine to minimize the risk of rebound HTN. Avoid use of nonselective beta-blockers in patients with asthma/COPD. For patients with asthma/COPD, use agents with beta-1 selectivity and monitor cautiously. Beta-1 selectivity diminishes at high doses. Avoid initiating beta-blocker therapy in acute decompensated heart failure, sick sinus syndrome without pacer, and severe peripheral artery disease. Agents with intrinsic sympathomimetic activity are contraindicated post acute MI. Patients with diabetes should be aware that beta-blockers may mask symptoms of hypoglycemic response. Concomitant amiodarone, digoxin, or nondihydropyridine calcium channel blockers may increase risk of bradycardia. Concomitant disopyramide may increase risk of bradycardia, asystole, and HF. Patients actively using cocaine should avoid beta-blockers with unopposed alpha-adrenergic vasoconstriction because this will promote coronary artery vasoconstriction/spasm (carvedilol or labetalol have additional alpha-1-blocking effects and are, therefore, safe). Do not routinely stop chronic beta-blocker therapy prior to surgery.*

ACEBUTOLOL (*Sectral*, ✦ *Rhotral*) HTN: Start 400 mg PO daily or 200 mg PO two times per day, maximum 1200 mg/day. Beta-1 receptor selective. [Generic/Trade: Caps 200, 400 mg.] ▶LK ♀B ▶− $$

ATENOLOL (*Tenormin*) Acute MI: 50 to 100 mg PO daily or in divided doses; or 5 mg IV over 5 min, repeat in 10 min. HTN: Start 25 to 50 mg PO daily or divided two times per day, maximum 100 mg/day. Beta-1 receptor selective. [Generic/Trade: Tabs unscored 25, 100 mg; scored, 50 mg.] ▶K ♀D ▶− $

BETAXOLOL (*Kerlone*) HTN: Start 5 to 10 mg PO daily, max 20 mg/day. Beta-1 receptor selective. [Generic: Tabs scored 10 mg, unscored 20 mg.] ▶LK ♀C ▶? $$

BISOPROLOL (*Zebeta*, ✦*Monocor*) HTN: Start 2.5 to 5 mg PO daily, max 20 mg/day. Beta-1 receptor selective. [Generic/Trade: Tabs scored 5 mg, unscored 10 mg.] ▶LK ♀C ▶? $$

CARVEDILOL (*Coreg, Coreg CR*) Heart failure, immediate-release: Start 3.125 mg PO two times per day, double dose every 2 weeks as tolerated up to max of 25 mg two times per day (for wt 85 kg or less) or 50 mg two times per day (for wt greater than 85 kg). Heart failure, sustained-release: Start 10 mg PO daily, double dose q 2 weeks as tolerated up to max of 80 mg/day. LV dysfunction following acute MI, immediate-release: Start 3.125 to 6.25 mg PO two times per day, double dose q 3 to 10 days as tolerated to max of 25 mg two times per day. LV dysfunction following acute MI, sustained-release: Start 10 to 20 mg PO daily, double dose q 3 to 10 days as tolerated to max of 80 mg/day. HTN, immediate-release: Start 6.25 mg PO two times per day, double dose q 7 to 14 days as tolerated to max 50 mg/day. HTN, sustained-release: Start 20 mg PO daily, double dose every 7 to 14 days as tolerated to max 80 mg/day. Take with food to decrease orthostatic hypotension. Give Coreg CR in the morning. Alpha-1, beta-1, and beta-2 receptor blocker. [Generic/Trade: Tabs immediate-release unscored 3.125, 6.25, 12.5, 25 mg. Trade only: Caps extended-release 10, 20, 40, 80 mg.] ▶L ♀C ▶? $$$$

ESMOLOL (*Brevibloc*) SVT/HTN emergency: Load 500 mcg/kg over 1 min (dilute 5 g in 500 mL to make a soln of 10 mg/mL and give 3.5 mL to deliver 35 mg bolus for 70 kg patient) then start infusion 50 to 200 mcg/kg/min (40 mL/h delivers 100 mcg/kg/min for 70 kg patient). Half-life is 9 min. Beta-1 receptor selective. ▶K ♀C ▶? $

LABETALOL (*Trandate*) HTN: Start 100 mg PO two times per day, max 2400 mg/day. HTN emergency: Start 20 mg IV slow injection, then 40 to 80 mg IV q 10 min prn up to 300 mg or IV infusion 0.5 to 2 mg/min. Peds: Start 0.3 to 1 mg/kg/dose (max 20 mg). May be used to manage BP during pregnancy. Alpha-1, beta-1, and beta-2 receptor blocker. [Generic/Trade: Tabs scored 100, 200, 300 mg.] ▶LK ♀C ▶+ $$$

METOPROLOL (*Lopressor, Toprol-XL*, ✦*Betaloc*) Acute MI: 50 to 100 mg PO q 12 h; or 5 mg increments IV q 5 to 15 min up to 15 mg followed by oral therapy. HTN, immediate-release: Start 100 mg PO daily or in divided doses, increase as necessary up to 450 mg/day; may require multiple daily doses to maintain 24 h BP control. HTN, extended-release: Start 25 to 100 mg PO daily, increase as necessary up to 400 mg/day. Heart failure: Start 12.5 to 25 mg (extended-release) PO daily, double dose every 2 weeks as tolerated to max 200 mg/day. Angina: Start 50 mg PO two times per day (immediate-release) or 100 mg PO daily (extended-release), increase prn up to 400 mg/day. Beta-1 receptor selective. IV to PO conversion: 1 mg IV is equivalent to 2.5 mg PO (divided four times per day). Immediate-release form is metoprolol tartrate; extended-release form is metoprolol succinate. Take with food. [Generic/Trade: Tabs scored 50, 100 mg, extended-release 25, 50, 100, 200 mg. Generic only: Tabs scored 25 mg.] ▶L ♀C ▶ $$

NADOLOL (*Corgard*) HTN: Start 20 to 40 mg PO daily, max 320 mg/day. Prevent rebleeding esophageal varices: 40 to 160 mg PO daily; titrate dose to reduce heart rate to 25% below baseline. Beta-1 and beta-2 receptor blocker. [Generic/Trade: Tabs scored 20, 40, 80, 120, 160 mg.] ▶K ♀C ▶– $$

NEBIVOLOL (*Bystolic*) HTN: Start 5 mg PO daily, maximum 40 mg/day. Beta-1 receptor selective at doses of 10 mg or less and in patients who extensively metabolize CYP2D6; otherwise, inhibits both beta-1 and beta-2 receptors. [Trade only: Tabs unscored 2.5, 5, 10, 20 mg.] ▶L ♀C ▶– $$$

PINDOLOL (✦ *Visken*) HTN: Start 5 mg PO two times per day, max 60 mg/ day. Beta-1 and beta-2 receptor blocker. [Generic only: Tabs, scored 5, 10 mg.] ▶K ♀B ▶? $$$

PROPRANOLOL (*Inderal, Inderal LA, InnoPran XL*) HTN: Start 20 to 40 mg PO two times per day or 60 to 80 mg PO daily, max 640 mg/day; extended-release (Inderal LA) max 640 mg/day; extended-release (InnoPran XL) 80 mg at bedtime (10 pm), max 120 mg at bedtime (chronotherapy). Supraventricular tachycardia or rapid atrial fibrillation/flutter: 1 mg IV q 2 min. Max of 2 doses in 4 h. Migraine prophylaxis: Start 40 mg PO two times per day or 80 mg PO daily (extended-release), max 240 mg/day. Prevent rebleeding esophageal varices: 20 to 180 mg PO two times per day; titrate dose to reduce heart rate to 25% below baseline. Beta-1 and beta-2 receptor blocker. [Generic/Trade: Tabs, scored 40, 60, 80. Caps, extended-release 60, 80, 120, 160 mg. Generic only: Soln 20, 40 mg/5 mL. Tabs, 10, 20 mg. Trade only: (InnoPran XL at bedtime) 80, 120 mg.] ▶L ♀C ▶+ $$

Calcium Channel Blockers (CCBs)—Dihydropyridines

NOTE: *See also antihypertensive combinations. May increase proteinuria, peripheral edema. Avoid concomitant grapefruit juice. Avoid in decompensated heart failure.*

AMLODIPINE (*Norvasc*) HTN: Start 5 mg PO daily, max 10 daily. Elderly, small, frail, or with hepatic insufficiency: Start 2.5 PO daily. [Generic/Trade: Tabs unscored 2.5, 5, 10 mg.] ▶L ♀C ▶? $

CLEVIDIPINE (*Cleviprex*) HTN: Start 1 to 2 mg/h IV, titrate q 1.5 to 10 min to BP response, usual maintenance dose 4 to 6 mg/h, max 32 mg/h IV. An increase of 1 to 2 mg/h will decrease SBP approximately 2 to 4 mm Hg. ▶KL ♀C ▶? $$$

FELODIPINE (*Plendil*, ✦ *Renedil*) HTN: Start 2.5 to 5 mg PO daily, maximum 10 mg/day. [Generic/Trade: Tabs extended-release, unscored 2.5, 5, 10 mg.] ▶L ♀C ▶? $$

ISRADIPINE (*DynaCirc, DynaCirc CR*) HTN: Start 2.5 mg PO two times per day, max 20 mg/day (max 10 mg/day in elderly). Controlled-release: 5 to 20 mg PO daily. [Trade only: Tabs controlled-release 5, 10 mg. Generic only: Immediate-release caps 2.5, 5 mg.] ▶L ♀C ▶? $$$$

NICARDIPINE (*Cardene, Cardene SR*) HTN emergency: Begin IV infusion at 5 mg/h, titrate to effect, max 15 mg/h. HTN: Start 20 mg PO three times per day, max 120 mg/day. Sustained-release: Start 30 mg PO two times per day, max 120 mg/day. <u>Short-term management of HTN, patient receiving PO nicardipine:</u> If using 20 mg PO q8h, give 0.5 mg/h IV; if using 30 mg PO q8h, give 1.2 mg/h IV; if using 40 mg PO q8h, give 2.2 mg/h. [Generic/Trade: Caps immediate-release 20, 30 mg. Trade only: Caps sustained-release 30, 45, 60 mg.] ▶L ♀C ▶? $$

NIFEDIPINE (*Procardia, Adalat, Procardia XL, Adalat CC, Afeditab CR, ◆ Adalat XL, Adalat PA*) <u>HTN/Angina:</u> Extended-release: 30 to 60 mg PO daily, max 120 mg/day. <u>Angina:</u> Immediate-release: Start 10 mg PO three times per day, max 120 mg/day. Avoid sublingual administration, may cause excessive hypotension, acute MI, CVA. Do not use immediate-release caps for treating HTN. <u>Preterm labor:</u> Loading dose: 10 mg PO q 20 to 30 min if contractions persist, up to 40 mg within the first h. Maintenance dose: 10 to 20 mg PO q 4 to 6 h or 60 to 160 mg extended-release PO daily. [Generic/Trade: Caps 10, 20 mg. Tabs extended-release (Adalat CC, Afeditab CR, Procardia XL) 30, 60 mg, (Adalat CC, Procardia XL) 90 mg.] ▶L ♀C ▶– $$

NISOLDIPINE (*Sular*) <u>HTN:</u> Start 17 mg PO daily, max 34 mg/day. Take on an empty stomach. [Trade only: Tabs extended-release 8.5, 17, 25.5, 34 mg. These replace the former 10, 20, 30, 40 mg tabs. Generic only: Tabs extended-release 20, 30, 40 mg.] ▶L ♀C ▶? $$$

Calcium Channel Blockers (CCBs)—Non-Dihydropyridines

NOTE: *See also antihypertensive combinations. Avoid in decompensated heart failure or 2nd/3rd degree heart block.*

DILTIAZEM (*Cardizem, Cardizem LA, Cardizem CD, Cartia XT, Dilacor XR, Diltiazem CD, Diltzac, Diltia XT, Tiazac, Taztia XT*) <u>Atrial fibrillation/ flutter, PSVT:</u> Bolus 20 mg (0.25 mg/kg) IV over 2 min. Rebolus 15 min later (if needed) 25 mg (0.35 mg/kg). Infusion 5 to 15 mg/h. <u>HTN, once daily, extended-release:</u> Start 120 to 240 mg PO daily, max 540 mg/day. <u>HTN, once daily, graded extended-release (Cardizem LA):</u> Start 180 to 240 mg PO daily, max 540 mg/day. <u>HTN, twice daily, sustained-release:</u> Start 60 to 120 mg PO two times per day, max 360 mg/day. <u>Angina, immediate-release:</u> Start 30 mg PO four times per day, max 360 mg/day divided three to four times per day; <u>Angina, extended-release:</u> start 120 to 240 mg PO daily, max 540 mg/day. <u>Angina, once daily, graded extended-release (Cardizem LA):</u> start 180 mg PO daily, doses more than 360 mg may provide no additional benefit. [Generic/Trade: Tabs immediate-release, unscored (Cardizem) 30, scored 60, 90, 120 mg; Caps extended-release (Cardizem CD, Cartia XT daily) 120, 180, 240, 300, 360 mg, (Diltzac, Taztia XT, Tiazac daily) 120, 180, 240, 300, 360, 420 mg, (Dilacor XR, Diltia XT) 120, 180, 240 mg. Trade only: Tabs extended-release graded (Cardizem LA daily) 120, 180, 240, 300, 360, 420 mg.] ▶L ♀C ▶+ $$

VERAPAMIL (*Isoptin SR, Calan, Covera-HS, Verelan, Verelan PM*) <u>SVT adults:</u> 5 to 10 mg IV over 2 min; <u>SVT peds</u> (age 1 to 15 yo): 2 to 5 mg (0.1 to

(cont.)

0.3 mg/kg) IV, max dose 5 mg. <u>Angina: Immediate-release</u>, start 40 to 80 mg PO three to four times per day, max 480 mg/day; <u>sustained to release</u>, start 120 to 240 mg PO daily, max 480 mg/day (use twice daily dosing for doses greater than 240 mg/day with Isoptin SR and Calan SR); (Covera-HS) 180 mg PO at bedtime, max 480 mg/day. <u>HTN</u>: Same as angina, except (Verelan PM) 100 to 200 mg PO at bedtime, max 400 mg/day; immediate-release tabs should be avoided in treating HTN. Use cautiously with impaired renal/hepatic function. [Generic/Trade: Tabs, immediate-release, scored (Calan) 40, 80, 120 mg; Tabs, sustained-release, unscored (Isoptin SR) 120, scored 180, 240 mg; Caps, sustained-release (Verelan) 120, 180, 240, 360 mg; Caps, extended-release (Verelan PM) 100, 200, 300 mg. Trade only: Tabs, extended-release (Covera-HS) 180, 240 mg.] ▶L ♀C ▶– $$

Diuretics—Carbonic Anhydrase Inhibitors

ACETAZOLAMIDE (*Diamox, Diamox Sequels*) <u>Glaucoma</u>: 250 mg PO up to four times per day (immediate-release) or 500 mg PO up to two times per day (sustained-release). Max 1 g/day. <u>Acute glaucoma</u>: 250 mg IV q 4 h or 500 mg IV initially with 125 to 250 mg q 4 h, followed by oral therapy. <u>Mountain sickness prophylaxis</u>: 125 to 250 mg PO two to three times per day, beginning 1 to 2 days prior to ascent and continuing at least 5 days at higher altitude. <u>Edema</u>: Rarely used, start 250 to 375 mg IV/PO q am given intermittently (every other day or 2 consecutive days followed by none for 1 to 2 days) to avoid loss of diuretic effect. <u>Urinary alkalinIzation</u>: 5 mg/kg IV, may repeat two or three times daily prn to maintain an alkaline diuresis. [Generic only: Tabs 125, 250 mg. Generic/Trade: Caps extended-release 500 mg.] ▶LK ♀C ▶+ $

Diuretics—Loop

BUMETANIDE (*Bumex, ✦Burinex*) <u>Edema</u>: 0.5 to 1 mg IV/IM; 0.5 to 2 mg PO daily. 1 mg bumetanide is roughly equivalent to 40 mg furosemide. [Generic/Trade: Tabs scored 0.5, 1, 2 mg.] ▶K ♀C ▶? $

ETHACRYNIC ACID (*Edecrin*) Can be safely used in patients with true sulfa allery. <u>Edema</u>: 0.5 to 1 mg/kg IV, max 100 mg/dose; 25 to 100 mg PO daily to two times per day. [Trade only: Tabs scored 25 mg.] ▶K ♀B ▶? $$$

FUROSEMIDE (*Lasix*) <u>HTN</u>: Start 10 to 40 mg PO twice daily, max 600 mg daily. <u>Edema</u>: Start 20 to 80 mg IV/IM/PO, increase dose by 20 to 40 mg in 6 to 8 h until desired response is achieved, max 600 mg/day. <u>Ascites</u>: 40 mg PO daily in combination with spironolactone; may increase dose after 2 to 3 days if no response. Use lower doses in elderly. [Generic/Trade: Tabs unscored 20, scored 40, 80 mg. Generic only: Oral soln 10 mg/mL, 40 mg/5 mL.] ▶K ♀C ▶? $

TORSEMIDE (*Demadex*) <u>HTN</u>: Start 5 mg PO daily, increase prn q 4 to 6 weeks, max 10 mg daily. <u>Edema</u>: 10 to 20 mg IV/PO daily, max 200 mg IV/PO daily. [Generic/Trade: Tabs scored 5, 10, 20, 100 mg.] ▶LK ♀B ▶? $

Diuretics—Thiazide Type

NOTE: *See also antihypertensive combinations.*

CHLORTHALIDONE (*Thalitone*) HTN: 12.5 to 25 mg PO daily, max 50 mg/day. Edema: 50 to 100 mg PO daily, max 200 mg/day. Nephrolithiasis (unapproved use): 25 to 50 mg PO daily. [Trade only: Tabs unscored (Thalitone) 15 mg. Generic only: Tabs unscored 25, 50 mg.] ▶L ♀B, D if used in pregnancy-induced HTN ▶+ $

HYDROCHLOROTHIAZIDE (*HCTZ, Esidrix, Oretic, Microzide, HydroDiuril*) HTN: 12.5 to 25 mg PO daily, max 50 mg/day. Edema: 25 to 100 mg PO daily, max 200 mg/day. [Generic/Trade: Tabs scored 25, 50 mg; Caps 12.5 mg.] ▶L ♀B, D if used in pregnancy-induced HTN ▶+ $

INDAPAMIDE (*Lozol, ◆Lozide*) HTN: 1.25 to 5 mg PO daily, max 5 mg/day. Edema: 2.5 to 5 mg PO q am. [Generic only: Tabs unscored 1.25, 2.5 mg.] ▶L ♀B, D if used in pregnancy-induced HTN ▶? $

METOLAZONE (*Zaroxolyn*) Edema: 5 to 10 mg PO daily, max 10 mg/day in heart failure, 20 mg/day in renal disease. If used with loop diuretic, start with 2.5 mg PO daily. [Generic/Trade: Tabs 2.5, 5, 10 mg.] ▶L ♀B, D if used in pregnancy-induced HTN ▶? $$$

Nitrates

NOTE: *Avoid in those who have received erectile dysfunction therapy in the last 24 (sildenafil, vardenafil) to 48 (tadalafil) hours.*

ISOSORBIDE DINITRATE (*Isordil, Dilatrate-SR*) Angina prophylaxis: 5 to 40 mg PO three times per day (7 am, noon, 5 pm), sustained-release: 40 to 80 mg PO two times per day (8 am, 2 pm). Acute angina, SL Tabs: 2.5 to 10 mg SL q 5 to 10 min prn, up to 3 doses in 30 min. [Generic/Trade: Tabs, scored 5, 10, 20, 30 mg. Trade only: Tabs, (Isordil) 40 mg, Caps, extended-release (Dilatrate-SR) 40 mg. Generic only: Tabs, sustained-release 40 mg, Tabs, sublingual 2.5, 5 mg.] ▶L ♀C ▶? $

ISOSORBIDE MONONITRATE (*ISMO, Monoket, Imdur*) Angina: 20 mg PO two times per day (8 am and 3 pm). Extended-release: Start 30 to 60 mg PO daily, maximum 240 mg/day. [Generic/Trade: Tabs unscored (ISMO, two times per day dosing) 20 mg, scored (Monoket, two times per day dosing) 10, 20 mg extended-release, scored (Imdur, daily dosing) 30, 60, unscored 120 mg.] ▶L ♀C ▶? $$

NITROGLYCERIN INTRAVENOUS INFUSION (*Tridil*) Perioperative HTN, acute MI/Heart failure, acute angina: Mix 50 mg in 250 mL D5W (200 mcg/mL), start at 10 to 20 mcg/min (3 to 6 mL/h), then titrate upward by 10 to 20 mcg/min prn. [Brand name "Tridil" no longer manufactured but retained herein for name recognition.] ▶L ♀C ▶? $

NITROGLYCERIN OINTMENT (*Nitro-BID*) Angina prophylaxis: Start 0.5 inch q 8 h, maintenance 1 to 2 inches q 8 h, maximum 4 inch q 4 to 6 h; 15 mg/inch. Allow for a nitrate-free period of 10 to 14 h to avoid nitrate tolerance. 1 inch ointment is ~15 mg. [Trade only: Ointment, 2%, tubes 1, 30, 60 g (Nitro-BID).] ▶L ♀C ▶? $

NITROGLYCERIN SPRAY (*Nitrolingual, NitroMist*) <u>Acute angina</u>: 1 to 2 sprays under the tongue prn, max 3 sprays in 15 min. [Trade only: Nitrolingual soln, 4.9, 12 mL. 0.4 mg/spray (60 or 200 sprays/canister); NitroMist aerosol 0.4 mg/spray (230 sprays/canister).] ▶L ♀C ▶? $$$$

NITROGLYCERIN SUBLINGUAL (*Nitrostat, NitroQuick*) <u>Acute angina</u>: 0.4 mg SL under tongue, repeat dose q 5 min prn up to 3 doses in 15 min. [Generic/Trade: Sublingual tabs unscored 0.3, 0.4, 0.6 mg; in bottles of 100 or package of 4 bottles with 25 tabs each.] ▶L ♀C ▶? $

NITROGLYCERIN TRANSDERMAL (*Minitran, Nitro-Dur, ✦ Trinipatch*) <u>Angina prophylaxis</u>: 1 patch 12 to 14 h each day. Allow for a nitrate-free period of 10 to 14 h each day to avoid nitrate tolerance. [Generic/Trade: Transdermal system 0.1, 0.2, 0.4, 0.6 mg/h. Trade only: (Nitro-Dur) 0.3, 0.8 mg/h.] ▶L ♀C ▶? $$

Pressors/Inotropes

DOBUTAMINE (*Dobutrex*) <u>Inotropic support</u>: 2 to 20 mcg/kg/min. Dilute 250 mg in 250 mL D5W (1 mg/mL); a rate of 21 mL/h delivers 5 mcg/kg/min for a 70 kg patient. ▶Plasma ♀D ▶− $

DOPAMINE (*Intropin*) <u>Pressor</u>: Start at 5 mcg/kg/min, increase prn by 5 to 10 mcg/kg/min increments at 10 min intervals, max 50 mcg/kg/min. Mix 400 mg in 250 mL D5W (1600 mcg/mL); a rate of 13 mL/h delivers 5 mcg/kg/min in a 70 kg patient. Doses in mcg/kg/min: 2 to 4 (traditional renal dose, apparently ineffective) dopaminergic receptors; 5 to 10 (cardiac dose) dopaminergic and beta 1 receptors; more than 10 dopaminergic, beta-1, and alpha-1 receptors. ▶Plasma ♀C ▶− $

EPHEDRINE <u>Pressor</u>: 10 to 25 mg slow IV, repeat q 5 to 10 min prn. ▶K ♀C ▶? $

EPINEPHRINE (*EpiPen, EpiPen Jr, Twinject*, adrenaline) <u>Cardiac arrest</u>: 1 mg IV q 3 to 5 min. <u>Anaphylaxis</u>: 0.1 to 0.5 mg SC/IM, may repeat SC dose q 10 to 15 min. <u>Acute asthma and hypersensitivity reactions</u>: Adults: 0.1 to 0.3 mg of 1:1000 soln SC or IM; Peds: 0.01 mg/kg (up to 0.3 mg) of 1:1000 soln SC or IM. [Soln for injection: 1:1000 (1 mg/mL in 1 mL amps or 10 mL vial). Trade only: EpiPen Auto-injector delivers one 0.3 mg (1:1000, 0.3 mL) IM dose. EpiPen Jr. Autoinjector delivers one 0.15 mg (1:2000, 0.3 mL) IM dose. Twinject Auto-injector delivers one 0.15 mg (1:1000, 0.15 mL) or 0.3 mg (1:1000, 0.3 mL) IM/SQ dose.] ▶Plasma ♀C ▶− $

INAMRINONE <u>Heart failure</u>: 0.75 mg/kg bolus IV over 2 to 3 min, then infusion 5 to 10 mcg/kg/min. Mix 100 mg in 100 mL NS (1 mg/mL) a rate of 21 mL/h delivers 5 mcg/kg/min for a 70 kg patient. ▶K ♀C ▶? $$$$$

MIDODRINE (*Orvaten, ProAmatine, ✦ Amatine*) <u>Orthostatic hypotension</u>: 10 mg PO three times per day while awake. [Generic/Trade: Tabs, scored 2.5, 5, 10 mg.] ▶LK ♀C ▶? $$$$$

MILRINONE (*Primacor*) <u>Systolic heart failure</u> (NYHA class III, IV): Load 50 mcg/kg IV over 10 min, then begin IV infusion of 0.375 to 0.75 mcg/kg/min. ▶K ♀C ▶? $$

```
CARDIAC PARAMETERS AND FORMULAS
Cardiac output (CO) = heart rate × CVA volume [normal 4 to 8 L/min]
Cardiac index (CI) = CO/BSA [normal 2.8 to 4.2 L/min/m²]
MAP (mean arterial press) = [(SBP − DBP)/3] + DBP [normal 80 to 100 mmHg]
SVR (systemic vasc resis) = (MAP − CVP) × (80)/CO [normal 800 to 1200 dynes × sec/cm⁵]
PVR (pulm vasc resis) = (PAM − PCWP) × (80)/CO [normal 45 to 120 dynes × sec/cm⁵]
QTc = QT/square root of RR [normal 0.38 to 0.42]
Right atrial pressure (central venous pressure) [normal 0 to 8 mmHg]
Pulmonary artery systolic pressure (PAS) [normal 20 to 30 mmHg]
Pulmonary artery diastolic pressure (PAD) [normal 10 to 15 mmHg]
Pulmonary capillary wedge pressure (PCWP) [normal 8 to 12 mmHg (post-MI ~16 mmHg)]
```

NOREPINEPHRINE *(Levophed)* <u>Acute hypotension:</u> start 8 to 12 mcg/min, adjust to maintain BP, average maintenance rate 2 to 4 mcg/min. Mix 4 mg in 500 mL D5W (8 mcg/mL), a rate of 22.5 mL/h delivers 3 mcg/min. Ideally through central line. ▶Plasma ♀C ▶? $

PHENYLEPHRINE—INTRAVENOUS *(Neo-Synephrine)* <u>Severe hypotension:</u> Infusion: 20 mg in 250 mL D5W (80 mcg/mL), start 100 to 180 mcg/min (75 to 135 mcg/min), usual dose once BP is stabilized 40 to 60 mcg/min. ▶Plasma ♀C ▶− $

Pulmonary Arterial Hypertension

SILDENAFIL *(Revatio)* <u>Pulmonary arterial hypertension:</u> 20 mg PO three times per day; or 10 mg IV three times per day. Contraindicated with nitrates. Coadministration is not recommended with ritonavir, potent CYP3A inhibitors, or other phosphodiesterase-5 inhibitors. Teach patients to seek medical attention for vision loss, hearing loss, or erections lasting longer than 4 h. [Trade only (Revatio): Tabs 20 mg.] ▶LK ♀B ▶− $$$$

TADALAFIL *(Adcirca)* <u>Pulmonary arterial hypertension:</u> 40 mg PO daily. Contraindicated with nitrates. Coadministration is not recommended with potent CYP3A inhibitors (itraconazole, ketoconazole), potent CYP3A inducers (rifampin), other phosphodiesterase-5 inhibitors. Caution with ritonavir, see prescribing information for specific dose adjustments. Teach patients to seek medical attention for vision loss, hearing loss, or erections lasting longer than 4 h. [Trade only (Adcirca): Tabs 20 mg.] ▶L ♀B ▶− $$$$

Thrombolytics

ALTEPLASE *(tpa, t-PA, Activase, Cathflo, ✦Activase rt-PA)* <u>Acute MI:</u> (dose for wt 67 kg or less) give 15 mg IV bolus, then 0.75 mg/kg (max 50 mg) over 30 min, then 0.5 mg/kg (max 35 mg) over the next 60 min; (dose for wt greater than 67 kg) give 15 mg IV bolus, then 50 mg over 30 min, then 35 mg over the next 60; use concurrent heparin infusion. <u>Acute ischemic stroke with symptoms 3 h or less:</u> 0.9 mg/kg (max 90 mg); give 10% of total dose as an IV bolus, and the remainder IV over 60 min. Multiple exclusion criteria. <u>Acute pulmonary embolism:</u> 100 mg IV over 2 h, then restart heparin when PTT twice normal or less. <u>Occluded central venous access device:</u> 2 mg/mL in catheter for 2 h. May use second dose if needed. ▶L ♀C ▶? $$$$$

THROMBOLYTIC THERAPY FOR ACUTE MI

Indications (if high-volume cath lab unavailable): Clinical history and presentation strongly suggestive of MI within 12 h plus at least 1 of the following: 1 mm ST elevation in at least 2 contiguous leads; new left BBB; or 2 mm ST depression in V1-4 suggestive of true posterior MI.

Absolute contraindications: Previous cerebral hemorrhage, known cerebral aneurysm or arteriovenous malformation, known intracranial neoplasm, recent (<3 months) ischemic CVA (except acute ischemic CVA <3 h), aortic dissection, active bleeding or bleeding diathesis (excluding menstruation), significant closed head or facial trauma (<3 months).

Relative contraindications: Severe uncontrolled HTN (>180/110 mm Hg) on presentation or chronic severe HTN; prior ischemic CVA (>3 months), dementia, other intracranial pathology; traumatic/prolonged (>10 min) cardiopulmonary resuscitation; major surgery (<3 weeks); recent (within 2–4 weeks) internal bleeding; puncture of noncompressible vessel; pregnancy; active peptic ulcer disease; current use of anticoagulants. For streptokinase/anistreplase: prior exposure (>5 days ago) or prior allergic reaction.

Reference: *Circulation* 2004;110:588–636

RETEPLASE *(Retavase)* Acute MI: 10 units IV over 2 min; repeat once in 30 min. ▶L ♀C ▶? $$$$$

STREPTOKINASE *(Streptase, Kabikinase)* Acute MI: 1.5 million units IV over 60 min. ▶L ♀C ▶? $$$$$

TENECTEPLASE *(TNKase)* Acute MI: Single IV bolus dose over 5 sec based on body wt; 30 mg for wt less than 60 kg, 35 mg for wt 60 to 69 kg, 40 mg for wt 70 to 79 kg, 45 mg for wt 80 to 89 kg, 50 mg for wt 90 kg or more. ▶L ♀C ▶? $$$$$

UROKINASE *(Kinlytic)* PE: 4400 units/kg IV loading dose over 10 min, followed by IV infusion 4400 units/kg/h for 12 h. Occluded IV catheter: 5000 units instilled into catheter, remove soln after 5 min. ▶L ♀B ▶? $$$$$

Volume Expanders

ALBUMIN *(Albuminar, Buminate, Albumarc, ✦Plasbumin)* Shock, burns: 500 mL of 5% soln IV infusion as rapidly as tolerated, repeat in 30 min if needed. ▶L ♀C ▶? $$$$$

DEXTRAN *(Rheomacrodex, Gentran, Macrodex)* Shock/hypovolemia: up to 20 mL/kg in first 24 h, then up to 10 mL/kg for 4 days. ▶K ♀C ▶? $$

HETASTARCH *(Hespan, Hextend)* Shock/hypovolemia: 500 to 1000 mL IV infusion, usually should not exceed 20 mL/kg/day (1500 mL) ▶K ♀C ▶? $$

PLASMA PROTEIN FRACTION *(Plasmanate, Protenate, Plasmatein)* Shock/hypovolemia: 5% soln 250 to 500 mL IV prn. ▶L ♀C ▶? $$$

Other

BIDIL (hydralazine + isosorbide dinitrate) Heart failure (adjunct to standard therapy in black patients): Start 1 tab PO three times per day, increase as tolerated to max 2 tabs three times per day. May decrease to ½ tab three times per day with intolerable side effects; try to increase dose

(cont.)

when side effects subside. [Trade only: Tabs, scored 37.5/20 mg.] ▶LK ♀C ▶? $$$$$

CILOSTAZOL (*Pletal*) Intermittent claudication: 100 mg PO two times per day on empty stomach. 50 mg PO two times per day with CYP3A4 inhibitors (eg, ketoconazole, itraconazole, erythromycin, diltiazem) or CYP2C19 inhibitors (eg, omeprazole). Contraindicated in heart failure of any severity due to decreased survival. [Generic/Trade: Tabs 50, 100 mg.] ▶L ♀C ▶? $$$$

NESIRITIDE (*Natrecor*) Hospitalized patients with decompensated heart failure with dyspnea at rest: 2 mcg/kg IV bolus over 60 sec, then 0.01 mcg/kg/ min IV infusion for up to 48 h. Do not initiate at higher doses. Limited experience with increased doses. Mix 1.5 mg vial in 250 mL D5W (6 mcg/mL) a bolus of 23.3 mL is 2 mcg/kg for a 70 kg patient, infusion set at rate 7 mL/h delivers a 0.01 mcg/kg/min for a 70 kg patient. Symptomatic hypotension. May increase mortality. Not indicated for outpatient infusion, for scheduled repetitive use, to improve renal function, or to enhance diuresis. ▶K, plasma ♀C ▶? $$$$$

PENTOXIFYLLINE (*Trental*) Intermittent claudication: 400 mg PO three times per day with meals. [Generic/Trade: Tabs, extended-release 400 mg.] ▶L ♀C ▶? $$$

RANOLAZINE (*Ranexa*) Chronic angina: 500 mg PO two times per day, max 1000 mg two times per day. Max 500 mg two times per day, if used with diltiazem, verapamil, or moderate CYP3A inhibitors. Baseline and follow-up ECGs; may prolong QT interval. Contraindicated with hepatic cirrhosis, potent CYP3A4 inhibitors, CYP3A inducers. May increase levels of cyclosporine, lovastatin, simvastatin, sirolimus, tacrolimus, antipsychotics, TCA(s). Swallow whole; do not crush, break, or chew. Instruct patients to report palpitations or fainting spells. [Trade only: Tabs extended-release 500, 1000 mg.] ▶LK ♀C ▶? $$$$$

CONTRAST MEDIA

MRI Contrast—Gadolinium-based

NOTE: *Avoid gadolinium-based contrast agents if severe renal insufficiency (GFR less than 30 mL/min/1.73 m^2) due to risk of nephrogenic systemic fibrosis/nephrogenic fibrosing dermopathy. Similarly avoid in acute renal insufficiency of any severity due to hepatorenal syndrome or during the perioperative phase of liver transplant.*

GADOBENATE (*MultiHance*) Non-iodinated, nonionic IV contrast for MRI. ▶K ♀C ▶? $$$$ ■

GADODIAMIDE (*Omniscan*) Non-iodinated, nonionic IV contrast for MRI. ▶K ♀C ▶? $$$$ ■

GADOPENTETATE (*Magnevist*) Non-iodinated IV contrast for MRI. ▶K ♀C ▶? $$$ ■

GADOTERIDOL (*Prohance*) Non-iodinated, nonionic IV contrast for MRI. ▶K ♀C ▶? $$$$ ■

GADOVERSETAMIDE (*OptiMARK*) Non-iodinated IV contrast for MRI. ▶K ♀C ▶– $$$$ ■

MRI Contrast—Other

FERUMOXIDES (*Feridex*) Non-iodinated, nonionic, iron-based IV contrast for hepatic MRI. ▶L ♀C ▶? $$$$
FERUMOXSIL (*GastroMARK*) Non-iodinated, nonionic, iron-based, oral GI contrast for MRI. ▶L ♀B ▶? $$$$
MANGAFODIPIR (*Teslascan*) Noniodinated manganese-based IV contrast for MRI. ▶L ♀– ▶– $$$$

Radiography Contrast

NOTE: *Beware of allergic or anaphylactoid reactions. Avoid IV contrast in renal insufficiency or dehydration. Hold metformin (Glucophage) prior to or at the time of iodinated contrast dye use and for 48 h after procedure. Restart after procedure only if renal function is normal.*

BARIUM SULFATE Non-iodinated GI (eg, oral, rectal) contrast. ▶Not absorbed ♀? ▶+ $
DIATRIZOATE (*Cystografin, Gastrografin, Hypaque, MD-Gastroview, RenoCal, Reno-DIP, Reno-60, Renografin*) Iodinated, ionic, high osmolality IV or GI contrast. ▶K ♀C ▶? $
IODIXANOL (*Visipaque*) Iodinated, nonionic, iso-osmolar IV contrast. ▶K ♀B ▶? $$$
IOHEXOL (*Omnipaque*) Iodinated, nonionic, low osmolality IV and oral/body cavity contrast. ▶K ♀B ▶? $$$
IOPAMIDOL (*Isovue*) Iodinated, nonionic, low osmolality IV contrast. ▶K ♀? ▶? $$
IOPROMIDE (*Ultravist*) Iodinated, nonionic, low osmolality IV contrast. ▶K ♀B ▶? $$$
IOTHALAMATE (*Conray, ✦Vascoray*) Iodinated, ionic, high osmolality IV contrast. ▶K ♀B ▶– $
IOVERSOL (*Optiray*) Iodinated, nonionic, low osmolality IV contrast. ▶K ♀B ▶? $$
IOXAGLATE (*Hexabrix*) Iodinated, ionic, low osmolality IV contrast. ▶K ♀B ▶– $$$
IOXILAN (*Oxilan*) Iodinated, nonionic, low osmolality IV contrast. ▶K ♀B ▶– $$$

DERMATOLOGY

Acne Preparations

ACANYA (clindamycin + benzoyl peroxide) Apply daily. [Trade only: Gel (clindamycin 1.2% + benzoyl peroxide 2.5%) 50 g.] ▶K ♀C ▶+ $$$$
ADAPALENE (*Differin*) Apply at bedtime. [Generic/Trade: Gel 0.1%. Cream 0.1% (45 g). Trade only: Gel 0.3% (45 g). Soln 0.1% (30 mL). Swabs 0.1% (60 ea).] ▶Bile ♀C ▶? $$$$
AZELAIC ACID (*Azelex, Finacea, Finevin*) Apply two times per day. [Trade only: Cream 20%, 30, 50 g (Azelex). Gel 15% 50 g (Finacea).] ▶K ♀B ▶? $$$$

BENZACLIN (clindamycin + benzoyl peroxide) Apply two times per day. [Generic/Trade: Gel (clindamycin 1% + benzoyl peroxide 5%) 50 g (jar). Trade only: 25, 35 g (jar) and 50 g (pump).] ►K ♀C ▶+ $$$$

BENZAMYCIN (erythromycin base + benzoyl peroxide) Apply two times per day. [Generic/Trade: Gel (erythromycin 3% + benzoyl peroxide 5%) 23.3, 46.6 g. Trade only: Benzamycin Pak, #60 gel pouches.] ►LK ♀C ▶? $$$

BENZOYL PEROXIDE (*Benzac, Benzagel 10%, Desquam, Clearasil, ✦ Solugel*) Apply once daily; increase to two to three times per day if needed. [OTC and Rx generic: Liquid 2.5, 5, 10%. Bar 5, 10%. Mask 5%. Lotion 4, 5, 8, 10%. Cream 5, 10%. Gel 2.5, 4, 5, 6, 10, 20%. Pad 3, 4, 6, 8, 9%. Other strengths available.] ►LK ♀C ▶? $

CLENIA (sulfacetamide + sulfur) Apply one to three times per day. [Generic only: Lotion (sodium sulfacetamide 10%/sulfur 5%) 25, 30, 45, 60 g. Trade only: Cream (sodium sulfacetamide 10%/sulfur 5%) 28 g. Generic/Trade: Foaming Wash 170, 340 g.] ►K ♀C ▶? $$$

CLINDAMYCIN—TOPICAL (*Cleocin T, Clindagel, ClindaMax, Evoclin, ✦ Dalacin T*) Apply daily (Evoclin, Clindagel, Clindamax) or two times per day (Cleocin T). [Generic/Trade: Gel 1% 30, 60 g. Lotion 1% 60 mL. Soln 1% 30, 60 mL. Trade only: Foam 1% 50, 100 g (Evoclin). Gel 1% 40, 75 mL (Clindagel).] ►L ♀B ▶– $

✦ DIANE-35 (cyproterone + ethinyl estradiol) Canada only. 1 tab PO daily for 21 consecutive days, stop for 7 days, repeat cycle. [Canada Generic/Trade: Blister pack of 21 tabs 2 mg cyproterone acetate/0.035 mg ethinyl estradiol.] ►L ♀X ▶– $$

DUAC (clindamycin + benzoyl peroxide, ✦ *Clindoxyl*) Apply at bedtime. [Trade only: Gel (clindamycin 1% + benzoyl peroxide 5%) 45 g.] ►K ♀C ▶+ $$$$

EPIDUO (adapalene + benzoyl peroxide) Apply daily. [Trade only: Gel (0.1% adapalene + benzoyl peroxide 2.5%) 45 g.] ►Bile, K ♀C ▶? $$$$$

ERYTHROMYCIN—TOPICAL (*Eryderm, Erycette, Erygel, A/T/S, ✦ Erysol*) Apply two times per day. [Generic/Trade: Soln 2% 60 mL. Pads 2%. Gel 2% 30, 60 g. Ointment 2% 25 g. Generic only: Soln 1.5% 60 mL.] ►L ♀B ▶? $

ISOTRETINOIN (*Amnesteem, Claravis, Sotret, ✦ Clarus*) 0.5 to 2 mg/kg/day PO divided two times per day for 15 to 20 weeks. Typical target dose is 1 mg/kg/day. Potent teratogen; use extreme caution. Can only be prescribed by healthcare professionals who are registered with the iPLEDGE program. May cause depression. Not for long-term use. [Generic: Caps 10, 20, 40 mg. Generic only (Sotret and Claravis): Caps 30 mg.] ►LK ♀X ▶– $$$$$ ■

SALICYLIC ACID (*Akurza, Clearasil Cleanser, Stridex Pads*) Apply/wash area up to three times per day. [OTC Generic/Trade: Pads, Gel, Lotion, Liquid, Mask scrub, 0.5%, 1%, 2%. Rx Trade only (Akurza): Cream 6% 340 g. Lotion 6%, 355 mL.] ►Not absorbed ♀? ▶? $

✦ SULFACET-R (sulfacetamide + sulfur) Canada only. Apply one to three times per day. [Generic/Trade: Lotion (sodium sulfacetamide 10%/sulfur 5%) 25 g.] ►K ♀C ▶? $$$

SULFACETAMIDE—TOPICAL *(Klaron)* Apply two times per day. [Generic/Trade: Lotion 10% 118 mL.] ▶K ♀C ▶? $$$$

TAZAROTENE *(Tazorac, Avage)* Acne (Tazorac): Apply 0.1% cream at bedtime. Psoriasis: Apply 0.05% cream at bedtime, increase to 0.1% prn. [Trade only (Tazorac): Cream 0.05% and 0.1% 30, 60 g. Gel 0.05% and 0.1% 30, 100 g. Trade only (Avage): Cream 0.1% 15, 30 g.] ▶L ♀X ▶? $$$$

TRETINOIN—TOPICAL *(Retin-A, Retin-A Micro, Renova, Retisol-A, ✦ Stieva-A, Rejuva-A, Vitamin A Acid Cream)* Apply at bedtime. [Generic/Trade: Cream 0.025% 20, 45 g, 0.05% 20, 45 g, 0.1% 20, 45 g. Gel 0.025% 15, 45 g, 0.1% 15, 45 g. Trade only: Renova cream 0.02% 40, 60 g. Retin-A Micro gel 0.04%, 0.1% 20, 45, 50 g.] ▶LK ♀C ▶? $$$

VELTIN *(clindamycin + tretinoin)* Acne: Apply at bedtime. [Trade: Gel clindamycin 1.2% + tretinoin 0/025%, 30 g.] ▶LK - ♀C ▶? $$$$

ZIANA *(clindamycin + tretinoin)* Apply at bedtime. [Trade only: Gel clindamycin 1.2% + tretinoin 0.025% 30, 60 g.] ▶LK ♀C ▶? $$$$

Actinic Keratosis Preparations

DICLOFENAC—TOPICAL *(Solaraze)* Solaraze. Actinic/solar keratoses: Apply two times per day to lesions for 60 to 90 days. [Trade only: Gel 3% 50 g (Solaraze), 100 g (Solaraze, Voltaren).] ▶L ♀B ▶? $$$$$

FLUOROURACIL—TOPICAL *(5-FU, Carac, Efudex, Fluoroplex)* Actinic keratoses: Apply two times per day for 2 to 6 weeks. Superficial basal cell carcinomas: Apply 5% cream/soln two times per day. [Trade only: Cream 0.5% 30 g (Carac), 5% 25 g (Efudex), 1% 30 g (Fluoroplex). Generic/Trade: Soln 2%, 5% 10 mL (Efudex). Cream 5% 40 g.] ▶L ♀X ▶– $$$ ■

METHYLAMINOLEVULINATE *(Metvix, Metvixia)* Apply cream to non-hyperkeratotic actinic keratoses lesion and surrounding area on face or scalp; cover with dressing for 3 h; remove dressing and cream and perform illumination therapy. Repeat in 7 days. [Trade only: Cream 16.8%, 2 g tube.] ▶Not absorbed ♀C ▶? ?

Antibacterials (Topical)

BACITRACIN Apply daily to three times per day. [OTC Generic/Trade: Ointment 500 units/g 1, 15, 30 g.] ▶Not absorbed ♀C ▶? $

FUSIDIC ACID—TOPICAL *(✦ Fucidin)* Canada only. Apply three to four times per day. [Canada trade only: Cream 2% fusidic acid 5, 15, 30 g. Ointment 2% sodium fusidate 5, 15, 30 g.] ▶L ♀? ▶? $

GENTAMICIN—TOPICAL *(Garamycin)* Apply three to four times per day. [Generic only: Ointment 0.1% 15, 30 g. Cream 0.1% 15, 30 g.] ▶K ♀D ▶? $

MAFENIDE *(Sulfamylon)* Apply one to two times per day. [Trade only: Cream 5% 57, 114, 454 g. Topical soln 50 g packets.] ▶LK ♀C ▶? $$

METRONIDAZOLE—TOPICAL *(Noritate, MetroCream, MetroGel, MetroLotion, ✦ Rosasol)* Rosacea: Apply daily (1%) or two times per day (0.75%). [Trade only: Gel (MetroGel) 1% 45, 60 g. Cream (Noritate) 1% 60 g. Generic/Trade: Gel 0.75% 45 g. Cream 0.75% 45 g. Lotion (MetroLotion) 0.75% 59 mL.] ▶KL ♀B(− in 1st trimester) ▶− $$$

MUPIROCIN (*Bactroban, Centany*) Impetigo/infected wounds: Apply three times per day. Nasal methicillin-resistant S. aureus eradication: 0.5 g in each nostril two times per day for 5 days. [Generic/Trade: Ointment 2% 22 g. Nasal ointment 1% 1 g single-use tubes (for MRSA eradication). Trade only: Cream 2% 15, 30 g.] ▶Not absorbed ♀B ▶? $$

NEOSPORIN CREAM (neomycin + polymyxin + bacitracin) Apply one to three times per day. [OTC Trade only: neomycin 3.5 mg/g + polymyxin 10,000 units/g 15 g and unit dose 0.94 g.] ▶K ♀C ▶? $

NEOSPORIN OINTMENT (bacitracin + neomycin + polymyxin) Apply one to three times per day. [OTC Generic/Trade: bacitracin 400 units/g + neomycin 3.5 mg/g + polymyxin 5000 units/g 15, 30 g and "to go" 0.9 g packets.] ▶K ♀C ▶? $

POLYSPORIN (bacitracin + polymyxin, ✚ *Polytopic*) Apply one to three times per day. [OTC Trade only: Ointment 15, 30 g and unit dose 0.9 g. Powder 10 g.] ▶K ♀C ▶? $

RETAPAMULIN (*Altabax*) Impetigo: Apply two times per day for 5 days. [Trade only: Ointment 1% 5, 10, 15 g.] ▶Not absorbed ♀B ▶? $$$

SILVER SULFADIAZINE (*Silvadene, ✚ Dermazin, Flamazine, SSD*) Apply one to two times per day. [Generic/Trade: Cream 1% 20, 50, 85, 400, 1000 g.] ▶LK ♀B ▶− $$

Antifungals (Topical)

BUTENAFINE (*Lotrimin Ultra, Mentax*) Apply one to two times per day. [Rx Trade only: Cream 1% 15, 30 g (Mentax). OTC Trade only: Cream 1% 12, 24 g (Lotrimin Ultra).] ▶L ♀B ▶? $

CICLOPIROX (*Loprox, Penlac, ✚ Stieprox shampoo*) Cream, lotion: Apply two times per day. Nail soln: Apply daily to affected nails; apply over previous coat; remove with alcohol q 7 days. Seborrheic dermatitis (Loprox shampoo): Shampoo two times per week for 4 weeks. [Trade only: Shampoo (Loprox) 1% 120 mL. Generic/Trade: Gel 0.77% 30, 45, 100 g. Nail soln (Penlac) 8% 6.6 mL. Cream (Loprox) 0.77% 15, 30, 90 g. Lotion (Loprox TS) 0.77% 30, 60 mL.] ▶K ♀B ▶? $$$$

CLOTRIMAZOLE—TOPICAL (*Lotrimin AF, Mycelex, ✚Canesten, Clotrimaderm*) Apply two times per day. [Note that Lotrimin brand cream, lotion, soln are clotrimazole, while Lotrimin powders and liquid spray are miconazole. Rx Generic only: Cream 1% 15, 30, 45 g. Soln 1% 10, 30 mL. OTC Trade only (Lotrimin AF): Cream 1% 12, 24 g. Soln 1% 10 mL.] ▶L ♀B ▶? $

ECONAZOLE Tinea pedis, tinea cruris, tinea corporis, tinea versicolor: Apply daily. Cutaneous candidiasis: Apply two times per day. [Generic only: Cream 1% 15, 30, 85 g.] ▶Not absorbed ♀C ▶? $$

KETOCONAZOLE—TOPICAL (*Extina, Nizoral, Xolegel, ✚ Ketoderm*) Tinea/candidal infections: Apply daily. Seborrheic dermatitis: Apply cream one to two

(cont.)

times per day for 4 weeks or gel daily for 2 weeks or foam two times per day for 4 weeks. Dandruff: Apply shampoo two times per week. Tinea versicolor: Apply shampoo to affected area, leave on for 5 min, rinse. [Generic/Trade: Cream 2% 15, 30, 60 g. Shampoo 2% 120 mL. Trade only: Shampoo 1% 120, 210 mL (OTC Nizoral). Gel 2% 15 g (Xolegel). Foam 2% 50, 100 g (Extina).] ▶L ♀C ▶? $$

MICONAZOLE—TOPICAL (*Micatin, Lotrimin AF, ZeaSorb AF*) Tinea, candida: Apply two times per day. [Note that Lotrimin brand cream, lotion, soln are clotrimazole, while Lotrimin powders and liquid spray are miconazole. OTC Trade only: Powder 2% 70, 160 g. Spray powder 2% 90, 100, 140 g. Spray liquid 2% 90, 105 mL. Gel 2% 24 g.] ▶L ♀+ ▶? $

NAFTIFINE (*Naftin*) Tinea: Apply daily (cream) or two times per day (gel). [Trade only: Cream 1% 15, 30, 60, 90 g. Gel 1% 20, 40, 60, 90 g.] ▶LK ♀B ▶? $$$

NYSTATIN—TOPICAL (*Mycostatin, ＋Nilstat, Nyaderm*) Candidiasis: Apply two to three times per day. [Generic/Trade: Cream, Ointment 100,000 units/g 15, 30 g. Powder 100,000 units/g 15, 30, 60 g.] ▶Not absorbed ♀C ▶? $

OXICONAZOLE (*Oxistat, Oxizole*) Tinea pedis, cruris, and corporis: Apply one to two times per day. Tinea versicolor (cream only): Apply daily. [Trade only: Cream 1% 15, 30, 60 g. Lotion 1% 30 mL.] ▶? ♀B ▶? $$$

SERTACONAZOLE (*Ertaczo*) Tinea pedis: Apply two times per day. [Trade only: Cream 2% 30, 60 g.] ▶Not absorbed ♀C ▶? $$$

TERBINAFINE—TOPICAL (*Lamisil, Lamisil AT*) Tinea: Apply one to two times per day. [OTC Trade only (Lamisil AT): Cream 1% 12, 24 g. Spray pump soln 1% 30 mL. Gel 1% 6, 12 g.] ▶L ♀B ▶? $$$

TOLNAFTATE (*Tinactin*) Apply two times per day. [OTC Generic/Trade: Cream 1% 15, 30 g. Soln 1% 10 mL. Powder 1% 45 g. OTC Trade only: Gel 1% 15 g. Powder 1% 90 g. Spray powder 1% 100, 133, 150 g. Spray liquid 1% 100, 113 mL.] ▶? ♀? ▶? $

Antiparasitics (Topical)

A-200 (pyrethrins + piperonyl butoxide, ＋*R&C*) Lice: Apply shampoo, wash after 10 min. Reapply in 5 to 7 days. [OTC Generic/Trade: Shampoo (0.33% pyrethrins, 4% piperonyl butoxide) 60, 120 mL.] ▶L ♀C ▶? $

BENZYL ALCOHOL (*Ulesfia*) Apply to dry hair to saturate scalp and hair. Rinse after 10 minutes. Reapply in 7 days, if necessary. [Lotion 5% 60 mL.] ▶Not absorbed - ♀B ▶? $$$$

CROTAMITON (*Eurax*) Scabies: Apply cream/lotion topically from chin to feet, repeat in 24 h, bathe 48 h later. Pruritus: Massage prn. [Trade only: Cream 10% 60 g. Lotion 10% 60, 480 mL.] ▶? ♀C ▶? $$$

LINDANE (＋*Hexit*) Other drugs preferred. Scabies: Apply 30 to 60 mL of lotion, wash after 8 to 12 h. Lice: 30 to 60 mL of shampoo, wash off after 4 min. Can cause seizures in epileptics or if overused/misused in children.

(cont.)

Not for infants. [Generic only: Lotion 1% 60, 480 mL. Shampoo 1% 60, 480 mL.] ▶L ♀B ▶? $ ■

MALATHION (*Ovide*) Apply to dry hair, let dry naturally, wash off in 8 to 12 h. Flammable. [Generic/Trade only: Lotion 0.5% 59 mL.] ▶? ♀B ▶? $$$$

PERMETHRIN (*Elimite, Acticin, Nix, ✦ Kwellada-P*) Scabies: Apply cream from head (avoid mouth/nose/eyes) to soles of feet and wash after 8 to 14 h. 30 g is typical adult dose. Lice: Saturate hair and scalp with 1% rinse, wash after 10 min. Do not use in age younger than 2 mo. May repeat therapy in 7 days, as necessary. [Generic/Trade: Cream (Elimite, Acticin) 5% 60 g. OTC Generic/Trade: Liquid creme rinse (Nix) 1% 60 mL.] ▶L ♀B ▶? $$

RID (pyrethrins + piperonyl butoxide) Lice: Apply shampoo/mousse, wash after 10 min. Reapply in 5 to 10 days, as necessary. [OTC Generic/Trade: Shampoo 60, 120, 240 mL. Trade only: Mousse 5.5 oz.] ▶L ♀C ▶– $$

SPINOSAD (*Natroba*) Lice: Apply to dry hair/scalp to cover. Leave on 10 min then rinse. Retreat, if necessary. [Topical susp, 0.9%, 120 mL.] ▶not absorbed – ♀B ▶? $$$$$

Antipsoriatics

ACITRETIN (*Soriatane*) 25 to 50 mg PO daily. Avoid pregnancy during therapy and for 3 years after discontinuation. [Trade only: Caps 10, 25 mg.] ▶L ♀X ▶– $$$$$ ■

ALEFACEPT (*Amevive*) 7.5 mg IV or 15 mg IM once a week for 12 doses. May repeat with 1 additional 12-week course after 12 weeks have elapsed since last dose. ▶? ♀B ▶? $$$$$

ANTHRALIN (*Drithocreme, ✦ Anthrascalp, Anthranol, Anthraforte, Dithranol*) Apply daily. Short contact periods (ie, 15 to 20 min) followed by removal may be preferred. [Trade only: Cream 0.5, 1% 50 g.] ▶? ♀C ▶– $$$

CALCIPOTRIENE (*Dovonex, Sorilux*) Apply two times per day. [Trade only: Ointment 0.005% 30, 60, 100 g (Dovonex). Cream 0.005% 30, 60, 100 g (Dovonex). Foam 0.005%60, 120 g (Sorilux). Generic/Trade: Scalp soln 0.005% 60 mL.] ▶L ♀C ▶? $$$$

TACLONEX (calcipotriene + betamethasone, ✦ *Dovobet, Xamiol*) Apply daily for up to 4 weeks. [Calcipotriene 0.005% + betamethasone dipropionate. Trade only: Ointment 15, 30, 60, 100 g. Topical susp 15, 30, 60 g.] ▶L ♀C ▶? $$$$$

USTEKINUMAB (*Stelara*) Severe plaque psoriasis: wt less than 100 kg, use 45 mg SC initially and again 4 weeks later, followed by 45 mg SC q 12 weeks. For wt greater than 100 kg, use 90 mg SC initially and again 4 weeks later, followed by 90 mg SC q 12 weeks. [Trade only: 45 and 90 mg prefilled syringe and vial.] ▶L – ♀B ▶? $$$$$

Antivirals (Topical)

ACYCLOVIR—TOPICAL (*Zovirax*) Herpes genitalis: Apply ointment q 3 h (6 times per day) for 7 days. Recurrent herpes labialis: Apply cream 5 times per day for 4 days. [Trade only: Ointment 5% 15 g. Cream 5% 2, 5 g.] ▶K ♀C ▶? $$$$$

DOCOSANOL (*Abreva*) Oral-facial herpes (cold sores): Apply 5 times per day until healed. [OTC Trade only: Cream 10% 2 g.] ▶Not absorbed ♀B ▶? $

IMIQUIMOD (*Aldara, Zyclara*) Genital/perianal warts: Apply once daily for up to 8 weeks. Wash off after 8 h. Non-hyperkeratotic, non-hypertrophic actinic keratoses on face/scalp in immunocompetent adults: Apply two times per week overnight for 16 weeks (Aldara) or once daily for 2 two-week periods separated by a 2 week break (Zyclara). Wash off after 8 h. Primary superficial basal cell carcinoma: Apply 5 times a week for 6 weeks (Aldara). Wash off after 8 h. [Generic/Trade: Cream 5% (Aldara) single-packets, 3.75% (Zyclara) single-use packets.] ▶Not absorbed ♀C ▶? $$$$$

PENCICLOVIR (*Denavir*) Herpes labialis (cold sores): Apply cream q 2 h while awake for 4 days. [Trade only: Cream 1% tube 1.5 g.] ▶Not absorbed ♀B ▶? $$

PODOFILOX (*Condylox*, ✦ *Condyline, Wartec*) External genital warts (gel and soln) and perianal warts (gel only): Apply two times per day for 3 consecutive days of the week and repeat for up to 4 weeks. [Generic/Trade: Soln 0.5% 3.5 mL. Trade only: Gel 0.5% 3.5 g.] ▶? ♀C ▶? $$$$

PODOPHYLLIN (*Podocon-25, Podofin, Podofilm*) Warts: Apply by physician. [Not to be dispensed to patients. For hospital/clinic use; not intended for outpatient prescribing. Trade only: Liquid 25% 15 mL.] ▶? ♀– ▶– $$$

SINECATECHINS (*Veregen*) Apply three times per day to external genital warts for up to 16 weeks. [Trade only: Ointment 15% 15, 30 g.] ▶Unknown ♀C ▶? $$$$$

Atopic Dermatitis Preparations

PIMECROLIMUS (*Elidel*) Atopic dermatitis: Apply two times per day. [Trade only: Cream 1% 30, 60, 100 g.] ▶L ♀C ▶? $$$$ ■

TACROLIMUS—TOPICAL (*Protopic*) Atopic dermatitis: Apply two times per day. [Trade only: Ointment 0.03%, 0.1% 30, 60, 100 g.] ▶Minimal absorption ♀C ▶? $$$$$

Corticosteroid/Antimicrobial Combinations

CORTISPORIN (neomycin + polymyxin + hydrocortisone) Apply two to four times per day. [Trade only: Cream 7.5 g. Ointment 15 g.] ▶LK ♀C ▶? $$$

✦ **FUCIDIN H** (fusidic acid + hydrocortisone) Canada only. Apply three times per day. [Canada Trade only: Cream (2% fusidic acid, 1% hydrocortisone acetate) 30 g.] ▶L ♀? ▶? $$

LOTRISONE (clotrimazole + betamethasone, ✦ *Lotriderm*) Apply two times per day. Do not use for diaper rash. [Generic/Trade: Cream (clotrimazole 1% + betamethasone 0.05%) 15, 45 g. Lotion (clotrimazole 1% + betamethasone 0.05%) 30 mL.] ▶L ♀C ▶? $$$

MYCOLOG II (nystatin + triamcinolone) Apply two times per day. [Generic only: Cream, Ointment 15, 30, 60, 120, 454 g.] ▶L ♀C ▶? $

CORTICOSTEROIDS—TOPICAL

Potency*	Generic	Trade Name	Forms	Frequency
Low	alclometasone dipropionate	Aclovate	0.05% C/O	bid-tid
Low	clocortolone pivalate	Cloderm	0.1% C	tid
Low	desonide	DesOwen, Tridesilon	0.05% C/L/O	bid-tid
Low	hydrocortisone	Hytone, others	0.5% C/L/O; 1% C/L/O; 2.5% C/O	bid-qid
Low	hydrocortisone acetate	Cortaid, Corticaine	0.5% C/O; 1% C/O/Sp	bid-qid
Medium	betamethasone valerate	Luxiq	0.1% C/L/O; 0.12% F (Luxiq)	daily-bid
Medium	desoximetasone‡	Topicort	0.05% C	bid
Medium	fluocinolone	Synalar	0.01% C/S; 0.025% C/O	bid-qid
Medium	flurandrenolide	Cordran	0.025% C/O; 0.05% C/L/O/T	bid-qid
Medium	fluticasone propionate	Cutivate	0.005% O; 0.05% C/L	daily-bid
Medium	hydrocortisone butyrate	Locoid	0.1% C/O/S	bid-tid
Medium	hydrocortisone valerate	Westcort	0.2% C/O	bid-tid
Medium	mometasone furoate	Elocon	0.1% C/L/O	daily
Medium	triamcinolone‡	Aristocort, Kenalog	0.025% C/L/O; 0.1% C/L/O/S	bid-tid
High	amcinonide	Cyclocort	0.1% C/L/O	bid-tid
High	betamethasone dipropionate‡	Maxivate, others	0.05% C/L/O (non-Diprolene)	daily-bid
High	desoximetasone‡	Topicort	0.05% G; 0.25% C/O	bid
High	diflorasone diacetate‡	Maxiflor	0.05% C/O	bid
High	fluocinonide	Lidex	0.05% C/G/O/S	bid-qid
High	halcinonide	Halog	0.1% C/O/S	bid-tid
High	triamcinolone‡	Aristocort, Kenalog	0.5% C/O	bid-tid
Very high	betamethasone dipropionate‡	Diprolene, Diprolene AF	0.05% C/G/L/O	daily-bid
Very high	clobetasol	Temovate, Cormax, Olux	0.05% C/G/O/L/S/Sp/F (Olux)	bid
Very high	diflorasone diacetate‡	Psorcon	0.05% C/O	daily-tid
Very high	halobetasol propionate	Ultravate	0.05% C/O	daily-bid

bid=two times per day; tid=three times per day; qid=four times per day.
*Potency based on vasoconstrictive assays, which may not correlate with efficacy. Not all available products are listed, including those lacking potency ratings. ‡These drugs have formulations in more than once potency category. C, cream; O, ointment; L, lotion; T, tape; F, foam; S, solution; G, gel; Sp, spray

Hemorrhoid Care

DIBUCAINE (*Nupercainal*) Apply three to four times per day prn. [OTC Trade only: Ointment 1% 30, 60 g.] ▶L ♀? ▶? $

PRAMOXINE (*Tucks Hemorrhoidal Ointment, Fleet Pain Relief, ProctoFoam NS*) Apply up to 5 times per day prn. [OTC Trade only: Ointment (Tucks Hemorrhoidal Ointment) 30 g. Pads (Fleet Pain Relief) 100 each. Aerosol foam (ProctoFoam NS) 15 g.] ▶Not absorbed ♀+ ▶+ $

STARCH (*Tucks Suppositories*) 1 suppository up to 6 times per day prn. [OTC Trade only: Suppository (51% topical starch; vegetable oil, tocopheryl acetate) 12, 24 each.] ▶Not absorbed ♀+ ▶+ $

WITCH HAZEL (*Tucks*) Apply to anus/perineum up to 6 times per day prn. [OTC Generic/Trade: Pads 50% 12, 40, 100 ea, generically available in various quantities.] ▶? ♀+ ▶+ $

Other Dermatologic Agents

ALITRETINOIN (*Panretin*) Apply two to four times per day to cutaneous Kaposi's lesions [Trade only: Gel 0.1% 60 g.] ▶Not absorbed ♀D ▶− $$$$$

ALUMINUM CHLORIDE (*Drysol, Certain Dri*) Apply at bedtime. [Rx Trade only: Soln 20% 37.5 mL bottle, 35, 60 mL bottle with applicator. OTC Trade only (Certain Dri): Soln 12.5% 36 mL bottle.] ▶K ♀? ▶? $

BECAPLERMIN (*Regranex*) Diabetic ulcers: Apply daily. [Trade only: Gel 0.01%, 2, 15 g.] ▶Minimal absorption ♀C ▶? $$$$$ ■

CALAMINE Apply three to four times per day prn for poison ivy/oak or insect bite itching. [OTC Generic only: Lotion 120, 240, 480 mL.] ▶? ♀? ▶? $

CAPSAICIN (*Zostrix, Zostrix-HP*) Arthritis, post-herpetic or diabetic neuralgia: Apply three to four times per day. [OTC Generic/Trade: Cream 0.025% 60 g, 0.075% (HP) 60 g. OTC Generic only: Lotion 0.025% 59 mL, 0.075% 59 mL.] ▶? ♀? ▶? $

COAL TAR (*Polytar, Tegrin, Cutar, Tarsum*) Apply shampoo at least two times per week, or for psoriasis apply one to four times per day. [OTC Generic/Trade: Shampoo, cream, ointment, gel, lotion, liquid, oil, soap.] ▶? ♀? ▶? $

DOXEPIN—TOPICAL (*Zonalon*) Pruritus: Apply four times per day for up to 8 days. [Trade only: Cream 5% 30, 45 g.] ▶L ♀B ▶− $$$$

EFLORNITHINE (*Vaniqa*) Reduction of facial hair: Apply two times per day. [Trade only: Cream 13.9% 30 g.] ▶K ♀C ▶? $$$

EMLA (prilocaine + lidocaine—topical) Topical anesthesia: Apply 2.5 g cream or 1 disc to region at least 1 h before procedure. Cover with occlusive dressing. [Generic/Trade: Cream (2.5% lidocaine + 2.5% prilocaine) 5, 30 g.] ▶LK ♀B ▶? $$

HYALURONIC ACID (*Bionect, Restylane, Perlane*) Moderate to severe facial wrinkles: Inject into wrinkle/fold (Restylane, Perlane). Protection of dermal ulcers: Apply gel/cream/spray two or three times per day (Bionect). [OTC Trade only: Cream 2% 15, 30 g. Rx Generic/Trade: Soln 3% 30 mL. Gel 4% 30 g. Cream 4% 15, 30, 60 g. Injectable gel 2%.] ▶? ♀? ▶? $$$

HYDROQUINONE (*Eldopaque, Eldoquin, Eldoquin Forte, EpiQuin Micro, Esoterica, Glyquin, Lustra, Melanex, Solaquin, Claripel, ✦Ultraquin*) Hyperpigmentation: Apply two times per day. [OTC Trade only: Cream 2% 15, 30 g. Rx Generic/Trade: Soln 3% 30 mL. Gel 4% 30 g. Cream 4% 15, 30, 60 g.] ▶? ♀C ▶? $

LACTIC ACID (*Lac-Hydrin, AmLactin, ✦Dermalac*) Apply two times per day. [Trade only: Lotion 12% 150, 360 mL. Generic/OTC: Cream 12% 140, 385 g. AmLactin AP is lactic acid (12%) with pramoxine (1%).] ▶? ♀? ▶? $$

LIDOCAINE—TOPICAL (*Xylocaine, Lidoderm, Numby Stuff, LMX, Zingo, ✦Maxilene*) Apply prn. Dose varies with anesthetic procedure, degree of anesthesia required, and individual patient response. Postherpetic neuralgia: Apply up to 3 patches to affected area at once for up to 12 h within a 24-h period. Apply 30 min prior to painful procedure (ELA-Max 4%). Discomfort with anorectal disorders: Apply prn (ELA-Max 5%). Intradermal powder injection for venipuncture/IV cannulation, 3 to 18 yo (Zingo): 0.5 mg to site 1 to 10 min prior. [For membranes of mouth and pharynx: Spray 10%, Ointment 5%, Liquid 5%, Soln 2%, 4%, Dental patch. For urethral use: Jelly 2%. Patch (Lidoderm) 5%. Intradermal powder injection system: 0.5 mg (Zingo). OTC Trade only: Liposomal lidocaine 4% (ELA-Max).] ▶LK ♀B ▶+ $$

MINOXIDIL—TOPICAL (*Rogaine, Women's Rogaine, Rogaine Extra Strength, Minoxidil for Men, Theroxidil Extra Strength*) Androgenetic alopecia in men or women: Apply 1 mL to dry scalp two times per day. [OTC Generic/Trade: Soln 2% 60 mL (Rogaine, Women's Rogaine). Soln 5% 60 mL (Rogaine Extra Strength, Theroxidil Extra Strength—for men only). Foam 5% 60 g (Rogaine Extra Strength).] ▶? ♀C ▶— $

MONOBENZONE (*Benoquin*) Extensive vitiligo: Apply two to three times per day. [Trade only: Cream 20% 35.4 g.] ▶Minimal absorption ♀C ▶? $$$

OATMEAL (*Aveeno*) Pruritus from poison ivy/oak, varicella: Apply lotion four times per day prn. Also bath packets for tub. [OTC Generic/Trade: Lotion. Bath packets.] ▶Not absorbed ♀? ▶? $

PANAFIL (*papain + urea + chlorophyllin copper complex*) Debridement of acute or chronic lesions: Apply to clean wound and cover one to two times per day. [Trade only: Ointment 6, 30 g. Spray 33 mL.] ▶? ♀? ▶? $$$

PRAMOSONE (*pramoxine + hydrocortisone, ✦Pramox HC*) Inflammatory and pruritic manifestations of corticosteroid-responsive dermatoses: Apply three to four times per day. [Trade only: 1% pramoxine/1% hydrocortisone acetate: Cream 30, 60 g. Ointment 30 g. Lotion 60, 120, 240 mL. 1% pramoxine/2.5% hydrocortisone acetate: Cream 30, 60 g. Ointment 30 g. Lotion 60, 120 mL.] ▶Not absorbed ♀C ▶? $$$

SELENIUM SULFIDE (*Selsun, Exsel, Versel*) Dandruff, seborrheic dermatitis: Apply 5 to 10 mL two times per week for 2 weeks then less frequently, thereafter. Tinea versicolor: Apply 2.5% to affected area daily for 7 days. [OTC Generic/Trade: Lotion/Shampoo 1% 120, 210, 240, 325 mL, 2.5% 120 mL. Rx Generic/Trade: Lotion/Shampoo 2.5% 120 mL.] ▶? ♀C ▶? $

SOLAG (*mequinol + tretinoin, ✦Solage*) Apply to solar lentigines two times per day. [Trade only: Soln 30 mL (mequinol 2% + tretinoin 0.01%).] ▶Not absorbed ♀X ▶? $$$$

SYNERA **(tetracaine + lidocaine—topical)** Apply 20 to 30 min prior to superficial dermatological procedure. [Trade only: Topical patch (lidocaine 70 mg + tetracaine 70 mg.] ▶Minimal absorption ♀B ▶? $$

TRI-LUMA **(fluocinolone + hydroquinone + tretinoin)** Melasma of the face: Apply at bedtime for 4 to 8 weeks. [Trade only: Cream 30 g (fluocinolone 0.01% + hydroquinone 4% + tretinoin 0.05%).] ▶Minimal absorption ♀C ▶? $$$$

VUSION **(miconazole—topical + zinc oxide + white petrolatum)** Apply to affected diaper area with each change for 7 days. [Trade only: Ointment 50 g.] ▶Minimal absorption ♀C ▶? $$$$$

ENDOCRINE & METABOLIC

Androgens / Anabolic Steroids

NOTE: *See OB/GYN section for other hormones.*

OXANDROLONE (*Oxandrin*) Weight gain: 2.5 mg/day to 20 mg/day PO divided two to four times per day for 2 to 4 weeks. [Generic/Trade: Tabs 2.5, 10 mg.] ▶L ♀X ▶?☺III $$$$$ ■

TESTOSTERONE (*Androderm, AndroGel, Axiron, Delatestryl, Depo-Testosterone, Striant, Testim, Testopel, TestroAQ, ✦Andriol*) Hypogonadism: Injectable enanthate or cypionate: 50 to 400 mg IM q 2 to 4 weeks. Transdermal: Androderm: 5 mg patch to nonscrotal skin at bedtime. AndroGel 1%: Apply 5 g from gel pack or 4 pumps (5 g) from dispenser daily to shoulders/upper arms/abdomen. Axiron: 60 mg (1 pump of 30 mg to each axilla) once daily. Testim: 1 tube (5 g) daily to shoulders/upper arms. Pellet: Testopel: 2 to 6 (150 to 450 mg testosterone) pellets SC q 3 to 6 months. Buccal: Striant: 30 mg q 12 h on upper gum above the incisor tooth; alternate sides for each application. [Trade only: Patch 2.5, 5 mg/24 h (Androderm). Gel 1% 2.5, 5 g packet, 75 g multidose pump (AndroGel, 1.25 g/actuation). Gel 1%, 5 g tube (Testim). Gel 110 mL multidose pump (Axiron, 30 mg/actuation). Pellet 75 mg (Testopel). Buccal: Blister packs: 30 mg (Striant). Generic/Trade: Injection 100, 200 mg/mL (cypionate), 200 mg/mL (ethanate).] ▶L ♀X ▶? $$$ ■

Bisphosphonates

ALENDRONATE (*Fosamax, Fosamax Plus D, ✦Fosavance*) Prevention of postmenopausal osteoporosis: 5 mg PO daily or 35 mg PO weekly. Treatment of postmenopausal osteoporosis: 10 mg daily, 70 mg PO weekly, 70 mg/vitamin D3 2800 international units PO weekly, or 70 mg/vitamin D3 5600 international units PO weekly. Treatment of glucocorticoid-induced osteoporosis: 5 mg PO daily in men and women or 10 mg PO daily in postmenopausal women not

(cont.)

taking estrogen. <u>Treatment of osteoporosis in men</u>: 10 mg PO daily, 70 mg PO weekly, or 70 mg/vitamin D3 2800 international units PO weekly, or 70 mg/vitamin D3 5600 international units PO weekly. <u>Paget's disease</u>: 40 mg PO daily for 6 months. [Generic/Trade (Fosamax): Tabs 5, 10, 35, 40, 70 mg. Trade only: Oral soln 70 mg/75 mL (single-dose bottle). Fosamax Plus D: 70 mg + either 2800 or 5600 units of vitamin D3.] ▶K ♀C ▶– $$

ETIDRONATE (**Didronel**) <u>Paget's disease</u>: 5 to 10 mg/kg PO daily for 6 months or 11 to 20 mg/kg daily for 3 months. [Generic/Trade: Tabs 400 mg. Generic only: Tabs 200 mg.] ▶K ♀C ▶? $$$$$

IBANDRONATE (**Boniva**) <u>Prevention and treatment of postmenopausal osteoporosis</u>: Oral: 2.5 mg PO daily or 150 mg PO once a month. IV: 3 mg IV q 3 months. [Trade only: Tabs 2.5, 150 mg. IV: 3 mg.] ▶K ♀C ▶? $$$$

PAMIDRONATE (**Aredia**) <u>Hypercalcemia of malignancy</u>: 60 to 90 mg IV over 2 to 24 h. Wait at least 7 days before considering retreatment. ▶K ♀D ▶? $$$$$

RISEDRONATE (**Actonel, Actonel Plus Calcium, Atelvia**) <u>Prevention and treatment of postmenopausal osteoporosis</u>: 5 mg PO daily, 35 mg PO weekly, or 150 mg once a month. <u>Treatment of osteoporosis in men</u>: 35 mg PO weekly. <u>Prevention and treatment of glucocorticoid-induced osteoporosis</u>: 5 mg PO daily. <u>Paget's disease</u>: 30 mg PO daily for 2 months. [Trade only: Tabs 5, 30, 35, 150 mg, Delayed-release tab (Atelvia): 35 mg. Trade only (Actonel + Calcium): Tabs 35/1250 mg combination package.] ▶K ♀C ▶? $$$$

ZOLEDRONIC ACID (**Reclast, Zometa, ✦Aclasta**) <u>Treatment of osteoporosis</u>: 5 mg (Reclast) once yearly IV infusion over 15 min or longer. <u>Prevention and treatment of glucocorticoid-induced osteoporosis</u>: 5 mg (Reclast) once a year IV infusion over 15 min or longer. <u>Hypercalcemia</u> (Zometa): 4 mg IV infusion over 15 min or longer. Wait at least 7 days before considering retreatment. <u>Paget's disease</u> (Reclast): 5 mg IV single dose infused over 15 min or longer. <u>Multiple myeloma and metastatic bone lesions from solid tumors</u> (Zometa): 4 mg IV infusion over 15 min or longer q 3 to 4 weeks. ▶K ♀D ▶? $$$$$

Corticosteroids

NOTE: *See also dermatology, ophthalmology.*

BETAMETHASONE (**Celestone, Celestone Soluspan, ✦Betaject**) <u>Anti-inflammatory/Immunosuppressive</u>: 0.6 to 7.2 mg/day PO/IV/IM divided two to four times per day; up to 9 mg/day IM. <u>Fetal lung maturation, maternal antepartum</u>: 12 mg IM q 24 h for 2 doses. [Trade only: Syrup 0.6 mg/5 mL.] ▶L ♀C ▶– $$$$$

CORTISONE (**Cortone**) 25 to 300 mg PO daily. [Generic only: Tabs 25 mg.] ▶L ♀D ▶– $

DEXAMETHASONE (**Decadron, Dexpak, ✦Dexasone**) <u>Anti-inflammatory/Immunosuppressive</u>: 0.5 to 9 mg/day PO/IV/IM, divided two to four times per day. <u>Cerebral edema</u>: 10 to 20 mg IV load, then 4 mg IM q 6 h (off-label IV use common) or 1 to 3 mg PO three times per day. <u>Bronchopulmonary dysplasia</u> in preterm infants: 0.5 mg/kg PO/IV divided q 12 h for 3 days, then taper.

(cont.)

CORTICO-STEROIDS	Approximate Equivalent Dose (mg)	Relative Anti-inflammatory Potency	Relative Mineralocorticoid Potency	Biological Half-life (h)
betamethasone	0.6–0.75	20–30	0	36–54
cortisone	25	0.8	2	8–12
dexamethasone	0.75	20–30	0	36–54
fludrocortisone	n/a	10	125	18–36
hydrocortisone	20	1	2	8–12
Methylprednisolone	4	5	0	18–36
prednisolone	5	4	1	18–36
prednisone	5	4	1	18–36
triamcinolone	4	5	0	12–36

n/a, not available.

Croup: 0.6 mg/kg PO or IM for one dose. Acute asthma: age older than 2 yo: 0.6 mg/kg to max 16 mg PO daily for 2 days. Fetal lung maturation, maternal antepartum: 6 mg IM q 12 h for 4 doses. Antiemetic, prophylaxis: 8 mg IV or 12 mg PO prior to chemotherapy; 8 mg PO daily for 2 to 4 days. Antiemetic, treatment: 10 to 20 mg PO/IV q 4 to 6 h. [Generic/Trade: Tabs 0.5, 0.75. Generic only: Tabs 0.25, 1.0, 1.5, 2, 4, 6 mg; elixir 0.5 mg/5 mL; Soln 0.5 mg/5 mL, 1 mg/1 mL (concentrate). Trade only: Dexpak 13 day (51 total 1.5 mg tabs for a 13-day taper), Dexpak 10 day (35 total 1.5 mg tabs for 10-day taper), Dexpak 6 days (21 total 1.5 mg tabs for 6-day taper).] ▶L ♀C ▶– $
FLUDROCORTISONE (*Florinef*) Mineralocorticoid activity: 0.1 mg PO three times per week to 0.2 mg PO daily. Postural hypotension: 0.05 to 0.4 mg PO daily. [Generic only: Tabs 0.1 mg.] ▶L ♀C ▶? $
HYDROCORTISONE (*Cortef, Cortenema, Solu-Cortef*) Adrenocortical insufficiency: 100 to 500 mg IV/IM q 2 to 6 h prn (sodium succinate) or 20 to 240 mg/day PO divided three to four times per day. Ulcerative colitis: 100 mg retention enema at bedtime (laying on side for 1 h or longer) for 21 days. [Generic/Trade: Tabs 5, 10, 20 mg; Enema 100 mg/60 mL.] ▶L ♀C ▶– $
METHYLPREDNISOLONE (*Solu-Medrol, Medrol, Depo-Medrol*) Anti-inflammatory/immunosuppressive: Oral (Medrol): Dose varies, 4 to 48 mg PO daily. Medrol Dosepak tapers 24 to 0 mg PO over / days. IM/Joints (Depo-Medrol): Dose varies, 4 to 120 mg IM q 1 to 2 weeks. Parenteral (Solu-Medrol): Dose varies, 10 to 250 mg IV/IM. Peds: 0.5 to 1.7 mg/kg PO/IV/IM divided q 6 to 12 h. [Trade only: Tabs 2, 16, 32 mg. Generic/Trade: Tabs 4, 8 mg. Medrol Dosepak (4 mg, 21 tabs).] ▶L ♀C ▶– $
PREDNISOLONE (*Flo-Pred, Prelone, Pediapred, Orapred, Orapred ODT*) 5 to 60 mg PO daily. [Generic/Trade: Syrup 15 mg/5 mL (Prelone; wild cherry flavor). Soln 5 mg/5 mL (Pediapred, raspberry flavor), 15 mg/5 mL (Orapred; grape flavor). Trade only: Orally disintegrating tabs 10, 15, 30 mg (Orapred ODT); Susp 5 mg/5 mL, 15 mg/5 mL (Flo-Pred; cherry flavor). Generic only: Tabs 5 mg. Syrup 5 mg/5 mL.] ▶L ♀C ▶+ $$

PREDNISONE (*Deltasone, Sterapred, ✦ Winpred*) 1 to 2 mg/kg or 5 to 60 mg PO daily. [Trade only: Sterapred (5 mg tabs: Tapers 30 to 5 PO over 6 days or 30 to 10 mg over 12 days), Sterapred DS (10 mg tabs: Tapers 60 to 10 mg over 6 days, or 60 to 20 mg PO over 12 days) taper packs. Generic only: Tabs 1, 2.5, 5, 10, 20, 50 mg. Soln 5 mg/5 mL, 5 mg/mL (Prednisone Intensol).] ▶L ♀C ▶+ $

TRIAMCINOLONE (*Aristospan, Kenalog, Trivaris*) 4 to 48 mg PO/IM daily. Intra-articular 2.5 to 40 mg (Kenalog, Trivaris), 2 to 20 mg (Aristospan). [Trade only: Injection 10 mg/mL, 40 mg/mL (Kenalog), 5 mg/mL, 20 mg/mL (Aristospan), 8 mg (80 mg/mL) syringe (Trivaris).] ▶L ♀C ▶– $

Diabetes-Related—Alpha-Glucosidase Inhibitors

ACARBOSE (*Precose, ✦ Glucobay*) DM, Type 2: Start 25 mg PO three times per day with meals, and gradually increase as tolerated to maintenance, 50 to 100 mg three times per day. [Generic/Trade: Tabs 25, 50, 100 mg.] ▶Gut/K ♀B ▶– $$$

MIGLITOL (*Glyset*) DM, Type 2: Start 25 mg PO three times per day with meals, maintenance 50 to 100 three times per day. [Trade only: Tabs 25, 50, 100 mg.] ▶K ♀B ▶– $$$

Diabetes-Related—Combinations

ACTOPLUS MET (pioglitazone + metformin) DM, Type 2: 1 tab PO daily or two times per day. If inadequate control with metformin monotherapy, start 15/500 or 15/850 PO one to two times per day. If inadequate control with pioglitazone monotherapy, start 15/500 two times per day or 15/850 daily. Max 45/2550 mg/day. Extended-release, start 1 tab (15/100 mg or 30/1000 mg) daily with evening meal. Max: 45/2000 mg/day. Obtain LFTs before therapy and periodically thereafter. [Trade only: Tabs 15/500, 15/850 mg, Extended-release, tabs: 15/1000 mg, 30/1000 mg.] ▶KL ♀C ▶? $$$$$ ■

AVANDAMET (rosiglitazone + metformin) DM, Type 2, initial therapy (drug-naive): Start 2/500 mg PO one or two times per day. If inadequate control with metformin alone, select tab strength based on adding 4 mg/day rosiglitazone to existing metformin dose. If inadequate control with rosiglitazone alone, select tab strength based on adding 1000 mg/day metformin to existing rosiglitazone dose. Max 8/2000 mg/day. Obtain LFTs before therapy and periodically thereafter. Due to potential for elevated cardiovascular risks, rosiglitazone products restricted by FDA to use in patients where other medications cannot control Type 2 DM. [Trade only: Tabs 2/500, 4/500, 2/1000, 4/1000 mg.] ▶KL ♀C ▶? $$$$$ ■

AVANDARYL (rosiglitazone + glimepiride) DM, Type 2, initial therapy (drug-naive): Start 4/1 mg PO daily. If switching from monotherapy with a sulfonylurea or glitazone, consider 4/2 mg PO daily. Max 8/4 mg/day. Obtain LFTs before therapy and periodically thereafter. Due to potential for elevated cardiovascular risks, rosiglitazone products restricted by FDA to use in

(cont.)

DIABETES NUMBERS*

Criteria for diagnosis:	*Self-monitoring glucose goals*	
Pre-diabetes: Fasting glucose 100–125 mg/dL or A1C 5.7–6.4%, or 140–199 mg/dL 2 h after 75 g oral glucose load	Preprandial	70–130 mg/dL
	Postprandial	< 180 mg/dL
Diabetes:† A1C ≥ 6.5% Fasting glucose ≥ 126 mg/dL, random glucose with symptoms: ≥ 200 mg/dL, or ≥ 200 mg/dL 2 h after 75 g oral glucose load	A1C goal < 7% for most non-pregnant adults, individualize based on comorbid conditions and hypoglycemia	

Critically ill glucose goal: 140–180 mg/dL
Non-critically ill glucose goal (hospitalized patients): premeal blood glucose < 140 mg/dL, random < 180 mg/dL.

Estimated average glucose (eAG): eAG (mg/dL) = $(28.7 \times A1C) - 46.7$

Complications prevention and management: ASA‡ (75–162 mg/day) in Type 1 and 2 adults for primary prevention if 10-year cardiovascular risk > 10% (includes most men > 50 yo or women > 60 yo with at least one other major risk factor) and secondary prevention (those with vascular disease); statin therapy to achieve good LDL regardless of baseline LDL (for those with vascular disease, those > 40 yo and additional risk factor, or those < 40 yo but LDL > 100 mg/dL), ACE inhibitor or ARB if hypertensive or micro-/macro-albuminuria; pneumococcal vaccine (revaccinate one time if age ≥ 65 and previously received vaccine at age < 65 and > 5 yr ago). *Every visit:* Measure wt & BP (goal < 130/80 mm Hg); visual foot exam; review self-monitoring glucose record; review/adjust meds; review self-management skills, dietary needs, and physical activity; smoking cessation counseling. *Twice a year:* A1C in those meeting treatment goals with stable glycemia (quarterly if not); dental exam. *Annually:* Fasting lipid profile** [goal LDL < 100 mg/dL; cardiovascular disease consider LDL < 70mg/dL, HDL > 40 mg/dL (> 50 mg/dL in women), TG < 150 mg/dL], q 2 yr with low-risk lipid values; creatinine; albumin to creatinine ratio spot collection; dilated eye exam; flu vaccine.

*See recommendations at: care.diabetesjournals.org. Reference: *Diabetes Care* 2011;34(Suppl 1):S11-61. Glucose values are plasma. †In the absence of symptoms, confirm diagnosis with glucose on subsequent day. ‡Avoid ASA if < 21 yo due to Reye's Syndrome risk; use if < 30 yo has not been studied.
**LDL is primary target of therapy, consider 30-40% LDL reduction from baseline as alternate goal if unable to reach targets on maximal tolerated statin.

patients where other medications cannot control Type 2 diabetes. [Trade only (restricted access): Tabs 4/1, 4/2, 4/4, 8/2, 8/4 mg rosiglitazone/glimepiride.] ▶LK ♀C ▸? $$$$ ■

DUETACT (pioglitazone + glimepiride) <u>DM, Type 2:</u> Start 30/2 mg PO daily. Start up to 30/4 mg PO daily if prior glimepiride therapy, or 30/2 mg PO daily if prior pioglitazone therapy; max 30/4 mg/day. Obtain LFTs before therapy and periodically thereafter. [Trade only: Tabs 30/2, 30/4 mg pioglitazone/glimepiride.] ▶LK ♀C ▸– $$$$ ■

GLUCOVANCE (glyburide + metformin) <u>DM, Type 2,</u> initial therapy (drug-naive): Start 1.25/250 mg PO daily or two times per day with meals; max 10/2000 mg daily. Inadequate control with a sulfonylurea or metformin alone: Start 2.5/500 or 5/500 mg PO two times per day with meals; max 20/2000 mg daily. [Generic/Trade: Tabs 1.25/250, 2.5/500, 5/500 mg.] ▶KL ♀B ▸? $$$ ■

JANUMET (sitagliptin + metformin) DM, Type 2: 1 tab PO two times per day. Individualize based on patient's current therapy. If inadequate control with metformin monotherapy, start 50/500 or 50/1000 two times per day based on current metformin dose. If inadequate control on sitagliptin, start 50/500 two times per day. Max 100/2000 mg/day. Give with meals. [Trade only: Tabs 50/500, 50/1000 mg sitagliptin/metformin.] ▶K ♀B ▶? $$$$ ■

KOMBIGLYZE XR (saxagliptin + metformin) DM, Type 2: Once daily with evening meal. Initial dose based on current dose of saxagliptin or metformin. Max: 5/2000 mg/day. [Trade only: Tabs 5/500, 2.5/1000, 5/1000 mg.] ♀B ▶? $$$$$ ■

METAGLIP (glipizide + metformin) DM, Type 2, initial therapy (drug-naive): Start 2.5/250 mg PO daily to 2.5/500 mg PO two times per day with meals; max 10/2000 mg daily. Inadequate control with a sulfonylurea or metformin alone: Start 2.5/500 or 5/500 mg PO two times per day with meals; max 20/2000 mg daily. [Generic/Trade: Tabs 2.5/250, 2.5/500, 5/500 mg.] ▶KL ♀C ▶? $$$ ■

PRANDIMET (repaglinide + metformin) DM, Type 2, initial therapy (drug-naive): Start 1/500 mg PO daily before meals; max 10/2500 mg daily or 4/1000 mg/meal. May start higher if already taking higher coadministered doses of repaglinide and metformin. [Trade: Tabs 1/500, 2/500 mg.] ▶KL ♀C ▶? $$$ ■

Diabetes-Related — "Gliptins" (DPP-4 inhibitors)

LINAGLIPTIN (*Tradjenta*) DM, Type 2: 5 mg PO once daily. [Trade only: Tab 5 mg.] ▶L – ♀B ▶? $$$$$

SAXAGLIPTIN (*Onglyza*) DM, Type 2: 2.5 or 5 mg PO daily. [Trade only: Tabs 2.5, 5 mg.] ▶LK ♀B ▶? $$$$$

SITAGLIPTIN (*Januvia*) DM, Type 2: 100 mg PO daily. [Trade only: Tabs 25, 50, 100 mg.] ▶K ♀B ▶? $$$$$

Diabetes-Related — GLP-1 agonists

EXENATIDE (*Byetta*) DM, Type 2, adjunctive therapy when inadequate control on metformin, a sulfonylurea, or a glitazone (alone or in combination): 5 mcg SC two times per day (within 1 h before the morning and evening meals, or 1 h before the two main meals of the day at least 6 h apart). May increase to 10 mcg SC two times per day after 1 month. [Trade only: Prefilled pen (60 doses each) 5 mcg/dose, 1.2 mL; 10 mcg/dose, 2.4 mL.] ▶K ♀C ▶? $$$$$

LIRAGLUTIDE (*Victoza*) DM, Type 2: Start 0.6 mg SC daily for 1 week, then increase to 1.2 mg SC daily. May increase to 1.8 mg SC daily. [Trade only: Multidose pen (18 mg/3 mL) delivers doses of 0.6 mg, 1.2 mg or 1.8 mg.] ♀C ▶? $$$$$ ■

Diabetes-Related—Insulins

INSULIN—INJECTABLE INTERMEDIATE/LONG-ACTING   (*Novolin N, Humulin N, Lantus, Levemir*)   Diabetes: Doses vary, but typically total insulin 0.3 to 0.5 unit/kg/day SC in divided doses (Type 1), and 1 to 1.5 unit/kg/day SC in divided doses (Type 2). Generally, 50 to 70% of insulin requirements are provided by rapid or short-acting insulin and the remainder from intermediate- or long-acting insulin. Lantus: Start 10 units SC daily (same time everyday) in insulin-naive patients. Levemir: Type 2 DM (inadequately controlled on oral meds): Start 0.1 to 0.2 units/kg once daily in evening or 10 units SC daily or two times per day. [Trade only: Injection NPH (Novolin N, Humulin N). Insulin detemir (Levemir). Insulin glargine (Lantus). Insulin available in pen form: Novolin N InnoLet, Humulin N Pen, Lantus OptiClik (reusable), Lantus SoloStar (prefilled-disposable), Levemir InnoLet, Levemir FlexPen. Premixed preparations of NPH and regular insulin also available.]
▶LK ♀B/C ▶+ $$$$

INSULIN—INJECTABLE SHORT/RAPID-ACTING   (*Apidra, Novolin R, NovoLog, Humulin R, Humalog, ✦NovoRapid*)   Diabetes: Doses vary, but typically total insulin 0.3 to 0.5 unit/kg/day SC in divided doses (Type 1) and 1 to 1.5 unit/kg/day SC in divided doses (Type 2). Generally, 50 to 70% of insulin requirements are provided by rapid or short-acting insulin and the remainder from intermediate- or long-acting insulin. Administer rapid-acting insulin (Humalog, NovoLog, Apidra) within 15 min before or immediately after a meal.

(cont.)

INJECTABLE INSULINS*		Onset (h)	Peak (h)	Duration (h)
Rapid/short-acting:	Insulin aspart (NovoLog)	<0.2	1–3	3–5
	Insulin glulisine (Apidra)	0.30 0.4	1	4–5
	Insulin lispro (Humalog)	0.25–0.5	0.5–2.5	≤5
	Regular (Novolin R, Humulin R)	0.5–1	2–3	3–6
Intermediate/long-acting:	NPH (Novolin N, Humulin N)	2–4	4–10	10–16
	Insulin detemir (Levemir)	n/a	flat action profile	up to 23†
	Insulin glargine (Lantus)	2 4	peakless	?4
Mixtures:	Insulin aspart protamine susp/ aspart (NovoLog Mix 70/30, NovoLog Mix 50/50)	0.25	1–4 (biphasic)	up to 24
	Insulin lispro protamine susp/ insulin lispro (HumaLog Mix 75/25, HumaLog Mix 50/50)	<0.25	1–3 (biphasic)	10–20
	NPH/Reg (Humulin 70/30, Humulin 50/50, Novolin 70/30)	0.5–1	2–10 (biphasic)	10–20

*These are general guidelines, as onset, peak, and duration of activity are affected by the site of injection, physical activity, body temperature, and blood supply. † Dose dependent duration of action, range from 6 to 23 h. n/a, not available.

Administer regular insulin 30 min before meals. <u>Severe hyperkalemia</u>: 5 to 10 units regular insulin plus concurrent dextrose IV. <u>Profound hyperglycemia</u> (eg, DKA): 0.1 unit regular/kg IV bolus, then initial infusion 100 units regular in 100 mL NS (1 unit/mL), at 0.1 units/kg/h. [Trade only: Injection regular (Novolin R, Humulin R). Insulin glulisine (Apidra). Insulin lispro (Humalog). Insulin aspart (NovoLog). Insulin available in pen form: Novolin R InnoLet, Humulin R, Apidra OptiClik, Humalog KwikPen, Novolog FlexPen.] ▶LK ♀B/C ▶+ $$$

INSULIN-INJECTABLE COMBINATIONS (*Humalog Mix 75/25, Humalog Mix 50/50, Humulin 70/30, Humulin 50/50, Novolin 70/30, Novolog Mix 70/30, Novolog Mix 50/50*) <u>Diabetes</u>: Doses vary, but typically total insulin 0.3 to 1 unit/kg/day SC in divided doses (Type 1), and 0.5 to 1.5 unit/kg/day SC in divided doses (Type 2). Administer rapid-acting insulin mixtures (Humalog, NovoLog) within 15 min before or immediately after a meal. Administer regular insulin mixtures 30 min before meals. [Trade only: Insulin lispro protamine susp/insulin lispro (Humalog Mix 75/25, Humalog Mix 50/50). Insulin aspart protamine/insulin aspart (Novolog Mix 70/30, Novolog Mix 50/50). NPH and regular mixtures (Humulin 70/30, Novolin 70/30 or Humulin 50/50). Insulin available in pen form: Novolin 70/30 InnoLet, Novolog Mix 70/30, Novolog Mix 50/50, FlexPen, Humulin 70/30, Humalog Mix 75/25 KwikPen, Humalog Mix 50/50 KwikPen.] ▶LK ♀B/C ▶+ $$$$

Diabetes-Related—Meglitinides

NATEGLINIDE (*Starlix*) <u>DM, Type 2</u>: 120 mg PO three times per day within 30 min before meals; use 60 mg PO three times per day in patients who are near goal A1C. [Generic/Trade: Tabs 60, 120 mg.] ▶L ♀C ▶? $$$

REPAGLINIDE (*Prandin, ✦ Gluconorm*) <u>DM, Type 2</u>: Start 0.5 to 2 mg PO three times per day before meals, maintenance 0.5 to 4 mg three to four times per day, max 16 mg/day. [Trade only: Tabs 0.5, 1, 2 mg.] ▶L ♀C ▶? $$$$$

Diabetes-Related—Sulfonylureas—2nd Generation

GLICLAZIDE (✦ *Diamicron, Diamicron MR*) Canada only. <u>DM, Type 2</u>, immediate-release: Start 80 to 160 mg PO daily, max 320 mg PO daily (160 mg or more per day should be in divided doses). Modified-release: Start 30 mg PO daily, max 120 mg PO daily. [Generic/Trade: Tabs 80 mg (Diamicron). Trade only: Tabs, modified-release 30 mg (Diamicron MR).] ▶KL ♀C ▶? $

GLIMEPIRIDE (*Amaryl*) <u>DM, Type 2</u>: Start 1 to 2 mg PO daily, usual 1 to 4 mg/day, max 8 mg/day. [Generic/Trade: Tabs 1, 2, 4 mg. Generic only: Tabs 3, 8 mg.] ▶LK ♀C ▶– $$

GLIPIZIDE (*Glucotrol, Glucotrol XL*) <u>DM, Type 2</u>: Start 5 mg PO daily, usual 10 to 20 mg/day, max 40 mg/day (divide two times per day if more than 15 mg/day). Extended-release: Start 5 mg PO daily, usual 5 to 10 mg/day, max 20 mg/day. [Generic/Trade: Tabs 5, 10 mg; Extended-release tabs 2.5, 5, 10 mg.] ▶LK ♀C ▶? $

GLYBURIDE (*DiaBeta, Glynase PresTab, ✦ Euglucon*) DM, Type 2: Start 1.25 to 5 mg PO daily, usual 1.25 to 20 mg daily or divided two times per day, max 20 mg/day. Micronized tabs: Start 1.5 to 3 mg PO daily, usual 0.75 to 12 mg/day divided two times per day, max 12 mg/day. [Generic/Trade: Tabs (scored) 1.25, 2.5, 5 mg. Micronized Tabs (scored) 1.5, 3, 4.5, 6 mg.] ▶LK ♀B ▶? $

Diabetes-Related—Thiazolidinediones

PIOGLITAZONE (*Actos*) DM, Type 2: Start 15 to 30 mg PO daily, max 45 mg/day. Monitor LFTs. [Trade only: Tabs 15, 30, 45 mg.] ▶L ♀C ▶– $$$$$ ■

ROSIGLITAZONE (*Avandia*) Type 2 DM monotherapy or in combination with metformin or sulfonylurea: Start 4 mg PO daily or divided two times per day, max 8 mg/day. Obtain LFTs before therapy and periodically thereafter. Due to potential for elevated cardiovascular risks, rosiglitazone products restricted by FDA to use in patients where other medications cannot control Type 2 DM. [Trade only (restricted access): Tabs 2, 4, 8 mg.] ▶L ♀C ▶– $$$$$ ■

Diabetes-Related—Other

DEXTROSE (*Glutose, B-D Glucose, Insta-Glucose, Dex-4*) Hypoglycemia: 0.5 to 1 g/kg (1 to 2 mL/kg) up to 25 g (50 mL) of 50% soln IV. Dilute to 25% for pediatric administration. [OTC Generic/Trade: Chewable tabs 4 g (Dex-4), 5 g (Glutose). Trade only: Oral gel 40%.] ▶L ♀C ▶? $

GLUCAGON (*GlucaGen*) Hypoglycemia: 1 mg IV/IM/SC, onset 5 to 20 min. Diagnostic aid: 1 mg IV/IM/SC. [Trade only: Injection 1 mg.] ▶LK ♀B ▶? $$$

METFORMIN (*Glucophage, Glucophage XR, Glumetza, Fortamet, Riomet*) DM, type 2, immediate-release: Start 500 mg PO one to two times per day or 850 mg PO daily with meals, may gradually increase to max 2550 mg/day. Extended-release: Glucophage XR: 500 mg PO daily with evening meal; increase by 500 mg once a week to max 2000 mg/day (may divide two times per day). Glumetza: 1000 mg PO daily with evening meal; increase by 500 mg once a week to max 2000 mg/day (may divide two times per day). Fortamet: 500 to 1000 mg daily with evening meal; increase by 500 mg once a week to max 2500 mg/day. Polycystic ovary syndrome (unapproved, immediate-release): 500 mg PO three times per day. DM prevention, Type 2 (with lifestyle modifications, unapproved): 850 mg PO daily for 1 month, then increase to 850 mg PO two times per day. [Generic/Trade: Tabs 500, 850, 1000 mg, extended-release 500, 750 mg. Trade only, extended-release: Fortamet 500, 1000 mg; Glumetza 500, 1000 mg. Trade only: Oral soln 500 mg/5 mL (Riomet).] ▶K ♀B ▶? $ ■

PRAMLINTIDE (*Symlin, Symlinpen*) DM, Type 1 with mealtime insulin therapy: Initiate 15 mcg SC immediately before major meals and titrate by 15 mcg increments (if significant nausea has not occurred for at least 3 days) to maintenance 30 to 60 mcg as tolerated. DM, Type 2 with mealtime insulin

(cont.)

therapy: Initiate 60 mcg SC immediately before major meals and increase to 120 mcg as tolerated (if significant nausea has not occurred for 3 to 7 days). Decrease initial premeal short-acting insulin doses by 50% including fixed-mix insulin (ie, 70/30). [Trade only: 600 mcg/mL in 5 mL vials, 1000 mcg/mL pen injector (Symlinpen) 1.5, 2.7 mL.] ▶K ♀C ▷? $$$$ ■

Gout-Related

ALLOPURINOL (*Aloprim, Zyloprim*) <u>Mild gout or recurrent calcium oxalate stones:</u> 200 to 300 mg PO daily to two times per day, max 800 mg/day. [Generic/Trade: Tabs 100, 300 mg.] ▶K ♀C ▷+ $

COLBENEMID (**colchicine + probenecid**) <u>Gout:</u> 1 tab PO daily for 1 week, then 1 tab two times per day. [Generic only: Tabs 0.5 mg colchicine + 500 mg probenecid.] ▶KL ♀C ▷? $

COLCHICINE (*Colcrys*) <u>Rapid treatment of acute gouty arthritis:</u> 1.2 mg (2 tab) PO at signs of attack then 0.6 mg (1 tab) 1h after initial administration. <u>Gout prophylaxis:</u> 0.6 mg PO two times per day if CrCl is 50 mL/min or greater, 0.6 mg PO daily if CrCl is 35 to 49 mL/min, 0.6 mg PO q 2 to 3 days if CrCl 10 to 34 mL/min. <u>Familial Mediterranean Fever:</u> 1.2 to 2.4 mg PO daily or divided two times per day. [Trade: Tabs 0.6 mg.] ▶L ♀C ▷? $$$$

FEBUXOSTAT (*Uloric*) <u>Hyperuricemia with gout:</u> Start 40 mg PO daily, max 80 mg daily. [Trade: Tabs 40, 80 mg.] ▶LK ♀C ▷? $$$$

PEGLOTICASE (*Krystexxa*) <u>Chronic gout (refractory):</u> 8 mg IV infusion q 2 weeks. [Trade only: single-use vial (8mg/mL)] ▶NA ♀C ▷? $$$$$ ■

PROBENECID (*✦Benuryl*) <u>Gout:</u> 250 mg PO two times per day for 7 days, then 500 mg two times per day. <u>Adjunct to penicillin injection:</u> 1 to 2 g PO in divided doses. [Generic only: Tabs 500 mg.] ▶KL ♀B ▷? $

Minerals

CALCIUM ACETATE (*PhosLo, Eliphos*) <u>Phosphate binder to reduce serum phosphorous in end stage renal disease:</u> Initially 2 tabs/caps PO with each meal. [Generic/Trade: Gelcaps 667 mg (169 mg elem Ca). Trade: Tab 667 mg (169 mg elem Ca).] ▶ ♀C ▷? $$$$

CALCIUM CARBONATE (*Caltrate, Mylanta Children's, Os-Cal, Oyst-Cal, Tums, Surpass, Viactiv, ✦Calsan*) <u>Supplement:</u> 1 to 2 g elemental Ca/day or more PO with meals divided two to four times per day. <u>Antacid:</u> 1000 to 3000 mg PO q 2 h prn or 1 to 2 pieces gum chewed prn, max 7000 mg/day. [OTC Generic/Trade: Tabs 500, 650, 750, 1000, 1250, 1500 mg, Chewable tabs 400, 500, 750, 850, 1000, 1177, 1250 mg, Caps 1250 mg, Gum 300, 450 mg, Susp 1250 mg/5 mL. Calcium carbonate is 40% elem Ca and contains 20 mEq of elem Ca/g calcium carbonate. Not more than 500 to 600 mg elem Ca/dose. Available in combination with sodium fluoride, vitamin D and/or vitamin K. Trade examples: Caltrate 600 + D = 600 mg elemental Ca/200 units vitamin D, Os-Cal 500 + D = 500 mg elemental Ca/200 units vitamin D, Os-Cal Extra D = 500 mg elemental Ca/400 units vitamin D, Tums

(cont.)

FLUORIDE SUPPLEMENTATION

Age	<0.3 ppm in drinking water	0.3–0.6 ppm in drinking water	>0.6 ppm in drinking water
0–0.5 yo	none	none	none
0.5–3 yo	0.25 mg PO daily	none	none
3–6 yo	0.5 mg PO daily	0.25 mg PO daily	none
6–16 yo	1 mg PO daily	0.5 mg PO daily	none

IV SOLUTIONS

Solution	Dextrose	Calories/ Liter	Na*	K*	Ca*	Cl*	Lactate*	Osm*
0.9 NS	0 g/L	0	154	0	0	154	0	310
LR	0 g/L	9	130	4	3	109	28	273
D5 W	50 g/L	170	0	0	0	0	0	253
D5 0.2 NS	50 g/L	170	34	0	0	34	0	320
D5 0.45 NS	50 g/L	170	77	0	0	77	0	405
D5 0.9 NS	50 g/L	170	154	0	0	154	0	560
D5 LR	50 g/L	179	130	4	2.7	109	28	527

* All given in mEq/L

(regular strength) = 200 mg elemental Ca, Tums (ultra) = 400 mg elemental Ca, Viactiv (chewable) 500 mg elemental Ca+ 100 units vitamin D + 40 mcg vitamin K.] ▶K ♀+ (? 1st trimester) ▶? $

CALCIUM CHLORIDE 500 to 1000 mg slow IV q 1 to 3 days. [Generic only: Injectable 10% (1000 mg/10 mL) 10 mL ampules, vials, syringes.] ▶K ♀+ ▶+ $

CALCIUM CITRATE (*Citracal*) 1 to 2 g elemental Ca/day or more PO with meals divided two to four times per day. [OTC Trade only (mg elem Ca): 200, 250 mg with 200 units vitamin D and 250 mg with 125 units vitamin D and 80 mg of magnesium. Chewable tabs 500 mg with 200 units vitamin D. OTC Generic/Trade: Tabs 200 mg, 315 mg with 200 units vitamin D.] ▶K ♀ ı ▶+ $

CALCIUM GLUCONATE 2.25 to 14 mEq slow IV. 500 to 2000 mg PO two to four times per day. [Generic only: Injectable 10% (1000 mg/10 mL, 4.65 mEq/10 mL) 1, 10, 50, 100, 200 mL. OTC Generic only: Tabs 50, 500, 650, 975, 1000 mg. Chewable tabs 650 mg.] ▶K ♀+ ▶+ $

FERRIC GLUCONATE COMPLEX (*Ferrlecit*) 125 mg elemental iron IV over 10 min or diluted in 100 mL NS IV over 1 h. Peds age 6 yo or older: 1.5 mg/kg (max 125 mg) elemental iron diluted in 25 mL NS and administered IV over 1 h. ▶K ♀ B ▶? $$$$$

FERROUS GLUCONATE (*Fergon*) 800 to 1600 mg ferrous gluconate PO divided three times per day. [OTC Generic/Trade: Tabs (ferrous gluconate) 240 mg (27 mg elemental iron). Generic only: Tabs 324, 325 mg.] ▶K ♀+ ▶+ $

POTASSIUM (oral forms)

Effervescent Granules:	20 mEq: Klorvess Effervescent, K-vescent
Effervescent Tabs:	10 mEq: Effer-K 20 mEq: Effer-K 25 mEq: Effer-K, K+Care ET, K-Lyte, K-Lyte/Cl, Klor-Con/EF 50 mEq: K-Lyte DS, K-Lyte/Cl 50
Liquids:	20 mEq/15 mL: Cena-K, Kaochlor S-F, K-G Elixir, Kaochlor 10%, Kay Ciel, Kaon, Kaylixir, Kolyum, Potasalan, Twin-K 30 mEq/15 mL: Rum-K 40 mEq/15 mL: Cena-K, Kaon-Cl 20% 45 mEq/15 mL: Tri-K
Powders:	15 mEq/pack: K+Care 20 mEq/pack: Gen-K, K+Care, Kay Ciel, K-Lor, Klor-Con 25 mEq/pack: K+Care, Klor-Con 25
Tabs/Caps:	8 mEq: K+8, Klor-Con 8, Slow-K, Micro-K 10 mEq: K+10, K-Norm, Kaon-Cl 10, Klor-Con M10 Klotrix, K-Tab, K-Dur 10, Micro-K 10 20 mEq: Klor-Con M20, K-Dur 20

FERROUS SULFATE (*Fer-in-Sol, Feosol, Slow FE, ✦ Ferodan, Slow-Fe*) 500 to 1000 mg ferrous sulfate (100 to 200 mg elemental iron) PO divided three times per day. [OTC Generic/Trade (mg ferrous sulfate): Tabs extended-release 160 mg. Tabs 200, 324, 325 mg. OTC Generic only (mg ferrous sulfate): Soln 75 mg/0.6 mL, Elixir 220 mg/5 mL.] ▶KL ♀+ ▶+ $ ■

FERUMOXYTOL (*Feraheme*) Iron deficiency in chronic kidney disease: Give 510 mg IV push, followed by 510 mg IV push once given 3 to 8 days after initial injection. ▶KL ♀C ▶? $$$$$

FLUORIDE (*Luride, ✦ Fluor-A-Day*) Adult dose: 10 mL of topical rinse swish and spit daily. Peds daily dose based on fluoride content of drinking water (table). [Generic only: Chewable tabs 0.5, 1 mg; Tabs 1 mg, gtts 0.125 mg, 0.25 mg, and 0.5 mg/dropperful, Lozenges 1 mg, Soln 0.2 mg/mL, Gel 0.1%, 0.5%, 1.23%, Rinse (sodium fluoride) 0.05, 0.1, 0.2%).] ▶K ♀? ▶? $

IRON DEXTRAN (*InFed, DexFerrum, ✦ Dexiron, Infufer*) 25 to 100 mg IM daily prn. Equations available to calculate IV dose based on wt and Hb. ▶KL ♀C ▶? $$$$ ■

IRON POLYSACCHARIDE (*Niferex, Niferex-150, Nu-Iron 150, Ferrex 150*) 50 to 200 mg PO divided one to three times per day. [OTC Trade only: Caps 60 mg (Niferex). OTC Generic/Trade: Caps 150 mg (Niferex-150, Nu-Iron 150, Ferrex-150), Elixir 100 mg/5 mL (Niferex). 1 mg iron polysaccharide = 1 mg elemental iron.] ▶K ♀+ ▶+ $$ ■

IRON SUCROSE (*Venofer*) Iron deficiency with hemodialysis: 5 mL (100 mg elemental iron) IV over 5 min or diluted in 100 mL NS IV over 15 min or longer. Iron deficiency in nondialysis chronic kidney disease: 10 mL (200 mg elemental iron) IV over 5 min. ▶KL ♀B ▶? $$$$$

MAGNESIUM CHLORIDE (*Slow-Mag*) 2 tabs PO daily. [OTC Trade only: Enteric coated tab 64 mg. 64 mg tab Slow-Mag = 64 mg elemental magnesium.] ▶K ♀A ▶+ $

MAGNESIUM GLUCONATE (*Almora, Magtrate, Maganate, ✦ Maglucate*) 500 to 1000 mg PO divided three times per day. [OTC Generic only: Tabs 500 mg (27 mg elemental Mg), liquid 54 mg elemental Mg/5 mL.] ▶K ♀A ▶+ $

MAGNESIUM OXIDE (*Mag-200, Mag-Ox 400*) 400 to 800 mg PO daily. [OTC Generic/Trade: Caps: 140 (84.5 mg elemental Mg), 250 (elemental), 400 (240 mg elemental Mg), 420 (253 mg elemental Mg), 500 mg (elemental).] ▶K ♀A ▶+ $

MAGNESIUM SULFATE Hypomagnesemia: 1 g of 20% soln IM q 6 h for 4 doses, or 2 g IV over 1 h (monitor for hypotension). Peds: 25 to 50 mg/kg IV/IM q 4 to 6 h for 3 to 4 doses, max single dose 2 g. Eclampsia: 4 to 6 g IV over 30 min, then 1 to 2 g/h. Drip: 5 g in 250 mL D5W (20 mg/mL), 2 g/h is a rate of 100 mL/h. Preterm labor: 6 g IV over 20 min, then 1 to 3 g/h titrated to decrease contractions. Monitor respirations and reflexes. If needed, may reverse toxic effects with calcium gluconate 1 g IV. Torsades de pointes: 1 to 2 g IV in D5W over 5 to 60 min. ▶K ♀A ▶+ $

PHOSPHORUS (*Neutra-Phos, K-Phos*) 1 cap/packet PO four times per day. 1 to 2 tabs PO four times per day. Severe hypophosphatemia (eg, less than 1 mg/dL): 0.08 to 0.16 mmol/kg IV over 6 h. [OTC Trade only: (Neutra-Phos, Neutra-Phos K) tab/cap/packet 250 mg (8 mmol) phosphorus. Rx: Trade only: (K-Phos) tab 250 mg (8 mmol) phosphorus.] ▶K ♀C ▶? $

POTASSIUM (*Cena-K, Effer-K, K+8, K+10, Kaochlor, Kaon, Kaon Cl, Kay Ciel, Kaylixir, K+Care, K+Care ET, K-Dur, K-G Elixir, K-Lease, K-Lor, Klor-con, Klorvess Effervescent, Klotrix, K-Lyte, K-Lyte Cl, K-Norm, Kolyum, K-Tab, K-vescent, Micro-K, Micro-K LS, Sl*) IV infusion 10 mEq/h (diluted). 20 to 40 mEq PO on or two times per day. [Injectable, many different products in a variety of salt forms (ie, chloride, bicarbonate, citrate, acetate, gluconate), available in tabs, caps, liquids, effervescent tabs, packets. Potassium gluconate is available OTC.] ▶K ♀C ▶? $

ZINC ACETATE (*Galzin*) Dietary supplement: 8 to 12 mg (elemental) daily. Zinc deficiency: 25 to 50 mg (elemental) daily. Wilson's disease: 25 to 50 mg (elemental) PO three times per day. [Trade only: Caps 25, 50 mg elemental zinc.] ▶Minimal absorption ♀A ▶− $$$

ZINC SULFATE (*Orazinc, Zincate*) Dietary supplement: 8 to 12 mg (elemental) daily. Zinc deficiency: 25 to 50 mg (elemental) PO daily. [OTC Generic/Trade: Tabs 66, 110, 200 mg. Rx Generic/Trade: Caps 220 mg.] ▶Minimal absorption ♀A ▶− $

Nutritionals

BANANA BAG Alcoholic malnutrition (one formula): Add thiamine 100 mg + folic acid 1 mg + IV multivitamins to 1 liter NS and infuse over 4 h. Magnesium sulfate 2 g may be added. "Banana bag" and "rally pack" are jargon and are not valid drug orders. Specify individual components. ▶KL ♀+ ▶+ $

FAT EMULSION (*Intralipid, Liposyn*) Dosage varies. ▶L ♀C ▶? $$$$$

FORMULAS—INFANT (*Enfamil, Similac, Isomil, Nursoy, ProSobee, Soyalac, Alsoy, Nutramigen Lipil*) Infant meals. [OTC: Milk-based (Enfamil, Similac, SMA) or soy-based (Isomil, Nursoy, ProSobee, Soyalac, Alsoy).] ▶L ♀+ ▶+ $

LEVOCARNITINE (*Carnitor*) 10 to 20 mg/kg IV at each dialysis session. [Generic/Trade: Tabs 330 mg, Oral soln 1 g/10 mL.] ▶KL ♀B ▶? $$$$$

OMEGA-3-ACID ETHYL ESTERS (*Lovaza, fish oil, omega-3 fatty acids*) Hypertriglyceridemia: 4 caps PO daily or divided two times per day. [Trade only: (Lovaza) 1 g cap (total 840 mg EPA + DHA).] ▶L ♀C ▶? $

Phosphate Binders

LANTHANUM CARBONATE (*Fosrenol*) Hyperphosphatemia in end stage renal disease: Start 1500 mg/day PO in divided doses with meals. Titrate dose q 2 to 3 weeks in increments of 750 mg/day until acceptable serum phosphate is reached. Most will require 1500 to 3000 mg/day to reduce phosphate less than 6.0 mg/dL. [Trade only: Chewable tabs 500, 750, 1000 mg.] ▶Not absorbed ♀C ▶? $$$$$

SEVELAMER (*Renagel, Renvela*) Hyperphosphatemia: 800 to 1600 mg PO three times per day with meals. [Trade only (Renagel—sevelamer hydrochloride): Tabs 400, 800 mg. (Renvela—sevelamer carbonate): Tabs 800 mg; Powder: 800, 2400 mg packets.] ▶Not absorbed ♀C ▶? $$$$$

Thyroid Agents

LEVOTHYROXINE (*L-Thyroxine, Levolet, Levo-T, Levothroid, Levoxyl, Novothyrox, Synthroid, Thyro-Tabs, Tirosint, Unithroid, T4, ✦ Eltroxin, Euthyrox*) Start 100 to 200 mcg PO daily (healthy adults) or 12.5 to 50 mcg PO daily (elderly or CV disease), increase by 12.5 to 25 mcg/day at 3 to 8 week intervals. Usual maintenance dose 100 to 200 mcg/day, max 300 mcg/day. [Generic/Trade: Tabs 25, 50, 75, 88, 100, 112, 125, 137, 150, 175, 200, 300 mcg. Trade only: Caps: 25, 50, 75, 100, 125, 150 mcg in 7 days blister packs, Tabs: 13 mcg (Tirosint).] ▶L ♀A ▶+ $ ■

LIOTHYRONINE (*T3, Cytomel, Triostat*) Start 25 mcg PO daily, max 100 mcg/day. [Generic/Trade: Tabs 5, 25, 50 mcg.] ▶L ♀A ▶? $$ ■

METHIMAZOLE (*Tapazole*) Start 5 to 20 mg PO three times per day or 10 to 30 mg PO daily, then adjust. [Generic/Trade: Tabs 5, 10. Generic only: Tabs 15, 20 mg.] ▶L ♀D ▶+ $$$

PROPYLTHIOURACIL (*PTU, ✦ Propyl-hyracil*) Hyperthyroidism: Start 100 mg PO three times per day, then adjust. Thyroid storm: 200 to 300 mg PO four times per day, then adjust. [Generic only: Tabs 50 mg.] ▶L ♀D (but preferred over methimazole in first trimester) ▶+ $ ■

SODIUM IODIDE I-131 (*Hicon, Iodotope, Sodium Iodide I-131 Therapeutic*) Specialized dosing for hyperthyroidism and thyroid carcinoma. [Generic/Trade: Caps/Oral soln: Radioactivity range varies at the time of calibration. Hicon is a kit containing caps and a concentrated oral soln for dilution and cap preparation.] ▶K ♀X ▶— $$$$$

Vitamins

ASCORBIC ACID (vitamin C, ✦ Redoxon) 70 to 1000 mg PO daily. [OTC Generic only: Tabs 25, 50, 100, 250, 500, 1000 mg, Chewable tabs 100, 250, 500 mg, Timed-release tabs 500, 1000, 1500 mg, Timed-release caps 500 mg, Lozenges 60 mg, Liquid 35 mg/0.6 mL, Oral soln 100 mg/mL, Syrup 500 mg/5 mL.] ▶K ♀C ▶? $

CALCITRIOL (*Rocaltrol, Calcijex*) 0.25 to 2 mcg PO daily. [Generic/Trade: Caps 0.25, 0.5 mcg. Oral soln 1 mcg/mL. Injection 1, 2 mcg/mL.] ▶L ♀C ▶? $$

CYANOCOBALAMIN (vitamin B12, *CaloMist, Nascobal*) Deficiency states: 100 to 200 mcg IM once a month or 1000 to 2000 mcg PO daily for 1 to 2 weeks followed by 1000 mcg PO daily, 500 mcg intranasal weekly (Nascobal: 1 spray 1 nostril once a week), or 50 to 100 mcg intranasal daily (CaloMist: 1 to 2 sprays each nostril daily). [OTC Generic only: Tabs 100, 500, 1000, 5000 mcg; Lozenges 100, 250, 500 mcg. Rx Trade only: Nasal spray 500 mcg/spray (Nascobal 2.3 mL), 25 mcg/spray (CaloMist, 18 mL).] ▶K ♀C ▶+ $

DOXERCALCIFEROL (*Hectorol*) Secondary hyperparathyroidism on dialysis: Oral: 10 mcg PO 3 times a week. May increase every 8 weeks by 2.5 mcg/dose; max 60 mcg/week. IV: 4 mcg IV 3 times a week. May increase dose q 8 weeks by 1 to 2 mcg/dose; max 18 mcg/week. Secondary hyperparathyroidism not on dialysis: Start 1 mcg PO daily, may increase by 0.5 mcg/dose q 2 weeks. Max 3.5 mcg/day. [Trade only: Caps 0.5, 2.5 mcg.] ▶L ♀B? $$$$$

ERGOCALCIFEROL (vitamin D2, *Calciferol, Drisdol*) Osteoporosis prevention and treatment (age 50 or older): 800 to 1000 units daily. Familial hypophosphatemia (Vitamin D resistant Rickets): 12,000 to 500,000 units PO daily. Hypoparathyroidism: 50,000 to 200,000 units PO daily. Vitamin D deficiency: 50,000 units PO weekly or biweekly for 8 to 12 weeks. Adequate daily intake: 1 to 70 yo: 600 units (15 mcg); older than 70 yo: 800 units (20 mcg). [OTC Generic only: Caps 400, 1000, 5000 units. Soln 8000 units/mL (Calciferol). Rx Generic/Trade: Caps 50,000 units. Rx Generic only: Caps 25,000 units.] ▶L ♀A (C if exceed RDA) ▶+ $

FOLIC ACID (folate, *Folvite*) 0.4 to 1 mg IV/IM/PO/SC daily. [OTC Generic only: Tabs 0.4, 0.8 mg. Rx Generic 1 mg.] ▶K ♀A ▶+ $

MULTIVITAMINS (**MVI**) Dose varies with product. Tabs come with and without iron. [OTC and Rx: Many different brands and forms available with and without iron (tabs, caps, chewable tabs, gtts, liquid).] ▶LK ♀+ ▶+ $

NEPHROCAP (ascorbic acid + folic acid + niacin + thiamine + riboflavin + pyridoxine + pantothenic acid + biotin + cyanocobalamin) 1 cap PO daily. If on dialysis, take after treatment. [Generic/Trade: Vitamin C 100 mg/folic acid 1 mg/niacin 20 mg/thiamine 1.5 mg/riboflavin 1.7 mg/pyridoxine 10 mg/pantothenic acid 5 mg/biotin 150 mcg/cyanocobalamin 6 mcg.] ▶K ♀? ▶? $

NEPHROVITE (ascorbic acid + folic acid + niacin + thiamine + riboflavin + pyridoxine + pantothenic acid + biotin + cyanocobalamin) 1 tab PO daily. If on dialysis, take after treatment. [Generic/Trade: Vitamin C 60 mg/folic acid 1 mg/niacin 20 mg/thiamine 1.5 mg/riboflavin 1.7 mg/pyridoxine 10 mg/pantothenic acid 10 mg/biotin 300 mcg/cyanocobalamin 6 mcg.] ▶K ♀? ▶? $

NIACIN (vitamin B3, nicotinic acid, *Niacor, Nicolar, Slo-Niacin, Niaspan*) Niacin deficiency: 10 to 500 mg PO daily. Hyperlipidemia: Start 50 to 100 mg PO two to three times per day with meals, increase slowly, usual maintenance range 1.5 to 3 g/day, max 6 g/day. Extended-release (Niaspan):

(cont.)

Start 500 mg at bedtime, increase monthly up to max 2000 mg. Extended-release formulations not listed here may have greater hepatotoxicity. Start with low doses and increase slowly to minimize flushing; 325 mg aspirin 30 to 60 min prior to niacin ingestion will minimize flush. [OTC Generic only: Tabs 50, 100, 250, 500 mg; Timed-release cap 125, 250, 400 mg; Timed-release tab 250, 500 mg; Liquid 50 mg/5 mL. Trade only: 250, 500, 750 mg (Slo-Niacin). Rx: Trade only: Tabs 500 mg (Niacor), Timed-release caps 500 mg, Timed-release tabs 500, 750, 1000 mg (Niaspan, $$$$).] ▶K ♀C ▶? $

PARICALCITOL (*Zemplar*) <u>Prevention/treatment of secondary hyperparathyroidism with renal insufficiency</u>: 1 to 2 mcg PO daily or 2 to 4 mcg PO 3 times a week; increase dose by 1 mcg/day or 2 mcg/week until desired PTH level is achieved. <u>Prevention/treatment of secondary hyperparathyroidism with renal failure</u> (CrCl less than 15 mL/min): PO: To calculate initial dose divide baseline iPTH by 80 and then administer this dose in mcg 3 times a week. To titrate dose based on response, divide recent iPTH by 80 then administer this dose in mcg 3 times a week. IV: 0.04 to 0.1 mcg/kg (2.8 to 7 mcg) IV 3 times a week at dialysis; increase dose by 2 to 4 mcg q 2 to 4 weeks until desired PTH level is achieved. Max dose 0.24 mcg/kg (16.8 mcg). [Trade only: Caps 1, 2, 4 mcg.] ▶L ♀C ▶? $$$$$

PHYTONADIONE (vitamin K, *Mephyton, AquaMephyton*) Single dose of 0.5 to 1 mg IM within 1 h after birth. <u>Excessive oral anticoagulation</u>: Dose varies based on INR. INR 5 to 9: 1 to 2.5 mg PO (up to 5 mg PO may be given if rapid reversal necessary); INR greater than 9 with no bleeding: 5 to 10 mg PO; serious bleeding and elevated INR: 10 mg slow IV infusion. <u>Adequate daily intake</u>: 120 mcg (males) and 90 mcg (females). [Trade only: Tabs 5 mg.] ▶L ♀C ▶+ $ ■

PYRIDOXINE (vitamin B6) 10 to 200 mg PO daily. <u>Prevention of deficiency due to isoniazid in high-risk patients</u>: 10 to 25 mg PO daily. <u>Treatment of neuropathies due to isoniazid</u>: 50 to 200 mg PO daily. <u>Hyperemesis of pregnancy</u>: 10 to 50 mg PO q 8 h. [OTC Generic only: Tabs 25, 50, 100 mg; Timed-release tab 100 mg.] ▶K ♀A ▶+ $

RIBOFLAVIN (vitamin B2) 5 to 25 mg PO daily. [OTC Generic only: Tabs 25, 50, 100 mg.] ▶K ♀A ▶+ $

THIAMINE (vitamin B1) 10 to 100 mg IV/IM/PO daily. [OTC Generic only: Tabs 50, 100, 250, 500 mg; Enteric-coated tab 20 mg.] ▶K ♀A ▶+ $

TOCOPHEROL (vitamin E, ✦*Aquasol E*) RDA: 22 units (natural, d-alpha-tocopherol) or 33 units (synthetic, d,l-alpha-tocopherol) or 15 mg (alpha-tocopherol). Max recommended 1000 mg alpha-tocopherol (1500 units) daily. <u>Antioxidant</u>: 400 to 800 units PO daily. [OTC Generic only: Tabs 200, 400 units; Caps 73.5, 100, 147, 165, 200, 330, 400, 500, 600, 1000 units; Gtts 50 mg/mL.] ▶L ♀A ▶? $

VITAMIN A RDA: 900 mcg RE (retinol equivalents) (males), 700 mcg RE (females). <u>Treatment of deficiency</u>: 100,000 units IM daily for 3 days, then 50,000 units IM daily for 2 weeks. 1 RE is equivalent to 1 mcg retinol or 6 mcg beta-carotene. Max recommended dose 3000 mcg. [OTC Generic only: Caps 10,000, 15,000 units. Trade only: Tabs 5000 units. Rx: Generic: 25,000 units. Trade only: Soln 50,000 units/mL.] ▶L ♀A (C if exceed RDA, X in high doses) ▶+ $

VITAMIN D3 (**cholecalciferol, _DDrops_**) Osteoporosis prevention and treatment (age 50 or older): 800 to 1000 units daily. Familial hypophosphatemia (Vitamin D–resistant Rickets): 12,000 to 500,000 units PO daily. Hypoparathyroidism: 50,000 to 200,000 units PO daily. Adequate daily intake: 1 to 70 yo: 600 units; older than 70 yo: 800 units. [OTC Generic: 200 units, 400 units, 800 units, 1000 units, 2000 units (cap/tab). Trade only: Soln 400 units/drop, 1000 units/drop, 2000 units/drop.] ▶L – ▶+ $

Other

BROMOCRIPTINE (**_Cycloset, Parlodel_**) Type 2 DM: 0.8 mg PO q am (within 2 h of waking), may increase weekly by 0.8 mg to max tolerated dose of 1.6 to 4.8 mg. Hyperprolactinemia: Start 1.25 to 2.5 mg PO at bedtime, then increase q 3 to 7 days to usual effective dose of 2.5 to 15 mg/day, max 40 mg/day. Acromegaly: Usual effective dose is 20 to 30 mg/day, max 100 mg/day. Doses greater than 20 mg/day can be divided two times per day. Also approved for Parkinson's disease, but rarely used. Take with food to minimize dizziness and nausea. [Generic/Trade: Tabs 2.5 mg. Caps 5 mg. Trade only: Tabs 0.8 mg (Cycloset).] ▶L ♀B ▶– $$$$$

CABERGOLINE (**_Dostinex_**) Hyperprolactinemia: 0.25 to 1 mg PO two times per week. [Generic/Trade: Tabs 0.5 mg.] ▶L ♀B ▶– $$$$$

CALCITONIN (**_Miacalcin, Fortical, ✦ Calcimar, Caltine_**) Osteoporosis: 100 units SC/IM every other day or 200 units (1 spray) intranasal daily (alternate nostrils). Paget's disease: 50 to 100 units SC/IM daily. Hypercalcemia: 4 units/kg SC/IM q 12 h. May increase after 2 days to max of 8 units/kg q 6 h. Skin test before using injectable product: 1 unit intradermally and observe for local reaction. [Generic/Trade: Nasal spray 200 units/activation in 3.7 mL bottle (minimum of 30 doses/bottle).] ▶Plasma ♀C ▶? $$$$

DENOSUMAB (**_Prolia_**) Postmenopausal osteoporosis: 60 mg SC q6 months. [Trade only: 60 mg/1 mL vial, prefilled syringe.] ▶? ♀C ▶? $$$$

DESMOPRESSIN (**_DDAVP, Stimate, ✦ Minlrin, Octostim_**) Diabetes insipidus: 10 to 40 mcg intranasally daily or divided two to three times per day, 0.05 to 1.2 mg/day PO or divided two to three times per day, or 0.5 to 1 mL/day SC/IV in 2 divided doses. Hemophilia A, von Willebrand's disease: 0.3 mcg/kg IV over 15 to 30 min, or 150 to 300 mcg intranasally. Enuresis: 0.2 to 0.6 mg PO at bedtime. Not for children younger than 6 yo. [Trade only: Stimate nasal spray 150 mcg/0.1 mL (1 spray), 2.5 mL bottle (25 sprays). Generic/Trade (DDAVP nasal spray): 10 mcg/0.1 mL (1 spray), 5 mL bottle (50 sprays). Note difference in concentration of nasal soln. Rhinal Tube: 2.5 mL bottle with 2 flexible plastic tube applicators with graduation marks for dosing. Generic only: Tabs 0.1, 0.2 mL.] ▶LK ♀B ▶? $$$$

SODIUM POLYSTYRENE SULFONATE (**_Kayexalate_**) Hyperkalemia: 15 g PO one to four times per day or 30 to 50 g retention enema (in sorbitol) q 6 h prn. Retain for 30 min to several hours. Irrigate with tap water after enema to prevent necrosis. [Generic only: Susp 15 g/60 mL. Powdered resin.] ▶Fecal excretion ♀C ▶? $$$$

SOMATROPIN (human growth hormone, *Genotropin, Humatrope, Norditropin, Norditropin NordiFlex, Nutropin, Nutropin AQ, Nutropin Depot, Omnitrope, Protropin, Serostim, Serostim LQ, Saizen, Tev-Tropin, Valtropin, Zorbtive*) Dosages vary by indication and product. [Single-dose vials (powder for injection with diluent). Tev-Tropin: 5 mg vial (powder for injection with diluent, stable for 14 days when refrigerated). Genotropin: 1.5, 5.8, 13.8 mg cartridges. Humatrope: 6, 12, 24 mg pen cartridges; 5 mg vial (powder for injection with diluent, stable for 14 days when refrigerated). Nutropin AQ: 10 mg multidose vial, 5, 10, 20 mg/pen cartridges. Norditropin: 5, 10, 15 mg pen cartridges. Norditropin NordiFlex: 5, 10, 15 mg prefilled pens. Omnitrope: 1.5, 5.8 mg vial (powder for injection with diluent). Saizen: Preassembled reconstitution device with autoinjector pen. Serostim: 4, 5, 6 mg single-dose vials; 4, 8.8 mg multidose vials; and 8.8 mg cartridges for autoinjector. Valtropin: 5 mg single-dose vials, 5 mg prefilled syringe. Zorbtive: 8.8 mg vial (powder for injection with diluent, stable for 14 days when refrigerated).] ▶LK ♀B/C ▶? $$$$$

TERIPARATIDE (*Forteo*) <u>Treatment of postmenopausal osteoporosis, treatment of men and women with glucocorticoid-induced osteoporosis or to increase bone mass in men with primary or hypogonadal osteoporosis and high risk for fracture:</u> 20 mcg SC daily in thigh or abdomen for no longer than 2 years. [Trade only: 28 dose pen injector (20 mcg/dose).] ▶LK ♀C ▶– $$$$$ ■

VASOPRESSIN (*Pitressin, ADH,* ✦ *Pressyn AR*) <u>Diabetes insipidus:</u> 5 to 10 units IM/SC two to four times per day prn. <u>Cardiac arrest:</u> 40 units IV; may repeat if no response after 3 min. <u>Septic shock:</u> 0.01 to 0.04 units/min. <u>Variceal bleeding:</u> 0.2 to 0.4 units/min initially (max 0.8 units/min). ▶LK ♀C ▶? $$$$$

ENT

Antihistamines—Non-Sedating

DESLORATADINE (*Clarinex,* ✦ *Aerius*) 5 mg PO daily for age older than 12 yo. Peds: 2 mL (1 mg) PO daily for age 6 to 11 mo, ½ tsp (1.25 mg) PO daily for age 12 mo to 5 yo, 1 tsp (2.5 mg) PO daily for age 6 to 11 yo. [Trade only: Tabs 5 mg. Fast-dissolve RediTabs 2.5, 5 mg. Syrup 0.5 mg/mL.] ▶LK ♀C ▶+ $$$

FEXOFENADINE (*Allegra*) 60 mg PO two times per day or 180 mg daily. Peds: 30 mg PO two times per day for age 2 to 11 yo. [Generic/Trade: Tabs 30, 60, 180 mg, Caps 60 mg. Trade only: Susp 30 mg/5 mL, orally disintegrating tab 30 mg.] ▶LK ♀C ▶+ $$$

LORATADINE (*Claritin, Claritin Hives Relief, Claritin RediTabs, Alavert, Tavist ND*) 10 mg PO daily for age older than 6 yo, 5 mg PO daily for age 2 to 5 yo. [OTC Generic/Trade: Tabs 10 mg. Fast-dissolve tabs (Alavert, Claritin RediTabs) 5, 10 mg. Syrup 1 mg/mL. Rx Trade only (Claritin): Chewable tabs 5 mg, Liqui-gel caps 10 mg.] ▶LK ♀B ▶+ $

Antihistamines—Other

CETIRIZINE (*Zyrtec, ♦ Reactine, Aller-Relief*) 5 to 10 mg PO daily for age older than 6 yo. Peds: give 2.5 mg PO daily for age 6 to 23 mo, give 2.5 mg PO daily to two times per day for age 2 to 5 yo. [OTC Generic/Trade: Tabs 5, 10 mg. Syrup 5 mg/5 mL. Chewable tabs, grape flavored 5, 10 mg.] ▶LK ♀B ▶—$$$

CHLORPHENIRAMINE (*Chlor-Trimeton, Aller-Chlor*) 4 mg PO q 4 to 6 h. Max 24 mg/day. Peds: give 2 mg PO q 4 to 6 h for age 6 to 11 yo. Max 12 mg/day. [OTC Generic only: Tabs extended-release 12 mg. Generic/Trade: Tabs 4 mg. Syrup 2 mg/5 mL. Tabs extended-release 8 mg.] ▶LK ♀B ▶—$

CLEMASTINE (*Tavist-1*) 1.34 mg PO two times per day. Max 8.04 mg/day. [OTC Generic/Trade: Tabs 1.34 mg. Rx: Generic/Trade: Tabs 2.68 mg, Syrup 0.67 mg/5 mL. Rx: Generic only: Syrup 0.5 mg/5 mL.] ▶LK ♀B ▶—$

CYPROHEPTADINE (*Periactin*) Start 4 mg PO three times per day. Max 32 mg/day. [Generic only: Tabs 4 mg. Syrup 2 mg/5 mL.] ▶LK ♀B ▶—$

DEXCHLORPHENIRAMINE (*Polaramine*) 2 mg PO q 4 to 6 h. Timed-release tabs: 4 or 6 mg PO at bedtime or q 8 to 10 h. [Generic only: Tabs immediate-release 2 mg, timed-release 4, 6 mg. Syrup 2 mg/5 mL.] ▶LK ♀? ▶—$$

DIPHENHYDRAMINE (*Benadryl, Banophen, Allermax, Diphen, Diphenhist, Dytan, Siladryl, Sominex, ♦ Allerdryl, Nytol*) Allergic rhinitis, urticaria, hypersensitivity reactions: 25 to 50 mg IV/IM/PO q 4 to 6 h. Peds: 5 mg/kg/day divided q 4 to 6 h. EPS: 25 to 50 mg PO three to four times per day or 10 to 50 mg IV/IM three to four times per day. Insomnia: 25 to 50 mg PO at bedtime. [OTC Trade only: Tabs 25, 50 mg, Chewable tabs 12.5 mg. OTC and Rx: Generic only: Caps 25, 50 mg, softgel cap 25 mg. OTC Generic/Trade: Soln 6.25 or 12.5 mg per 5 mL. Rx: Trade only: (Dytan) Susp 25 mg/5 mL, Chewable tabs 25 mg.] ▶LK ♀B ▶—$

HYDROXYZINE (*Atarax, Vistaril*) 25 to 100 mg IM/PO one to four times per day or prn. [Generic only: Tabs 10, 25, 50, 100 mg; Caps 100 mg; Syrup 10 mg/5 mL. Generic/Trade: Caps 25, 50 mg, Susp 25 mg/5 mL (Vistaril). (Caps = Vistaril, Tabs = Atarax).] ▶L ♀C ▶—$$

LEVOCETIRIZINE (*Xyzal*) 5 mg PO daily for age 12 yo or older. Peds: give 2.5 mg PO daily for age 6 to 11 yo. [Trade only: Tabs scored 5 mg; Oral soln 2.5 mg/5 mL (148 mL).] ▶K ♀B ▶—$$$

MECLIZINE (*Antivert, Bonine, Medivert, Meclicot, Meni-D, ♦ Bonamine*) Motion sickness: 25 to 50 mg PO 1 h prior to travel, then 25 to 50 mg PO daily. Vertigo: 25 mg PO q 6 h prn. [Rx/OTC/Generic/Trade: Tabs 12.5, 25 mg; Chewable tabs 25 mg. Rx/Trade only: Tabs 50 mg.] ▶L ♀B ▶? $

Antitussives / Expectorants

BENZONATATE (*Tessalon, Tessalon Perles*) 100 to 200 mg PO three times per day. Swallow whole. Do not chew. Numbs mouth; possible choking hazard. [Generic/Trade: Softgel caps: 100, 200 mg.] ▶L ♀C ▶? $$

DEXTROMETHORPHAN (*Benylin, Delsym, DexAlone, Robitussin Cough, Vick's 44 Cough*) 10 to 20 mg PO q 4 h or 30 mg PO q 6 to 8 h. Sustained action liquid 60 mg PO q 12 h. [OTC Trade only: Caps 15 mg (Robitussin), 30 mg (DexAlone), Susp, extended-release 30 mg/5 mL (Delsym). Generic/Trade: Syrup 5, 7.5, 10, 15 mg/5 mL. Generic only: Lozenges 5, 10 mg.] ▶L ♀+ ▶+ $

GUAIFENESIN (*Robitussin, Hytuss, Guiatuss, Mucinex*) 100 to 400 mg PO q 4 h. 600 to 1200 mg PO q 12 h (extended-release). Peds: 50 to 100 mg/dose for age 2 to 5 yo, give 100 to 200 mg/dose for age 6 to 11 yo. [Rx Generic/Trade: Extended-release tabs 600, 1200 mg. OTC Generic/Trade: Liquid, Syrup 100 mg/5 mL. OTC Trade only: Caps 200 mg (Hytuss), extended-release tabs 600 mg (Mucinex). OTC Generic only: Tabs 100, 200, 400 mg.] ▶L ♀C ▶+ $

Decongestants

NOTE: See ENT—Nasal Preparations for nasal spray decongestants (oxymetazoline, phenylephrine). Deaths have occurred in children younger than 2 yo attributed to toxicity from cough and cold medications; the FDA does not recommend their use in this age group.

PHENYLEPHRINE (*Sudafed PE*) 10 mg PO q 4 h. [OTC Trade only: Tabs 10 mg.] ▶L ♀C ▶+ $

PSEUDOEPHEDRINE (*Sudafed, Sudafed 12 Hour, Efidac/24, Dimetapp Decongestant Infant Drops, PediaCare Infants' Decongestant Drops, Triaminic Oral Infant Drops, ✦ Pseudofrin*) Adult: 60 mg PO q 4 to 6 h. Extended release tabs: 120 mg PO two times per day or 240 mg PO daily. Peds: give 15 mg PO q 4 to 6 h for age 2 to 5 yo, give 30 mg PO q 4 to 6 h for age 6 to 12 yo. [OTC Generic/Trade: Tabs 30, 60 mg, Tabs, extended-release 120 mg (12 h). Soln 15, 30 mg/5 mL. Trade only: Chewable tabs 15 mg, Tabs, extended-release 240 mg (24 h).] ▶L ♀C ▶+ $

Ear Preparations

AURALGAN † (benzocaine + antipyrine) 2 to 4 gtts in ear(s) three to four times per day prn. [Generic/Trade: Otic soln 10, 15 mL.] ▶Not absorbed ♀C ▶? $

CARBAMIDE PEROXIDE (*Debrox, Murine Ear*) 5 to 10 gtts in ear(s) two times per day for 4 days. [OTC Generic/Trade: Otic soln 6.5%, 15, 30 mL.] ▶Not absorbed ♀? ▶? $

CIPRO HC OTIC † (ciprofloxacin + hydrocortisone) 3 gtts in ear(s) two times per day for 7 days for age 1 yo to adult. [Trade only: Otic susp 10 mL.] ▶Not absorbed ♀C ▶– $$$$

CIPRODEX OTIC (ciprofloxacin + dexamethasone) 4 gtts in ear(s) two times per day for 7 days for age 6 mo to adult. [Trade only: Otic susp 5, 7.5 mL.] ▶Not absorbed ♀C ▶– $$$$

CIPROFLOXACIN (*Cetraxal*) 1 single-use container in ear(s) two times per day for 7 days for age 1 yo to adult. [Trade only: 0.25 mL single-use containers with 0.2% ciprofloxacin soln, #14.] ▶Not absorbed ♀C ▶– $$$$

ENT COMBINATIONS (selected)	Decon-gestant	Antihis-tamine	Anti-tussive	Typical Adult Doses
OTC				
Actifed Cold & Allergy	PE	CH	-	1 tab 4–6 h
Actifed Cold & Sinus‡	PS	CH		2 tabs q 6 h
Allerfrim, Aprodine	PS	TR	-	1 tab or 10 mL q 4–6 h
Benadryl Allergy/Cold‡	PE	DPH		2 tabs q 4 h
Benadryl-D Allergy/Sinus Tablets	PE	DPH	-	1 tab q 4 h
Claritin-D 12-h, Alavert D-12	PS	LO	-	1 tab q 12 h
Claritin-D 24-h	PS	LO	-	1 tab daily
Dimetapp Cold & Allergy Elixir	PE	BR	-	20 mL q 4 h
Dimetapp DM Cold & Cough	PE	BR	DM	20 mL q 4 h
Drixoral Cold & Allergy	PS	DBR	-	1 tab q 12 h
Mucinex-DM Extended-Release	-	-	GU,DM	1–2 tabs q 12 h
Robitussin CF	PE	-	GU, DM	10 mL q 4 h*
Robitussin DM, Mytussin DM	-	-	GU, DM	10 mL q 4 h*
Robitussin PE, Guiatuss PE	PE	-	GU	10 mL q 4 h*
Triaminic Cold & Allergy	PE	CH	-	10 mL q 4 h
Rx Only				
Allegra-D 12-h	PS	FE	-	1 tab q 12 h
Allegra-D 24-h	PS	FE	-	1 tab daily
Bromfenex	PS	BR	-	1 cap q 12 h
Clarinex-D 24-h	PS	DL	-	1 tab daily
Deconamine	PS	CH	-	1 tab or 10 mL tid-qid
Deconamine SR, Chlordrine SR	PS	CH	-	1 tab q 12 h
Deconsal I	PE	-	GU	1-2 tabs q 12 h
Dimetane-DX	PS	BR	DM	10 mL PO q 4 h
Duratuss	PS	-	GU	1 tab q 12 h
Duratuss HD©III	PE	-	GU, HY	5-10 mL q 4–6 h
Entex PSE, Guaifenex PSE 120	PS	-	GU	1 tab q 12 h
Histussin D ©III	PS	-	HY	5 mL qid
Histussin HC ©III	PE	CH	HY	10 mL q 4 h
Humibid DM	-	-	GU, DM	1 tab q 12 h
Hycotuss ©III	-	-	GU, HY	5 mL pc & qhs
Phenergan/Dextromethorphan	-	PR	DM	5 mL q 4–6 h
Phenergan VC	PE	PR	-	5 mL q 4–6 h
Phenergan VC w/codeine©V	PE	PR	CO	5 mL q 4–6 h
Robitussin AC ©V (generic only)	-	-	GU, CO	10 mL q 4 h*
Robitussin DAC ©V (generic only)	PS	-	GU, CO	10 mL q 4 h*
Rondec Syrup	PE	CH	-	5 mL qid†
Rondec DM Syrup	PE	CH	DM	5 mL qid†
Rondec Oral Drops	PE	CH	-	0.75 to 1 mL qid
Rondec DM Oral Drops	PE	CH	DM	0.75 to 1 mL qid
Rynatan	PE	CH	-	1–2 tabs q 12 h
Rynatan-P Pediatric	PE	CH	-	2.5–5 mL q 12 h*
Semprex-D	PS	AC	-	1 cap q 4–6 h
Tanafed (generic only)	PS	CH	-	10–20 mL q 12 h*
Tussionex ©III	-	CH	HY	5 mL q 12 h

©=class   DL=desloratadine   FE=fexofenadine   PE=phenylephrine
AC=acrivastine   DM=dextromethorphan   GU=guaifenesin   PR=promethazine
BR=brompheniramine   DBR=dexbrompheniramine   HY=hydrocodone   PS=pseudoephedrine
CH=chlorpheniramine   DPH=diphenhydramine   LO=loratadine   TR=triprolidine
CO=codeine

*5 mL/dose if 6–11 yo. 2.5 mL if 2–5 yo. †2.5 mL/dose if 6–11 yo. 1.25 mL if 2–5 yo. ‡Also contains acetaminophen.

tid=three times per day; qid=four times per day; qhs=at bedtime.

CORTISPORIN OTIC (hydrocortisone + polymyxin + neomycin, Pediotic) 4 gtts in ear(s) three to four times per day up to 10 days of soln or susp. Peds: 3 gtts in ear(s) three to four times per day up to 10 days. Caution with perforated TMs or tympanostomy tubes as this increases the risk of neomycin ototoxicity, especially if use prolonged or repeated. Use susp rather than acidic soln. [Generic only: Otic soln or susp 7.5, 10 mL.] ▶Not absorbed ♀? ▶? $

CORTISPORIN TC OTIC (hydrocortisone + neomycin + thonzonium + colistin) 4 to 5 gtts in ear(s) three to four times per day up to 10 days. [Trade only: Otic susp, 10 mL.] ▶Not absorbed ♀? ▶? $$$

DOMEBORO OTIC (acetic acid + aluminum acetate) 4 to 6 gtts in ear(s) q 2 to 3 h. Peds: 2 to 3 gtts in ear(s) q 3 to 4 h. [Generic only: Otic soln 60 mL.] ▶Not absorbed ♀? ▶? $

FLUOCINOLONE-OTIC (*DermOtic*) 5 gtts in affected ear(s) two times per day for 7 to 14 days for age 2 yo to adult. [Trade only: Otic oil 0.01% 20 mL.] ▶L ♀C ▶? $$

OFLOXACIN-OTIC (*Floxin Otic*) Otitis externa: 5 gtts in ear(s) daily for age 1 to 12 yo, 10 gtts in ear(s) daily for age 12 or older. [Generic/Trade: Otic soln 0.3% 5, 10 mL. Trade only: "Singles": Single-dispensing containers 0.25 mL (5 gtts), 2 per foil pouch.] ▶Not absorbed ♀C ▶– $$$

SWIM-EAR (isopropyl alcohol + anhydrous glycerins) 4 to 5 gtts in ears after swimming. [OTC Trade only: Otic soln 30 mL.] ▶Not absorbed ♀? ▶? $

VOSOL HC (acetic acid + propylene glycol + hydrocortisone) 5 gtts in ear(s) three to four times per day. Peds age older than 3 yo: 3 to 4 gtts in ear(s) three to four times per day. [Generic/Trade: Otic soln 2%/3%/1% 10 mL.] ▶Not absorbed ♀? ▶? $

Mouth and Lip Preparations

AMLEXANOX (*Aphthasol, OraDisc A*) Aphthous ulcers: Apply ¼ inch paste or mucoadhesive patch to affected area four times per day after oral hygiene for up to 10 days. Up to 3 patches may be applied at one time. [Trade only: Oral paste 5% (Aphthasol), 3, 5 g tube. Mucoadhesive patch (OraDisc) 2 mg, #20.] ▶LK ♀B ▶? $

CEVIMELINE (*Evoxac*) Dry mouth due to Sjögren's syndrome: 30 mg PO three times per day. [Trade only: Caps 30 mg.] ▶L ♀C ▶– $$$$$

CHLORHEXIDINE GLUCONATE (*Peridex, Periogard, ✚ Denticare*) Rinse with 15 mL of undiluted soln for 30 sec two times per day. Do not swallow. Spit after rinsing. [Generic/Trade: Oral rinse 0.12% 473 to 480 mL bottles.] ▶Fecal excretion ♀B ▶? $

DEBACTEROL (sulfuric acid + sulfonated phenolics) Aphthous stomatitis, mucositis: Apply to dry ulcer. Rinse with water. [Trade only: 1 mL prefilled, single-use applicator.] ▶Not absorbed ♀C ▶+ $$

GELCLAIR (maltodextrin + propylene glycol) Aphthous ulcers, mucositis, stomatitis: Rinse mouth with 1 packet three times per day or prn. Do not eat or drink for 1 h after treatment. [Trade only: 21 packets/box.] ▶Not absorbed ♀+ ▶+ $$$

LIDOCAINE—VISCOUS (*Xylocaine*) <u>Mouth or lip pain</u> in adults only: 15 to 20 mL topically or swish and spit q 3 h. [Generic/Trade: Soln 2%, 20 mL unit dose, 100 mL bottle.] ▶LK ♀B ▶+ $

MAGIC MOUTHWASH (**diphenhydramine + Mylanta + sucralfate**) 5 mL PO swish and spit or swish and swallow three times per day before meals and prn. [Compounded susp. A standard mixture is 30 mL diphenhydramine liquid (12.5 mg/5 mL)/60 mL Mylanta or Maalox/4 g sucralfate.] ▶LK ▶– $$$

PILOCARPINE (*Salagen*) <u>Dry mouth due to radiation of head and neck or Sjögren's syndrome</u>: 5 mg PO three to four times per day. [Generic/Trade: Tabs 5, 7.5 mg.] ▶L ♀C ▶– $$$$

Nasal Preparations—Corticosteroids

BECLOMETHASONE (*Vancenase, Vancenase AQ Double Strength, Beconase AQ*) Vancenase: 1 spray per nostril two to four times per day. Beconase AQ: 1 to 2 sprays per nostril two times per day. Vancenase AQ Double Strength: 1 to 2 sprays per nostril daily. [Trade only: Vancenase 42 mcg/spray, 80 or 200 sprays/bottle. Beconase AQ 42 mcg/spray, 200 sprays/bottle. Vancenase AQ Double Strength 84 mcg/spray, 120 sprays/bottle.] ▶L ♀C ▶? $$$$

BUDESONIDE—NASAL (*Rhinocort Aqua*) 1 to 4 sprays per nostril daily. [Trade only: Nasal inhaler 120 sprays/bottle.] ▶L ♀B ▶? $$$$

CICLESONIDE (*Omnaris*) 2 sprays per nostril daily. [Trade only: Nasal spray, 50 mcg/spray, 120 sprays/bottle.] ▶L ♀C ▶? $$$

FLUNISOLIDE (*Nasalide, Nasarel, ✦ Rhinalar*) Start 2 sprays per nostril two times per day. Max 8 sprays/nostril/day. [Generic/Trade: Nasal soln 0.025%, 200 sprays/bottle. Nasalide with pump unit. Nasarel with meter pump and nasal adapter.] ▶L ♀C ▶? $$$

FLUTICASONE—NASAL (*Flonase, Veramyst*) 2 sprays per nostril daily. [Generic/Trade: Flonase. Nasal spray 0.05%, 120 sprays/bottle. Trade only: (Veramyst): Nasal spray susp: 27.5 mcg/spray, 120 sprays/bottle.] ▶L ♀C ▶? $$$

MOMETASONE—NASAL (*Nasonex*) Adult: 2 sprays/nostril daily. Peds 2 to 11 yo: 1 spray/nostril daily. [Trade only: Nasal spray, 120 sprays/bottle.] ▶L ♀C ▶? $$$$

TRIAMCINOLONE—NASAL (*Nasacort AQ, Nasacort HFA, Tri-Nasal, AllerNaze*) Nasacort HFA, Tri-Nasal, AllerNaze: 2 sprays per nostril daily to two times per day. Max 4 sprays/nostril/day. Nasacort AQ: 1 to 2 sprays per nostril daily. [Trade only: Nasal inhaler 55 mcg/spray, 100 sprays/bottle (Nasacort HFA). Nasal spray, 55 mcg/spray, 120 sprays/bottle (Nasacort AQ). Nasal spray 50 mcg/spray, 120 sprays/bottle (Tri-Nasal, AllerNaze).] ▶L ♀C ▶– $$$$

Nasal Preparations—Other

AZELASTINE—NASAL (*Astelin, Astepro*) 1 to 2 sprays per nostril two times per day. [Generic: Nasal spray, 200 sprays/bottle.] ▶L ♀C ▶? $$$$

CROMOLYN—NASAL (*NasalCrom*) 1 spray per nostril three to four times per day. [OTC Generic/Trade: Nasal inhaler 200 sprays/bottle 13, 26 mL.] ▶LK ♀B ▶+ $

IPRATROPIUM—NASAL (*Atrovent Nasal Spray*) 2 sprays per nostril two to four times per day. [Generic/Trade: Nasal spray 0.03%, 345 sprays/bottle, 0.06%, 165 sprays/bottle.] ▶L ♀B ▶? $$

+ LEVOCABASTINE—NASAL Canada only. 2 sprays per nostril two times per day, increase prn to three to four times per day. [Trade only: Nasal spray 0.5 mg/mL, plastic bottles of 15 mL. 50 mcg/spray.] ▶L (but minimal absorption) ♀C ▶– $$

OLOPATADINE—NASAL (*Patanase*) 2 sprays per nostril two times per day. [Trade only: Nasal spray, 240 sprays/bottle.] ▶L ♀C ▶? $$$

OXYMETAZOLINE (*Afrin, Dristan 12 Hr Nasal, Nostrilla, Vicks Sinex 12 Hr*) 2 to 3 gtts/sprays per nostril two times per day prn nasal congestion for no more than 3 days. [OTC Generic/Trade: Nasal spray 0.05% 15, 30 mL; Nose gtts 0.025%, 0.05% 20 mL with dropper.] ▶L ♀C ▶? $

PHENYLEPHRINE—NASAL (*Neo-Synephrine, Vicks Sinex*) 2 to 3 sprays or gtts per nostril q 4 h prn × 3 days. [OTC Generic/Trade: Nasal gtts/spray 0.25, 0.5, 1% (15 mL).] ▶L ♀C ▶? $

SALINE NASAL SPRAY (*SeaMist, Entsol, Pretz, NaSal, Ocean, + HydraSense*) <u>Nasal dryness:</u> 1 to 3 sprays or gtts per nostril prn. [Generic/Trade: Nasal spray 0.4, 0.5, 0.65, 0.75%, Nasal gtts 0.4, 0.65%. Trade only: Preservative-free nasal spray 3% (Entsol).] ▶Not metabolized ♀A ▶+ $

GASTROENTEROLOGY

Antidiarrheals

BISMUTH SUBSALICYLATE (*Pepto-Bismol, Kaopectate*) 2 tabs or caps or 30 mL (262 mg/15 mL) PO q 30 min to 1 h up to 8 doses per day for up to 2 days. Peds: 5 mL (262 mg/15 mL) or ⅓ tab or cap PO for age 3 to 6 yo, 10 mL (262 mg/15 mL) or ⅔ tab or cap PO for age 6 to 9 yo. Risk of Reye's syndrome in children. [OTC Generic/Trade: Chewable tabs 262 mg. Susp 262, 525, 750 mg/15 mL. OTC Trade only: Caps 262 mg (Pepto-Bismol). Susp 87 mg/5 mL (Kaopectate Children's Liquid).] ▶K ♀D ▶? $

IMODIUM MULTI-SYMPTOM RELIEF (**loperamide + simethicone**) 2 tabs or caps PO initially, then 1 tab or cap PO after each unformed stool to a max of 4 tabs/caps per day. Peds: 1 tab or cap PO initially, then ½ cap PO after each unformed stool (up to 2 tabs or caps PO per day for age 6 to 8 yo or wt 48 to 59 lbs or up to 3 tabs or caps PO per day for age 9 to 11 yo or wt 60 to 95 lbs). [OTC Generic/Trade: Caps, chewable tabs 2 mg loperamide/125 mg simethicone.] ▶L ♀C ▶– $

LOMOTIL (**diphenoxylate + atropine**) 2 tabs or 10 mL PO four times per day. [Generic/Trade: Oral soln or tab 2.5 mg/0.025 mg diphenoxylate/atropine per 5 mL or tab.] ▶L ♀C ▶–©V $

LOPERAMIDE (*Imodium, Imodium AD,* ✦*Diarr-eze*) 4 mg PO initially, then 2 mg PO after each unformed stool to a maximum of 16 mg per day. Peds: 1 mg PO three times per day for wt 13 to 20 kg, 2 mg PO two times per day for wt 21 to 30 kg, 2 mg PO three times per day for wt greater than 30 kg. [OTC Generic/Trade: Tabs 2 mg. Oral soln 1 mg/5 mL. OTC Trade only: Oral soln 1 mg/7.5 mL.] ▶L ♀C ▶+ $

MOTOFEN (**difenoxin + atropine**) 2 tabs PO initially, then 1 tab after each loose stool q 3 to 4 h prn (up to 8 tabs per day). [Trade only: Tabs difenoxin 1 mg + atropine 0.025 mg.] ▶L ♀C ▶–©IV $$

OPIUM (**opium tincture, paregoric**) 5 to 10 mL paregoric PO daily (up to four times) or 0.6 mL (range 0.3 to 1 mL) opium tincture PO q 2 to 6 h prn to max 6 mL per day. [Trade only: Opium tincture 10% (deodorized opium tincture, 10 mg morphine equivalent/mL). Generic only: Paregoric (camphorated opium tincture, 2 mg morphine equivalent/5 mL).] ▶L ♀B (D with long-term use) ▶?©II (opium tincture), III (paregoric) $$

Antiemetics—5-HT3 Receptor Antagonists

DOLASETRON (*Anzemet*) Nausea with chemo: 1.8 mg/kg (up to 100 mg) PO single dose. Post-op nausea: 12.5 mg IV in adults and 0.35 mg/kg IV in children as single dose. Alternative for prevention: 100 mg (adults) PO or 1.2 mg/kg (children) PO 2 h before surgery. [Trade only: Tabs 50, 100 mg. Injectable no longer available in Canada.] ▶LK ♀B ▶? $$$

GRANISETRON (*Kytril, Sancuso*) Nausea with chemo: 10 mcg/kg IV over 5 min, 30 min prior to chemo. Oral: 1 mg PO two times per day or 2 mg PO once for 1 day only. Transdermal (Sancuso): 1 patch to upper outer arm at least 24 h (but up to 48 h) before chemotherapy. Remove 24 h after completion of chemotherapy. Can be worn up to 7 days depending on the duration of chemo. Radiation-induced nausea and vomiting: 2 mg PO 1 h before first irradiation fraction of each day. [Generic/Trade: Tabs 1 mg. Trade only: Oral soln 2 mg/10 mL (30 mL). : Transdermal patch (Sancuso) 34.3 mg of granisetron delivering 3.1 mg/24 h.] ▶L ♀B ▶? $$$$

ONDANSETRON (*Zofran*) Nausea with chemo: IV: 32 mg IV over 15 min, or 0.15 mg/kg dose 30 min prior to chemo and repeated at 4 and 8 h after 1st dose for age 6 mo or older. PO: 4 mg PO 30 min prior to chemo and repeat at 4 and 8 h for age 4 to 11 yo, 8 mg PO and repeated 8 h later for age 12 yo or older. Prevention of post-op nausea: 4 mg IV over 2 to 5 min or 4 mg IM or 16 mg PO 1 h before anesthesia. Give 0.1 mg/kg IV over 2 to 5 min as a single dose for age 1 mo to 12 yo if wt 40 kg or less; 4 mg IV over 2 to 5 min as a single dose if wt greater than 40 kg. Prevention of N/V associated with radiotherapy: 8 mg PO three times per day. [Generic/Trade: Tabs 4, 8, 24 mg. Orally disintegrating tab 4, 8 mg. Oral soln 4 mg/5 mL. Generic only: Tabs 16 mg.] ▶L ♀B ▶? $$$$$

PALONOSETRON (*Aloxi*) Nausea with chemo: 0.25 mg IV over 30 sec, 30 min prior to chemo. Prevention of post-op N/V: 0.075 mg IV over 10 sec just prior to anesthesia. [Trade only: injectable.] ▶L ♀B ▶? $$$$$

Antiemetics—Other

APREPITANT (*Emend, fosaprepitant*) <u>Prevention of nausea with moderately to highly emetogenic chemo, in combination with a corticosteroid and a 5-HT3 antagonist:</u> 125 mg PO on day 1 (1 h prior to chemo), then 80 mg PO q am on days 2 and 3. Alternative for 1st dose only is 115 mg IV (fosaprepitant) over 15 min given 30 min prior to chemo. Alternatively, 150 mg IV (fosaprepitant) over 20 to 30 minutes, with a corticosteroid and a 5-HT3 antagonist. <u>Prevention of post-op N/V:</u> 40 mg PO within 3 h prior to anesthesia. [Trade only (aprepitant): Caps 40, 80, 125 mg. IV prodrug form is fosaprepitant.] ▶L ♀B ▶? $$$$$

+DICLECTIN (**doxylamine + pyridoxine**) Canada only. 2 tabs PO at bedtime. May add 1 tab in am and 1 tab in afternoon, if needed. [Canada Trade only: Delayed-release tabs doxylamine 10 mg + pyridoxine 10 mg.] ▶LK ♀A ▶? $

DIMENHYDRINATE (*Dramamine, + Gravol*) 50 to 100 mg PO/IM/IV q 4 to 6 h prn (max 400 mg/24 h PO, 600 mg/day IV/IM). [OTC Generic/Trade: Tabs 50 mg. Trade only: Chewable tabs 50 mg. Generic only: Oral soln 12.5 mg/5 mL. Canada only: Supp 25, 50, 100 mg.] ▶LK ♀B ▶– $

+ DOMPERIDONE Canada only. <u>Postprandial dyspepsia:</u> 10 to 20 mg PO three to four times per day, 30 min before a meal. <u>Nausea and vomiting:</u> 20 mg PO three to four times per day. [Canada only. Generic: Tabs 10, 20 mg.] ▶L ♀? ▶– $$

DOXYLAMINE (*Unisom Nighttime Sleep Aid,* **others**) 12.5 mg PO two to four times per day; often used in combination with pyridoxine. [Generic/Trade: Tabs 25 mg.] ▶L ♀A ▶? $

DRONABINOL (*Marinol*) <u>Nausea with chemo:</u> 5 mg/m² PO 1 to 3 h before chemo then 5 mg/m²/dose q 2 to 4 h after chemo for 4 to 6 doses/day. <u>Anorexia associated with AIDS:</u> initially 2.5 mg PO two times per day before lunch and dinner. [Generic/Trade: Caps 2.5, 5, 10 mg.] ▶L ♀C ▶–©III $$$$$

DROPERIDOL (*Inapsine*) 0.625 to 2.5 mg IV or 2.5 mg IM. May cause fatal QT prolongation, even in patients with no risk factors. Monitor ECG before. ▶L ♀C ▶? $

METOCLOPRAMIDE (*Reglan, Metozolv ODT, + Maxeran*) 10 mg IV/IM q 2 to 3 h prn. 10 to 15 mg PO four times per day, 30 min before meals and at bedtime. Caution with long-term (more than 3 months) use. [Generic/Trade: Tabs 5, 10 mg. Trade: Orally disintegrating tabs 5, 10 mg (Metozolv). Generic only: Oral soln 5 mg/5 mL.] ▶K ♀B ▶? $

NABILONE (*Cesamet*) 1 to 2 mg PO two times per day, 1 to 3 h before chemotherapy. [Trade only: Caps 1 mg.] ▶L ♀C ▶–©III $$$$$

PHOSPHORATED CARBOHYDRATES (*Emetrol*) 15 to 30 mL PO q 15 min prn, max 5 doses. Peds: 5 to 10 mL per dose. [OTC Generic/Trade: Soln containing dextrose, fructose, and phosphoric acid.] ▶L ♀A ▶+ $

PROCHLORPERAZINE (*Compazine*) 5 to 10 mg IV over at least 2 min. 5 to 10 mg PO/IM three to four times per day. 25 mg PR q 12 h. Sustained-

(cont.)

release: 15 mg PO q am or 10 mg PO q 12 h. Peds: 0.1 mg/kg/dose PO/PR three to four times per day or 0.1 to 0.15 mg/kg/dose IM three to four times per day. [Generic only: Tabs 5, 10, 25 mg. Supp 25 mg.] ▶LK ♀C ▶? $

PROMETHAZINE (*Phenergan*) Adults: 12.5 to 25 mg PO/IM/PR q 4 to 6 h. Peds: 0.25 to 1 mg/kg PO/IM/PR q 4 to 6 h. Contraindicated if age younger than 2 yo; caution in older children. IV use common but not approved. [Generic only: Tabs/Supp 12.5, 25, 50 mg. Syrup 6.25 mg/5 mL.] ▶LK ♀C ▶– $ ■

SCOPOLAMINE (*Transderm-Scop, Scopace, ✦ Transderm-V*) <u>Motion sickness:</u> Apply 1 disc (1.5 mg) behind ear 4 h prior to event; replace q 3 days. Tab: 0.4 to 0.8 mg PO 1 h before travel and q 8 h prn. [Trade only: Topical disc 1.5 mg/72 h, box of 4. Oral tab 0.4 mg.] ▶L ♀C ▶+ $$

THIETHYLPERAZINE (*Torecan*) 10 mg PO/IM one to three times per day. [Trade only: Tabs 10 mg.] ▶L ♀? ▶? $

TRIMETHOBENZAMIDE (*Tigan*) 300 mg PO q 6 to 8 h, 200 mg IM q 6 to 8 h. [Generic/Trade: Cap 300 mg.] ▶LK ♀C ▶? $

Antiulcer—Antacids

ALKA-SELTZER (acetylsalicylic acid + citrate + bicarbonate) 2 regular-strength tabs in 4 oz water q 4 h PO prn (up to 8 tabs daily for age younger than 60 years, up to 4 tabs daily for age 60 years or older) or 2 extra-strength tabs in 4 oz water q 6 h PO prn (up to 7 tabs daily for age younger than 60 years, up to 3 tabs daily for age 60 years or older). [OTC Trade only: Regular-strength, original: aspirin 325 mg + citric acid 1000 mg + sodium bicarbonate 1916 mg. Regular-strength lemon lime and cherry: 325 mg + 1000 mg + 1700 mg. Extra-strength: 500 mg + 1000 mg + 1985 mg. Not all forms of Alka Seltzer contain aspirin (eg, Alka Seltzer Heartburn Relief).] ▶LK ♀? (- 3rd trimester) ▶? $

ALUMINUM HYDROXIDE (*Alternagel, Amphojel, Alu-Tab, Alu-Cap, ✦ Basalgel, Mucaine*) 5 to 10 mL or 300 to 600 mg PO up to 6 times per day. Constipating. [OTC Generic/Trade: Susp 320, 600 mg/ 5 mL.] ▶LK ♀C ▶? $

CITROCARBONATE (bicarbonate + citrate) 1 to 2 teaspoons in cold water PO 15 min to 2 h after meals prn. [OTC Trade only: Sodium bicarbonate 0.78 g + sodium citrate anhydrous 1.82 g in each 1 teaspoonful 150, 300 g.] ▶K ♀? ▶? $

GAVISCON (aluminum hydroxide + magnesium carbonate) 2 to 4 tabs or 15 to 30 mL (regular-strength) or 10 mL (extra-strength) PO four times per day prn. [OTC Trade only: Tabs: Regular-strength (Al hydroxide 80 mg + Mg carbonate 20 mg), Extra-strength (Al hydroxide 160 mg + Mg carbonate 105 mg). Liquid: Regular-strength (Al hydroxide 95 mg + Mg carbonate 358 mg per 15 mL), Extra-strength (Al hydroxide 254 mg + Mg carbonate 237.5 mg per 5 mL).] ▶K ♀? ▶? $

MAALOX (aluminum hydroxide + magnesium hydroxide) 10 to 20 mL or 1 to 2 tabs PO prn. [OTC Generic/Trade: Regular-strength chewable tabs (Al hydroxide + Mg hydroxide 200/200 mg), susp (225/200 mg per 5 mL). Other strengths available.] ▶K ♀C ▶? $

MAGALDRATE   *(Riopan Plus)* 5 to 10 mL PO prn. [OTC Trade only: Riopan Plus (with simethicone) available as susp 540/20 mg/5 mL.] ▶K ♀C ▶? $

MYLANTA   (aluminum hydroxide + magnesium hydroxide + simethicone) 10 to 20 mL PO between meals and at bedtime prn. [OTC Generic/Trade: Liquid (various concentrations, eg, regular-strength, maximum-strength, supreme, etc).] ▶K ♀C ▶? $

ROLAIDS   (calcium carbonate + magnesium hydroxide) 2 to 4 tabs PO q 1 h prn, max 12 tabs/day (regular-strength) or 10 tabs/day (extra-strength). [OTC Trade only: Tabs: Regular-strength (Ca carbonate 550 mg, Mg hydroxide 110 mg), Extra-strength (Ca carbonate 675 mg, Mg hydroxide 135 mg).] ▶K ♀? ▶? $

Antiulcer—H2 Antagonists

CIMETIDINE   *(Tagamet, Tagamet HB)* 300 mg IV/IM/PO q 6 to 8 h, 400 mg PO two times per day, or 400 to 800 mg PO at bedtime. <u>Erosive esophagitis:</u> 800 mg PO two times per day or 400 mg PO four times per day. Continuous IV infusion 37.5 to 50 mg/h (900 to 1200 mg/day). [Tabs 200, 300, 400, 800 mg. Rx Generic only: Oral soln 300 mg/5 mL. OTC Generic/Trade: Tabs 200 mg.] ▶LK ♀B ▶+ $

FAMOTIDINE   *(Pepcid, Pepcid AC, Maximum Strength Pepcid AC)* 20 mg IV q 12 h, 20 to 40 mg PO at bedtime, or 20 mg PO two times per day. [Generic/Trade: Tabs 10 mg (OTC, Pepcid AC Acid Controller), 20 mg (Rx and OTC, Maximum Strength Pepcid AC), 40 mg. Rx Generic/Trade: Susp 40 mg/5 mL.] ▶LK ♀B ▶? $

NIZATIDINE   *(Axid, Axid AR)* 150 to 300 mg PO at bedtime, or 150 mg PO two times per day. [OTC Trade only (Axid AR): Tabs 75 mg. Rx Trade only: Rx Generic/Trade: Caps 150 mg. Oral soln 15 mg/mL (120, 480 mL). Generic: Caps 300 mg.] ▶LK ♀B ▶? $$$$

PEPCID COMPLETE   (famotidine + calcium carbonate + magnesium hydroxide) <u>Treatment of heartburn:</u> 1 tab PO prn. Max 2 tabs/day. [OTC trade/generic: Chewable tab, famotidine 10 mg with calcium carbonate 800 mg and magnesium hydroxide 165 mg.] ▶LK ♀B ▶? $

RANITIDINE   *(Zantac, Zantac Efferdose, Zantac 75, Zantac 150, Peptic Relief)* 150 mg PO two times per day or 300 mg PO at bedtime. 50 mg IV/IM q 8 h, or continuous infusion 6.25 mg/h (150 mg/day). [Generic/Trade: Tabs 75 mg (OTC: Zantac 75), 150 mg (OTC and Rx: Zantac 150), 300 mg. Syrup 75 mg/5 mL. Rx Trade only: Effervescent tabs 25 mg. Rx Generic only: Caps 150, 300 mg.] ▶K ♀B ▶? $$$

Antiulcer—Helicobacter pylori Treatment

HELIDAC   (bismuth subsalicylate + metronidazole + tetracycline) 1 dose PO four times per day for 2 weeks. To be given with an H2 antagonist. [Trade only: Each dose consists of bismuth subsalicylate 524 mg (2 × 262 mg) chewable tab + metronidazole 250 mg tab + tetracycline 500 mg cap.] ▶LK ♀D ▶− $$$$$

HELICOBACTER PYLORI THERAPY

- Triple therapy PO for 10 to 14 days: clarithromycin 500 mg two times per day + amoxicillin 1 g two times per day (or metronidazole 500 mg two times per day) + PPI*
- Quadruple therapy PO for 14 days: bismuth subsalicylate 525 mg (or 30 mL) three to four times per day plus metronidazole 500 mg three to four times per day plus tetracycline 500 mg three to four times per day plus a PPI* or a H2 blocker†
- PPI or H2 blocker may need to be continued past 14 days to heal the ulcer.

*PPIs include esomeprazole 40 mg daily, lansoprazole 30 mg two times per day, omeprazole 20 mg two times per day, pantoprazole 40 mg two times per day, rabeprazole 20 mg two times per day. †H₂ blockers include cimetidine 400 mg two times per day, famotidine 20 mg two times per day, nizatidine 150 mg two times per day, ranitidine 150 mg two times per day. Adapted from *Medical Letter Treatment Guidelines* 2008:55.

PREVPAC (lansoprazole + amoxicillin + clarithromycin, ✦HP-Pac) 1 dose PO two times per day for 10 to 14 days. [Trade only: Each dose consists of lansoprazole 30 mg cap + amoxicillin 1 g (2 × 500 mg cap), + clarithromycin 500 mg tab.] ▶LK ♀C ▶? $$$$$

PYLERA (bismuth subcitrate potassium + metronidazole + tetracycline) 3 caps PO four times per day (after meals and at bedtime) for 10 days. Use with omeprazole 20 mg PO two times per day. [Trade only: Each cap contains biskalcitrate 140 mg + metronidazole 125 mg + tetracycline 125 mg.] ▶LK ♀D ▶– $$$$$

Antiulcer—Proton Pump Inhibitors

NOTE: *May increase levels of diazepam, warfarin, and phenytoin. May decrease absorption of ketoconazole, itraconazole, iron, ampicillin, and digoxin. Reduces plasma levels of atazanavir. Avoid administration with sucralfate.*

DEXLANSOPRAZOLE (*Dexilant*) Erosive esophagitis: 60 mg PO daily for up to 8 weeks. Maintenance therapy after healing of erosive esophagitis: 30 mg PO daily for up to 6 months. GERD: 30 mg PO daily for up to 4 weeks. [Trade only: Cap 30, 60 mg.] ▶L ♀B ▶? $$$$

ESOMEPRAZOLE (*Nexium*) Erosive esophagitis: 20 to 40 mg PO daily for 4 to 8 weeks. Maintenance of erosive esophagitis: 20 mg PO daily. Zollinger-Ellison: 40 mg PO two times per day for 4 to 8 weeks. GERD: 20 mg PO daily for 4 weeks. GERD with esophagitis: 20 to 40 mg IV daily for 10 days until taking PO. Prevention of NSAID-associated gastric ulcer: 20 to 40 mg PO daily for up to 6 months. H. pylori eradication: 40 mg PO daily with amoxicillin 1000 mg PO two times per day and clarithromycin 500 mg PO two times per day for 10 days. [Trade only: Cap delayed-release 20, 40 mg. Delayed-release granules for oral susp 10, 20, 40 mg per packet.] ▶L ♀B ▶? $$$$

LANSOPRAZOLE (*Prevacid*) Heartburn: 15 mg PO daily. Duodenal ulcer or maintenance therapy after healing of duodenal ulcer: 15 mg PO daily for up to 12 months. NSAID-induced gastric ulcer: 30 mg PO daily for 8 weeks (treatment), 15 mg PO daily for up to 12 weeks (prevention). GERD: 15 mg PO daily. Gastric ulcer: 30 mg PO daily. Erosive esophagitis: 30 mg PO daily for up to 8 weeks or 30 mg IV daily for 7 days or until taking PO. [OTC

(cont.)

Trade only: Caps 15 mg. Rx Generic/Trade: 15, 30 mg. Rx Trade only: Orally disintegrating tab 15, 30 mg. Prevacid NapraPac: 7 lansoprazole 15 mg caps packaged with 14 naproxen tabs 375 mg or 500 mg.] ▶L ♀B ▶? $$$

OMEPRAZOLE (*Prilosec,* ✦ *Losec*) GERD, duodenal ulcer, erosive esophagitis: 20 mg PO daily. Heartburn (OTC): 20 mg PO daily for 14 days. Gastric ulcer: 40 mg PO daily. Hypersecretory conditions: 60 mg PO daily. [Rx Generic/Trade: Caps 10, 20, 40 mg. Trade only: Granules for oral susp 2.5 mg, 10 mg. OTC Trade only: Cap 20 mg.] ▶L ♀C ▶? OTC $, Rx $$$$

PANTOPRAZOLE (*Protonix,* ✦ *Pantoloc*) GERD: 40 mg PO daily. Zollinger-Ellison syndrome: 80 mg IV q 8 to 12 h for 7 days until taking PO. GERD associated with a history of erosive esophagitis: 40 mg IV daily for 7 to 10 days until taking PO. [Generic/Trade: Tabs 20, 40 mg. Trade only: Granules for susp 40 mg/packet.] ▶L ♀B ▶? $$$$

RABEPRAZOLE (*AcipHex,* ✦ *Pariet*) 20 mg PO daily. [Trade: Tabs 20 mg.] ▶L ♀B ▶? $$$$

ZEGERID (**omeprazole + bicarbonate**) Duodenal ulcer, GERD, erosive esophagitis: 20 mg PO daily for 4 to 8 weeks. Gastric ulcer: 40 mg PO once daily for 4 to 8 weeks. Reduction of risk of upper GI bleed in critically ill (susp only): 40 mg PO, then 40 mg 6 to 8 h later, then 40 mg once daily thereafter for up to 14 days. [OTC Trade only: omeprazole/sodium bicarbonate caps 20 mg/1 g. Rx Trade only: 20 mg/1.1 g and 40 mg/1.68 g, powder packets for susp 20 mg/1.1 g and 40 mg/1.68 g.] ▶L ♀C ▶? $$$$$

Antiulcer—Other

DICYCLOMINE (*Bentyl,* ✦ *Bentylol*) 10 to 20 mg PO/IM four times per day up to 40 mg PO four times per day. [Generic/Trade: Tabs 20 mg. Caps 10 mg. Syrup 10 mg/5 mL.] ▶LK ♀B ▶– $

DONNATAL (**phenobarbital + hyoscyamine + atropine + scopolamine**) 1 to 2 tabs/caps or 5 to 10 mL PO three to four times per day. 1 extended-release tab PO q 8 to 12 h. [Generic/trade: Phenobarbital 16.2 mg + hyoscyamine 0.1 mg + atropine 0.02 mg + scopolamine 6.5 mcg in each tab or 5 mL. Trade only: Extended-release tab 48.6 + 0.3111 + 0.0582 + 0.0195 mg.] ▶LK ♀C ▶– $$$

GI COCKTAIL (**"green goddess"**) Acute GI upset: Mixture of Maalox/Mylanta 30 mL + viscous lidocaine (2%) 10 mL + Donnatal 10 mL administered PO in a single dose. ▶LK ♀See individual ▶See individual $

HYOSCINE (✦ *Buscopan*) Canada only: GI or bladder spasm: 10 to 20 mg PO/IV up to 60 mg daily (PO) or 100 mg daily (IV). [Canada Trade only: Tabs 10 mg.] ▶LK ♀C ▶? $$

HYOSCYAMINE (*Anaspaz, A-spaz, Cystospaz, ED Spaz, Hyosol, Hyospaz, Levbid, Levsin, Levsinex, Medispaz, NuLev, Spacol, Spasdel, Symax*) Bladder spasm, control gastric secretion, GI hypermotility, irritable bowel syndrome: 0.125 to 0.25 mg PO/SL q 4 h or prn. Extended-release: 0.375 to 0.75 mg PO q 12 h. Max 1.5 mg/day. [Generic/Trade: Tabs 0.125. Sublingual tabs 0.125 mg. Chewable tabs 0.125 mg. Extended-release tabs 0.375 mg. Elixir 0.125 mg/5 mL. Gtts 0.125 mg/1 mL.] ▶LK ♀C ▶– $

MEPENZOLATE (*Cantil*) 25 to 50 mg PO four times per day, with meals and at bedtime. [Trade only: Tabs 25 mg.] ▶K + gut ♀B ▶? $$$$$

MISOPROSTOL (*PGE1, Cytotec*) <u>Prevention of NSAID–induced gastric ulcers:</u> Start 100 mcg PO two times per day, then titrate as tolerated up to 200 mcg PO four times per day. <u>Cervical ripening:</u> 25 mcg intravaginally q 3 to 6 h (or 50 mcg q 6 h). <u>First trimester pregnancy failure:</u> 800 mcg intravaginally, repeat on day 3 if expulsion incomplete. [Generic/Trade: Oral tabs 100, 200 mcg.] ▶LK ♀X ▶– $$$$ ■

PROPANTHELINE (*Pro-Banthine*) 7.5 to 15 mg PO 30 min after meals and 30 mg at bedtime. [Generic only: Tabs 15 mg.] ▶LK ♀C ▶– $$$

SIMETHICONE (*Mylicon, Gas-X, Phazyme, ✦ Ovol*) 40 to 360 mg PO four times per day prn, max 500 mg/day. Infants: 20 mg PO four times per day prn. [OTC Generic/Trade: Chewable tabs 80, 125 mg. Gtts 40 mg/0.6 mL. Trade only: Softgels 166 mg (Gas-X) 180 mg (Phazyme). Strips, oral (Gas-X) 62.5 mg (adults), 40 mg (children).] ▶Not absorbed ♀C but + ▶? $

SUCRALFATE (*Carafate, ✦ Sulcrate*) 1 g PO 1 h before meals (2 h before other medications) and at bedtime. [Generic/Trade: Tabs 1 g. Susp 1 g/10 mL.] ▶Not absorbed ♀B ▶? $$

Laxatives—Bulk-Forming

METHYLCELLULOSE (*Citrucel*) 1 heaping tbsp in 8 oz water PO daily (up to three times per day). [OTC Trade only: Regular and sugar-free packets and multiple-use canisters, Clear-mix soln, Caps 500 mg.] ▶Not absorbed ♀+ ▶? $

POLYCARBOPHIL (*FiberCon, Konsyl Fiber, Equalactin*) <u>Laxative:</u> 2 tabs (1250 mg) PO four times per day prn. <u>Diarrhea:</u> 2 tabs (1250 mg) PO q 30 min. Max daily dose 6 g. [OTC Generic/Trade: Tabs/Caps 625 mg. OTC Trade only: Chewable tabs 625 mg (Equalactin).] ▶Not absorbed ♀+ ▶? $

PSYLLIUM (*Metamucil, Fiberall, Konsyl, Hydrocil, ✦ Prodium Plain*) 1 tsp in liquid, 1 packet in liquid, or 1 to 2 wafers with liquid PO daily (up to three times per day). [OTC Generic/Trade: Regular and sugar-free powder, Granules, Caps, Wafers, including various flavors and various amounts of psyllium.] ▶Not absorbed ♀+ ▶? $

Laxatives—Osmotic

GLYCERIN (*Fleet*) 1 adult or infant supp or 5 mL to 15 mL as an enema PR prn. [OTC Generic/Trade: Supp infant and adult, Soln (Fleet Babylax) 4 mL/applicator.] ▶Not absorbed ♀C ▶? $

LACTULOSE (*Enulose, Kristalose*) <u>Constipation:</u> 15 to 30 mL (syrup) or 10 to 20 g (powder for oral soln) PO daily. <u>Hepatic encephalopathy:</u> 30 to 45 mL (syrup) PO three to four times per day, or 300 mL retention enema. [Generic/Trade: Syrup 10 g/15 mL. Trade only (Kristalose): 10, 20 g packets for oral soln.] ▶Not absorbed ♀B ▶? $$

MAGNESIUM CITRATE (✤ *Citro-Mag*) 150 to 300 mL PO once or in divided doses. 2 to 4 mL/kg/day once or in divided doses for age younger than 6 yo. [OTC Generic only: Soln 300 mL/bottle. Low-sodium and sugar-free available.] ▶K ♀B ▶? $

MAGNESIUM HYDROXIDE (*Milk of Magnesia*) Laxative: 30 to 60 mL regular-strength (400 mg per 5 mL) liquid PO. Antacid: 5 to 15 mL regular-strength liquid or 622 to 1244 mg PO four times per day prn. [OTC Generic/Trade: Susp 400 mg/5 mL. Trade only: Chewable tabs 311, 400 mg. Generic only: Susp 800 mg/5 mL, (concentrated) 1200 mg/5 mL, sugar-free 400 mg/5 mL.] ▶K ♀+ ▶? $

POLYETHYLENE GLYCOL (*MiraLax, GlycoLax*) 17 g (1 heaping tablespoon) in 4 to 8 oz water, juice, soda, coffee, or tea PO daily. [OTC Trade only: Powder for oral soln 17 g/scoop. Rx Generic/Trade: Powder for oral soln 17 g/scoop.] ▶Not absorbed ♀C ▶? $

POLYETHYLENE GLYCOL WITH ELECTROLYTES (*GoLytely, Colyte, TriLyte, NuLytely, Moviprep, HalfLytely, and Bisacodyl Tablet Kit, ✤ Klean-Prep, Electropeg, Peg-Lyte*) Bowel prep: 240 mL q 10 min PO or 20 to 30 mL/min per NG until 4 L is consumed. Moviprep: Follow specific instructions. [Generic/Trade: Powder for oral solution in disposable jug 4 L or 2 L (Moviprep). Also, as a kit of 2 L of polyethylene glycol with electrolytes and 2 or 4 bisacodyl tabs 5 mg (HalfLytely and Bisacodyl Tablet Kit). Trade only (GoLytely): Packet for oral solution to make 3.785 L.] ▶Not absorbed ♀C ▶? $

SODIUM PHOSPHATE (*Fleet enema, Fleet Phospho-Soda, Fleet EZ-Prep, Accu-Prep, Osmoprep, Visicol, ✤ Enemol, Phoslax*) 1 adult or pediatric enema PR or 20 to 30 mL of oral soln PO prn (max 45 mL/24 h). Visicol: Evening before colonoscopy: 3 tabs with 8 oz clear liquid q 15 min until 20 tabs are consumed. Day of colonoscopy: Starting 3 to 5 h before procedure, 3 tabs with 8 oz clear liquid q 15 min until 20 tabs are consumed. Osmoprep: 32 tabs PO with total of 2 quarts clear liquids as follows: pm before procedure: 4 tabs PO with 8 oz of clear liquids q 15 min for a total of 20 tabs; day of procedure: 3 to 5 h before procedure, 4 tabs with 8 oz of clear liquids q 15 min for a total of 12 tabs. [OTC Generic/Trade: Adult enema, oral soln. OTC Trade only: Pediatric enema, bowel prep. Rx Trade only: Visicol, Osmoprep tab ($$$$) 1.5 g.] ▶Not absorbed ♀C ▶? $ ■

SORBITOL 30 to 150 mL (of 70% soln) PO or 120 mL (of 25 to 30% soln) PR as a single dose. Cathartic: 4.3 mL/kg PO. [Generic only: Soln 70%.] ▶Not absorbed ♀C ▶? $

Laxatives—Stimulant

BISACODYL (*Correctol, Dulcolax, Feen-a-Mint, Fleet*) 5 to 15 mg PO prn, 10 mg PR prn, 5 to 10 mg PR prn if 2 to 11 yo. [OTC Generic/Trade: Tabs 5 mg, suppository 10 mg. OTC Trade only (Fleet): Enema, 10 mg/30 mL.] ▶L ♀C ▶? $

CASCARA 325 mg PO at bedtime prn or 5 mL of aromatic fluid extract PO at bedtime prn. [OTC Generic only: Tabs 325 mg, liquid aromatic fluid extract.] ▶L ♀C ▶+ $

CASTOR OIL Children: 5 to 15 mL/dose of castor oil PO or 7.5 to 30 mL emulsified castor oil PO once per day. Adult: 15 to 60 mL of castor oil or 30 to 60 mL emulsified castor oil PO once per day. [OTC Generic only: Oil 60, 120, 180, 480 mL.] ▶Not absorbed ♀− ▶? $

SENNA (*Senokot, SenokotXTRA, Ex-Lax, Fletcher's Castoria, ✦ Glysennid*) 2 tabs or 1 teaspoon granules or 10 to 15 mL syrup PO. Max 8 tabs, 4 teaspoon granules, 30 mL syrup/day. Take granules with full glass of water. [OTC Generic/Trade (All dosing is based on sennosides content; 1 mg sennosides is equivalent to 21.7 mg standardized senna concentrate): Syrup 8.8 mg/5 mL, Liquid 33.3 mg senna concentrate/mL (Fletcher's Castoria), Tabs 8.6, 15, 17, 25 mg, Chewable tabs 10, 15 mg.] ▶L ♀C ▶+ $

Laxatives—Stool Softener

DOCUSATE (*Colace, Surfak, Kaopectate Stool Softener, Enemeez*) Docusate calcium: 240 mg PO daily. Docusate sodium: 50 to 500 mg/day PO divided in 1 to 4 doses. Peds: 10 to 40 mg/day for age younger than 3 yo, give 20 to 60 mg/day for age 3 to 6 yo, give 40 to 150 mg/day for age 6 to 12 yo. In all cases doses are divided up to four times per day. Cerumen impaction: 1 mL in affected ear. [Docusate calcium OTC Generic/Trade: Caps 240 mg. Docusate sodium OTC Generic/Trade: Caps 50, 100, 250 mg. Liquid 50 mg/5 mL. Syrup 20 mg/5 mL. Docusate sodium OTC Trade only (Enemeez): Enema, rectal 283 mg/5 mL.] ▶L ♀C ▶? $

Laxatives—Other or Combinations

LUBIPROSTONE (*Amitiza*) Chronic idiopathic constipation: 24 mcg PO two times per day with food and water. Irritable bowel syndrome with constipation in women age 18 yo or older: 8 mcg PO two times per day. [Trade only: Cap 8, 24 mcg.] ▶Gut ♀C ▶? $$$$$

MINERAL OIL (*Kondremul, Fleet Mineral Oil Enema, Liqui-Doss, ✦ Lansoyl*) 15 to 45 mL PO. Peds: 5 to 15 mL/dose PO. Mineral oil enema: 60 to 150 mL PR. Peds: 30 to 60 mL PR. [OTC Generic/Trade: Oil (30, 480 mL), Enema (Fleet). OTC Trade only: Oral liquid (Liqui-Doss) 13.5 mg/15 mL. Oral microemulsion (Kondremul) 2.5 mg/5 mL.] ▶Not absorbed ♀C ▶? $

PERI-COLACE (docusate + sennosides) 2 to 4 tabs PO once daily or in divided doses prn. [OTC Generic/Trade: Tabs 50 mg docusate + 8.6 mg sennosides.] ▶L ♀C ▶? $

SENOKOT-S (senna + docusate) 2 tabs PO daily. [OTC Generic/Trade: Tabs 8.6 mg senna concentrate + 50 mg docusate.] ▶L ♀C ▶+ $

Ulcerative Colitis

BALSALAZIDE (*Colazal*) 2.25 g PO three times per day for 8 to 12 weeks. [Generic/Trade: Caps 750 mg.] ▶Minimal absorption ♀B ▶? $$$$$

MESALAMINE (5-aminosalicylic *acid, Apriso, 5-Aspirin, Asacol, Lialda, Pentasa, Canasa, Rowasa, ✦ Mesasal, Salofalk*) Apriso: 1.5 g (4 caps) PO q am. Asacol: 800 to 1600 mg PO three times per day. Pentasa: 1000 mg PO four times per day. Lialda: 2.4 to 4.8 g PO daily with a meal. Canasa: 500 mg PR two to three times per day or 1000 mg PR at bedtime Susp: 4 g enema PR at bedtime (retain 8 h) for 3 to 6 weeks. [Trade only: Delayed-release tab 400 mg (Asacol), 800 mg (Asacol HD). Controlled-release cap 250, 500 mg (Pentasa). Delayed-release tab 1200 mg (Lialda). Rectal suppository 1000 mg (Canasa). Controlled-release cap 0.375 g (Apriso). Generic/Trade: Rectal susp 4 g/60 mL (Rowasa).] ▶Gut ♀C ▶? $$$$$

OLSALAZINE (*Dipentum*) Ulcerative colitis: 500 mg PO two times per day with food. [Trade only: Caps 250 mg.] ▶L ♀C ▶– $$$$$

SULFASALAZINE (*Azulfidine, Azulfidine EN-tabs, ✦ Salazopyrin En-tabs, S.A.S.*) Colitis: 500 to 1000 mg PO four times per day. Peds: 30 to 60 mg/kg/day divided q 4 to 6 h. RA: 500 mg PO two times per day after meals up to 1 g PO two times per day. May turn body fluids, contact lenses, or skin orange-yellow. [Generic/Trade: Tabs 500 mg, scored. Enteric-coated, Delayed-release (EN-tabs) 500 mg.] ▶L ♀D ▶– $$

Other GI Agents

ALOSETRON (*Lotronex*) Diarrhea-predominant irritable bowel syndrome in women who have failed conventional therapy: 0.5 mg PO two times per day for 4 weeks; discontinue in patients who become constipated. If well tolerated and symptoms not controlled after 4 weeks, may increase to 1 mg PO two times per day. Discontinue if symptoms not controlled in 4 weeks on 1 mg PO two times per day. [Trade only: Tabs 0.5, 1 mg.] ▶L ♀B ▶? $$$$$ ■

ALPHA-GALACTOSIDASE (*Beano*) 5 gtts or 1 tab per ½ cup gassy food, 2 to 3 tabs PO (chew, swallow, crumble) or 1 melt-away tab or 10 gtts per typical meal. [OTC Trade only: Oral gtts, tabs, melt-away tabs.] ▶Minimal absorption ♀? ▶? $

ALVIMOPAN (*Entereg*) Short-term (up to 15 doses) in hospitalized patients undergoing partial large or small bowel resection surgery with primary anastomosis: 12 mg PO 30 min to 5 h prior to surgery, then 12 mg PO two times per day starting the day after surgery for up to 7 days. [Trade only: Caps 12 mg.] ▶Intestinal flora ♀B ▶? ? ■

BUDESONIDE (*Entocort EC*) Crohn's: 9 mg PO daily for up to 8 weeks (remission induction) or 6 mg PO daily for 3 months (maintenance). [Trade only: Caps 3 mg.] ▶L ♀C ▶? $$$$$

CERTOLIZUMAB (*Cimzia*) Crohn's: 400 mg SC at 0, 2, and 4 weeks. If response occurs, then 400 mg SC q 4 weeks. Rheumatoid arthritis: 400 mg SC at 0, 2, and 4 weeks. [Trade only: 400 mg kit.] ▶Plasma, K ♀B ▶? $$$$$ ■

CHLORDIAZEPOXIDE-CLIDINIUM (*Librax*) 1 cap PO three to four times per day. [Generic/Trade: Caps, chlordiazepoxide 5 mg + clidinium 2.5 mg.] ▶K ♀D ▶– $$$

GLYCOPYRROLATE *(Robinul, Robinul Forte, Cuvposa)* <u>Peptic ulcer disease</u>: 1 to 2 mg PO two to three times per day. <u>Chronic drooling in children</u> (Cuvposa): 0.02 mg/kg PO three times per day. [Trade: Solution 1 mg/5 mL (480 mL, Cuvposa). Generic/Trade: Tabs 1, 2 mg.] ▶K ♀B ▶? $$$$

LACTASE *(Lactaid)* Swallow or chew 3 caps (Original strength), 2 caps (Extra strength), 1 cap (Ultra) with first bite of dairy foods. Adjust dose based on response. [OTC Generic/Trade: Caps, Chewable tabs.] ▶Not absorbed ♀+ ▶+ $

METHYLNALTREXONE *(Relistor)* <u>Opioid-induced constipation</u>: Less than 38 kg: 0.15 mg/kg SC every other day; 38 kg to 61 kg: 8 mg SC every other day; 62 kg to 114 kg: 12 mg SC every other day. 0.15 mg/kg SC every other day. [Injectable soln 12 mg/0.6 mL.] ▶unchanged ♀B ▶? $$$$$

NEOMYCIN—ORAL *(Neo-Fradin)* <u>Hepatic encephalopathy</u>: 4 to 12 g/day PO divided q 4 to 6 h. Peds: 50 to 100 mg/kg/day PO divided q 6 to 8 h. [Generic only: Tabs 500 mg. Trade only: Soln 125 mg/5 mL.] ▶Minimally absorbed ♀D ▶? $$$

OCTREOTIDE *(Sandostatin, Sandostatin LAR)* <u>Variceal bleeding</u>: Bolus 25 to 50 mcg IV followed by infusion 25 to 50 mcg/h. <u>AIDS diarrhea</u>: 25 to 250 mcg SC three times per day. [Generic/Trade: Injection vials 0.05, 0.1, 0.2, 0.5, 1 mg. Trade only: Long-acting injectable susp (Sandostatin LAR) 10, 20, 30 mg.] ▶LK ♀B ▶? $$$$$

ORLISTAT *(Alli, Xenical)* <u>Weight loss</u>: 60 to 120 mg PO three times per day with meals. [OTC Trade only (Alli): Caps 60 mg. Rx Trade only (Xenical): Caps 120 mg.] ▶Gut ♀R ▶? $$$

PANCREATIN *(Creon, Ku-Zyme, ✦ Entozyme)* 8000 to 24,000 units lipase (1 to 2 tabs/caps) PO with meals and snacks. [Tabs, Caps with varying amounts of lipase, amylase, and protease.] ▶Gut ♀C ▶? $$$

PANCRELIPASE *(Creon, Pancreaze, Viokase, Pancrease, Pancrecarb, Cotazym, Ku-Zyme HP, Zenpep)* Varies by weight. Initial infant dose 2000 to 4000 lipase units per 120 mL formula or breast milk. 12 mo or older to younger than 4 yo: 1000 lipase units/kg PO. 4 yo or older: 500 lipase units/kg per meal PO, max 2500 lipase units/kg per meal. [Tabs, Caps, Powder with varying amounts of lipase, amylase, and protease.] ▶Gut ♀C ▶? $$$

PINAVERIUM *(✦ Dicetel)* Canada only. <u>IBS</u>: 50 to 100 mg PO three times per day. [Trade only: tabs 50, 100 mg.] ▶? ♀C ▶– $$$

SECRETIN *(SecreFlo, ChiRhoStim)* Test dose 0.2 mcg IV. If tolerated, 0.2 to 0.4 mcg/kg IV over 1 min. ▶Serum ♀C ▶? $$$$$

URSODIOL *(Actigall, URSO, URSO Forte)* <u>Gallstone solution</u> (Actigall): 8 to 10 mg/kg/day PO divided two to three times per day. <u>Prevention of gallstones associated with rapid wt loss</u> (Actigall): 300 mg PO two times per day. <u>Primary biliary cirrhosis</u> (URSO): 13 to 15 mg/kg/day PO divided in 2 to 4 doses. [Generic/Trade: Caps 300 mg, Tabs 250, 500 mg.] ▶Bile ♀B ▶? $$$$

HEMATOLOGY

Anticoagulants—Direct Thrombin Inhibitors

NOTE: *See cardiovascular section for antiplatelet drugs and thrombolytics*

ARGATROBAN HIT: Start 2 mcg/kg/min IV infusion. Get PTT at baseline and 2 h after starting infusion. Adjust dose (max dose: 10 mcg/kg/min) until PTT is 1.5 to 3 times baseline (not more than 100 sec). ACCP recommends starting at lower doses of 0.5 to 1.2 mcg/kg/min in patients with heart failure, multiorgan failure, anasarca, or post-cardiac surgery. ▶L ♀B ▶– $$$$$

BIVALIRUDIN (*Angiomax*) Anticoagulation during PCI (patients with or at risk of HIT): 0.75 mg/kg IV bolus prior to intervention, then 1.75 mg/kg/h for duration of procedure (with provisional GPIIb/IIIa inhibition). For CrCl less than 30 mL/min, reduce infusion dose to 1 mg/kg/h after bolus. Use with aspirin 300 to 325 mg PO daily. Additional bolus of 0.3 mg/kg if activated clotting time less than 225 sec. ▶proteolysis/K ♀B ▶? $$$$$

DABIGATRAN (*Pradaxa*) Stroke prevention in atrial fibrillation: 150 mg PO two times per day (if CrCl 15 to 30 mL/min: 75 mg PO two times per day). ▶K ♀ C ▶? $$$$$

DESIRUDIN (*Iprivask*) DVT prophylaxis (hip replacement surgery): 15 mg SC q 12 h (if CrCl 31 to 60 mL/min give 5 mg SC q 12 h). ▶K ♀C ▶? ■

LEPIRUDIN (*Refludan*) Anticoagulation in HIT and associated thromboembolic disease: Bolus 0.4 mg/kg up to 44 mg IV over 15 to 20 sec, then infuse 0.15 mg/kg/h up to 16.5 mg/h. Alternate initial dosing recommended by ACCP: Bolus 0.2 mg/kg IV (bolus only if life- or limb-threatening thrombosis) then infuse 0.05 to 0.1 mg/kg/h. Adjust dose to maintain PTT ratio of 1.5 to 2.5. ▶K ♀B ▶? $$$$$

Anticoagulants—Factor Xa Inhibitors

FONDAPARINUX (*Arixtra*) DVT prophylaxis, hip/knee replacement or hip fracture surgery, abdominal surgery: 2.5 mg SC daily starting 6 to 8 h post-op. DVT/PE treatment based on wt: 5 mg (if wt less than 50 kg), 7.5 mg (if 50 to 100 kg), 10 mg (if wt greater than 100 kg) SC daily for at least 5 days and therapeutic oral anticoagulation. [Trade/generic: Prefilled syringes 2.5 mg/0.5 mL, 5 mg/0.4 mL, 7.5 mg/0.6 mL, 10 mg/0.8 mL.] ▶K ♀B ▶? $$$$$

RIVAROXABAN (*Xarelto*) DVT prophylaxis in knee or hip replacement: 10 mg PO daily. [Trade only: Tabs 10 mg.] ▶K– ♀C ▶?

Anticoagulants—Low Molecular Weight Heparins (LMWH)

DALTEPARIN (*Fragmin*) DVT prophylaxis, acute medical illness with restricted mobility: 5000 units SC daily. DVT prophylaxis, abdominal surgery: 2500 units SC 1 to 2 h pre-op and daily post-op. DVT prophylaxis, abdominal surgery in patients with malignancy: 5000 units SC evening before surgery and daily post-op, or 2500 units 1 to 2 h pre-op and 12 h later, then 5000 units daily. DVT prophylaxis, hip replacement: Pre-op start (day of surgery): 2500 units SC

(cont.)

given 2 h pre-op, 4 to 8 h post-op, then 5000 units daily starting at least 6 h after 2nd dose, or 5000 units 10 to 14 h pre-op, 4 to 8 h post-op, then daily (approximately 24 h between doses). Pre-op start (evening before surgery): 5000 units SC given evening before surgery then 5000 units daily starting at least 4 to 8 h post-op (approximately 24 h between doses). Post-op start: 2500 units 4 to 8 h post-op, then 5000 units daily starting at least 6 h after first dose. <u>Treatment of DVT/PE in cancer:</u> 200 units/kg SC daily for 1 month, then 150 units/kg SC daily for 5 months; max 18,000 units/day. <u>Unstable angina or non-Q-wave MI:</u> 120 units/kg up to 10,000 units SC q 12 h with aspirin (75 to 165 mg/day PO) until clinically stable. [Trade only: Single-dose syringes 2500, 5000 units/0.2 mL, 7500 units/0.3 mL, 10,000 units/1 mL, 12,500 units/0.5 mL, 15,000 units/0.6 mL, 18,000 units/0.72 mL; multidose vial 10,000 units/mL, 9.5 mL and 25,000 units/mL, 3.8 mL.] ▶KL ♀B ▶+ $$$$$ ■

ENOXAPARIN (Lovenox) <u>DVT prophylaxis, acute medical illness with restricted mobility:</u> 40 mg SC daily (if CrCl < 30 mL/min: give 30 mg SC daily). <u>DVT prophylaxis, hip/knee replacement:</u> 30 mg SC q 12 h starting 12 to 24 h post-op (if CrCl < 30 mL/min: give 30 mg SC daily). <u>Hip replacement, pre-op start:</u> 40 mg SC daily starting 12 h pre-op. <u>Abdominal surgery:</u> 40 mg SC daily starting 2 h pre-op (if CrCl < 30 mL/min: give 30 mg SC daily). <u>Outpatient treatment of DVT without pulmonary embolus:</u> 1 mg/kg SC q 12 h. Continue for at least 5 days and until therapeutic oral anticoagulation. <u>Inpatient treatment of DVT with/without pulmonary embolus:</u> 1 mg/kg SC q 12 h or 1.5 mg/kg SC q 24 h (CrCl < 30 mL/min). Continue for at least 5 days and until therapeutic oral anticoagulation. <u>Unstable angina or non-Q-wave MI:</u> 1 mg/kg SC q 12 h with aspirin (100 to 325 mg PO daily) for at least 2 days and until clinically stable (if CrCl < 30 mL/min: give 1 mg/kg SC daily). <u>Acute ST-elevation MI:</u> For age 75 yo or younger: give 30 mg IV bolus, followed 15 min later by 1 mg/kg SC, then 1 mg/kg SC (max 100 mg/dose for the first two doses) q 12 h (if CrCl < 30 mL/min: give 30 mg IV bolus followed 15 min later by 1 mg/kg SC dose then 1 mg/kg SC daily); or if older than 75 yo: 0.75 mg/kg (max 75 mg/dose for the first two doses, no bolus) SC q 12 h (CrCl < 30 mL/min: 1 mg/kg SC daily, no bolus). [Trade only: Multidose vial 300 mg; Syringes 30, 40 mg; graduated syringes 60, 80, 100, 120, 150 mg. Concentration is 100 mg/mL except for 120, 150 mg, which are 150 mg/mL.] ▶KL ♀B ▶+ $$$$$ ■

TINZAPARIN (Innohep) <u>DVT with/without pulmonary embolus:</u> 175 units/kg SC daily for at least 6 days and until therapeutic oral anticoagulation. [Trade only: 20,000 anti-Xa units/mL, 2 mL multidose vial.] ▶K ♀B ▶+ $$$$$ ■

Anticoagulants—Other

HEPARIN (✦ Hepalean) <u>Venous thrombosis/pulmonary embolus treatment:</u> Load 80 units/kg IV, then initiate infusion at 18 units/kg/h. Adjust based on coagulation testing (PTT)—see Table on next page. <u>DVT prophylaxis:</u> 5000 units SC q 8 to 12 h. <u>Acute coronary syndromes with or without PCI:</u> see Table. Peds: Load 50 units/kg IV, then infuse 25 units/kg/h. [Generic only: 1000, 5000, 10,000, 20,000 units/mL in various vial and syringe sizes.] ▶Reticuloendothelial system ♀C but + ▶+ $$ ■

HEPARIN DOSING FOR ACUTE CORONARY SYNDROME (ACS)

ST elevation myocardial infarction (STEMI)	Adjunct to thrombolytics: For use with alteplase, reteplase, or tenecteplase: Bolus 60 units/kg IV load (max 4000 units), then initial infusion 12 units/kg/h (max 1000 units/h) adjusted to achieve goal PTT 1.5 to 2× control.
Unstable angina/Non-ST elevation myocardial infarction (UA/NSTEMI)	Initial Treatment: Bolus 60 units/kg IV load (max 4000 units), then initiate infusion at 12 to 15 units/kg/h (max 1000 units/h) and adjust to achieve goal PTT 1.5 to 2.5× control.
Percutaneous coronary intervention (PCI)	With initial medical treatment but without concurrent GPIIb/IIIa inhibitor planned: target ACT 250-300 seconds for HemoTec or 300-350 seconds for Hemochron.
	With initial medical treatment and with planned concurrent GPIIb/IIIa inhibitor: target 200-250 seconds.
	Without initial medical treatment and without concurrent GPIIb/IIIa inhibitor planned: Bolus 70-100 units/kg with target ACT 250-300 seconds for HemoTec or 300-350 seconds for Hemochron.
	Without initial medical treatment and with planned concurrent GPIIb/IIIa inhibitor: Bolus 50-70 units/kg with target ACT 200-250 seconds

References: *CHEST* 2008;133:145S. Circulation 2004;110:e82-292. *J Am Coll Cardiol* 2007;50:e37. *J Am Coll Cardiol* 2009;54:2235. *J Am Coll Cardiol* 2011;57:1946.

WEIGHT-BASED HEPARIN DOSING FOR DVT/PE*

Initial dose: 80 units/kg IV bolus, then 18 units/kg/h. Check PTT in 6 h.

PTT less than 35 sec (less than 1.2 × control): 80 units/kg IV bolus, then increase infusion rate by 4 units/kg/h.

PTT 35–45 sec (1.2–1.5 × control): 40 units/kg IV bolus, then increase infusion by 2 units/kg/h.

PTT 46–70 sec (1.5–2.3 × control): No change.

PTT 71–90 sec (2.3–3 × control): decrease infusion rate by 2 units/kg/h.

PTT greater than 90 sec (greater than 3 × control): Hold infusion for 1 h, then decrease infusion rate by 3 units/kg/h.

*PTT = Activated partial thromboplastin time. Reagent-specific target PTT may differ; use institutional nomogram when available. Consider establishing a max bolus dose/max initial infusion rate or use an adjusted body wt in obesity. Monitor PTT 6 h after heparin initiation and 6 h after each dosage adjustment. When PTT is stable within therapeutic range, monitor every morning. Therapeutic PTT range corresponds to anti-factor Xa activity of 0.3–0.7 units/mL. Check platelets between days 3 and 5. Can begin warfarin on first day of heparin; continue heparin for ≈ 4 to 5 days of combined therapy. Adapted from *Ann Intern Med* 1993;119:874; *Chest* 2008:133:463S–464S, *Circulation* 2001; 103:2994.

WARFARIN (*Coumadin, Jantoven*) Start 2 to 5 mg PO daily for 1 to 2 days, then adjust dose to maintain therapeutic PT/INR. [Generic/Trade: Tabs 1, 2, 2.5, 3, 4, 5, 6, 7.5, 10 mg.] ▶L ♀X ▶+ $ ■

Colony Stimulating Factors

DARBEPOETIN *(Aranesp, NESP)* <u>Anemia of chronic renal failure:</u> 0.45 mcg/kg IV/SC once a week, or 0.75 mcg/kg q 2 weeks in some nondialysis patients. <u>Cancer chemo anemia:</u> 2.25 mcg/kg SC weekly, or 500 mcg SC every 3 weeks. Adjust dose based on Hb. [Trade only: All forms are available with or without albumin. Single-dose vials: 25, 40, 60, 100, 200, 300, 500 mcg/1 mL, and 150 mcg/0.75 mL. Single-dose prefilled syringes or autoinjectors: 25 mcg/0.42 mL, 40 mcg/0.4 mL, 60 mcg/0.3 mL, 100 mcg/0.5 mL, 150 mcg/0.3 mL, 200 mcg/0.4 mL, 300 mcg/0.6 mL, 500 mcg/1 mL.] ▶cellular sialidases, L ♀C ▶? $$$$$ ■

FILGRASTIM *(G-CSF, Neupogen)* <u>Neutropenia:</u> 5 mcg/kg SC/IV daily. <u>Bone marrow transplant:</u> 10 mcg/kg/day SC/IV infusion. [Trade only: Single-dose vials: 300 mcg/1 mL, 480 mcg/1.6 mL. Single-dose syringes: 300 mcg/0.5 mL, 480 mcg/0.8 mL.] ▶L ♀C ▶? $$$$$

OPRELVEKIN *(Neumega)* <u>Chemotherapy-induced thrombocytopenia in adults:</u> 50 mcg/kg SC daily. [Trade only: 5 mg single-dose vials with diluent.] ▶K ♀C ▶? $$$$$ ■

PEGFILGRASTIM *(Neulasta)* 6 mg SC once each chemo cycle. [Trade only: Single-dose syringes 6 mg/0.6 mL.] ▶Plasma ♀C ▶? $$$$$

SARGRAMOSTIM *(GM-CSF, Leukine)* Specialized dosing for bone marrow transplant. ▶L ♀C ▶? $$$$$

Other Hematological Agents

AMINOCAPROIC ACID *(Amicar)* <u>Hemostasis:</u> 4 to 5 g PO/IV over 1 h, then 1 g/h prn. [Generic/Trade: Syrup 250 mg/mL, Tabs 500 mg. Trade only: Tabs 1000 mg.] ▶K ♀D ▶? $ IV $$$$$ Oral

DEFERASIROX *(Exjade)* <u>Chronic iron overload:</u> 20 mg/kg PO daily; adjust dose q 3 to 6 months based on ferritin trends. Max 40 mg/kg/day. [Trade only: Tabs for dissolving into oral susp 125, 250, 500 mg.] ▶L ♀B ▶? $$$$$ ■

HYDROXYUREA *(Hydrea, Droxia)* <u>Sickle cell anemia (Droxia):</u> Start 15 mg/kg PO daily while monitoring CBC q 2 weeks. If no marrow depression, then

(cont.)

THERAPEUTIC GOALS FOR ANTICOAGULATION

INR Range[a]	Indication
2.0–3.0	Atrial fibrillation, deep venous thrombosis†, pulmonary embolism†, bio-prosthetic heart valve, mechanical prosthetic heart valve (aortic position, bileaflet or tilting disk with normal sinus rhythm and normal left atrium)
2.5–3.5	Mechanical prosthetic heart valve: (1) mitral position, (2) aortic position with atrial fibrillation, (3) caged ball or caged disk

[a]Aim for an INR in the middle of the INR range (e.g, 2.5 for range of 2 to 3 and 3.0 for range of 2.5 to 3.5). Adapted from: *Chest* 2008; 133: 456-7S, 459S, 547S, 594-5S; see this manuscript for additional information and other indications. †For first-event unprovoked DVT/PE, after 3 months of therapy at goal INR 2 to 3, may consider low-intensity therapy (INR range 1.5 to 2.0) in patients with strong preference for less frequent INR testing.

increase dose q 12 weeks by 5 mg/kg/day (max 35 mg/kg/day). <u>Solid tumors</u> (Hydrea): Intermittent therapy: 80 mg/kg PO for a single dose q 3 days. Continuous therapy: 20 to 30 mg/kg PO daily. <u>Head and neck cancer</u> with radiation (Hydrea): 80 mg/kg PO for a single dose q 3 days. <u>Resistant chronic myelocytic leukemia</u>: 20 to 30 mg/kg PO daily. Give concomitant folic acid. [Generic/Trade: Caps 500 mg. Trade only: (Droxia) Caps 200, 300, 400 mg.] ▶LK ♀D ▶– $ varies by therapy ■

PROTAMINE <u>Reversal of heparin</u>: Within 30 minutes of IV heparin: 1 mg antagonizes about 100 units heparin. If greater than 30 minutes since IV heparin: 0.5 mg antagonizes about 100 units heparin. Due to short half-life of heparin (60 to 90 min), use IV heparin doses only from last several hours to calculate dose of protamine. SC heparin may require prolonged administration of protamine. <u>Reversal of low-molecular-weight heparin</u>: If within 8 h of LMWH dose: give 1 mg protamine per 100 anti-Xa units of dalteparin or tinzaparin or 1 mg protamine per 1 mg enoxaparin. Smaller doses advised if greater than 8 h since LMWH administration. Give IV (max 50 mg) over 10 min. May cause allergy/anaphylaxis. ▶Plasma ♀C ▶? $ ■

HERBAL & ALTERNATIVE THERAPIES

NOTE: *In the United States, herbal and alternative therapy products are regulated as dietary supplements, not drugs. Premarketing evaluation and FDA approval are not required unless specific therapeutic claims are made. Since these products are not required to demonstrate efficacy, it is unclear whether many of them have health benefits. In addition, there may be considerable variability in content from lot to lot or between products.*

ALOE VERA (*acemannan, burn plant*) Topical: Efficacy unclear for seborrheic dermatitis, psoriasis, genital herpes, skin burns. Gel possibly effective for oral lichen planus. Do not apply to surgical incisions; impaired healing reported. Oral: Efficacy unclear for mild to moderate active ulcerative colitis, type 2 diabetes. OTC laxatives containing aloe were removed from US market due to possible increased risk of colon cancer. [Not by prescription.] ▶LK ♀oral– topical+? ▶oral– topical+? $

ARNICA (*Arnica montana, leopard's bane, wolf's bane*) Do not take by mouth or use on open wounds. Topical promoted for treatment of bruises, aches, and sprains; but insufficient data to assess efficacy. [Not by prescription.] ▶? ♀– ▶– $

ARTICHOKE LEAF EXTRACT (*Cynara scolymus*) May reduce total cholesterol, but clinical significance is unclear. Possibly effective for functional dyspepsia. [Not by prescription.] ▶? ♀? ▶? $

ASTRAGALUS (*Astragalus membranaceus, huang qi, Jin Fu Kang, vetch*) Used in combination with other herbs in traditional Chinese medicine for CAD, CHF, chronic liver disease, kidney disease, viral infections, and upper respiratory tract infection. Possibly effective for improving survival and performance status with platinum-based chemotherapy for non-small-cell lung cancer. However, astragalus-based herbal formula (Jin Fu Kang) did not affect survival or pharmacokinetics of docetaxel in phase II study of patients with non-small-cell lung cancer. [Not by prescription.] ▶? ♀? ▶? $

BILBERRY (*Vaccinium myrtillus, huckleberry, Tegens, VMA extract*) Insufficient data to evaluate efficacy for macular degeneration or prevention of cataracts. Does not appear to improve night vision. [Not by prescription.] ▶Bile, K ♀– ▶– $

BITTER MELON (*Momordica charantia, ampalaya, karela*) Efficacy unclear for type 2 diabetes. Hypoglycemic coma reported in 2 children ingesting tea. Seeds can cause hemolytic anemia in G6PD deficiency. [Not by prescription.] ▶? ♀– ▶– $$

BUTTERBUR (*Petasites hybridus, Petadolex*) Migraine prophylaxis (possibly effective): Petadolex 50 to 75 mg PO two times per day. Allergic rhinitis prophylaxis (possibly effective): Petadolex 50 mg PO two times per day. Efficacy unclear for asthma. [Not by prescription. Standardized pyrrolizidine-free extracts: Petadolex caps 50, 75 mg.] ▶? ♀– ▶– $$

CESIUM CHLORIDE Can cause life-threatening QT interval prolongation and torsades. Health Canada and FDA are taking action against Internet sellers promoting cesium chloride as alternative treatment of late-stage cancer. Evidence for benefit as cancer treatment is lacking. [Not by prescription.] ▶K ♀– ▶– $$$

CHAMOMILE (*Matricaria recutita—German chamomile, Anthemis nobilis—Roman chamomile*) Promoted as a sedative or anxiolytic, to relieve GI distress, for skin infections or inflammation, many other indications. Efficacy unclear for any indication. [Not by prescription.] ▶? ♀– ▶? $

CHASTEBERRY (*Vitex agnus castus fruit extract, Femaprin*) Premenstrual syndrome (possibly effective): 20 mg PO daily of extract ZE 440. [Not by prescription.] ▶? ♀– ▶– $

CHONDROITIN Does not appear effective for relief of OA pain overall. Chondroitin 400 mg PO three times per day + glucosamine may improve pain in subgroup of patients with moderate to severe knee OA. [Not by prescription.] ▶K ♀? ▶? $

COENZYME Q10 (*CoQ-10, ubiquinone*) Heart failure: 100 mg/day PO divided two to three times per day (conflicting clinical trials; AHA does not recommend). Statin induced myalgia. 100 to 200 mg PO daily (efficacy unclear, conflicting clinical trials). Parkinson's disease: 1200 mg/day PO divided four times per day ($$$$; efficacy unclear; might slow progression slightly, but the American Academy of Neurology does not recommend). Efficacy unclear for hypertension and improving athletic performance. Appears ineffective for diabetes. [Not by prescription.] ▶Bile ♀– ▶– $

CRANBERRY (*Cranactin, Vaccinium macrocarpon*) Prevention of UTI (possibly effective): 300 mL/day PO cranberry juice cocktail. Usual dose of cranberry juice extract caps/tabs is 300 to 400 mg PO two times per day. Insufficient data to assess efficacy for treatment of UTI. Potential increase in INR with warfarin. [Not by prescription.] ▶? ♀+ in food, – in supplements ▶+ in food, – in supplements $

CREATINE Promoted to enhance athletic performance. No benefit for endurance exercise; modest benefit for intense anaerobic tasks lasting less than 30 sec. Usual loading dose of 20 g/day PO for 5 days, then 2 to 5 g/day divided two times per day. [Not by prescription.] ▶LK ♀– ▶– $

DEHYDROEPIANDROSTERONE (*DHEA, Aslera, Fidelin, Prasterone*) Does not improve cognition, quality of life, or sexual function in elderly. Not recommended as androgen replacement in late-onset male hypogonadism. To improve well-being in women with adrenal insufficiency: 50 mg PO daily (possibly effective; conflicting clinical trials). [Not by prescription.] ▶Peripheral conversion to estrogens and androgens ♀–▶– $

DEVIL'S CLAW (*Harpagophytum procumbens, Doloteffin, Harpadol*) <u>OA,</u> <u>acute exacerbation of chronic low-back pain</u> (possibly effective): 2400 mg extract/day (50 to 100 mg harpagoside/day) PO divided two to three times per day. [Not by prescription. Extracts standardized to harpagoside (iridoid glycoside) content.] ▶? ♀–▶– $

DONG QUAI (*Angelica sinensis*) Appears ineffective for postmenopausal symptoms; North American Menopause Society recommends against use. May increase bleeding risk with warfarin; avoid concurrent use. [Not by prescription.] ▶? ♀–▶– $

ELDERBERRY (*Sambucus nigra, Rubini, Sambucol, Sinupret*) Efficacy unclear for influenza, sinusitis, and bronchitis. [Not by prescription.] ▶? ♀–▶– $

EVENING PRIMROSE OIL (*Oenothera biennis*) Appears ineffective for premenstrual syndrome, postmenopausal symptoms, atopic dermatitis. Inadequate data to evaluate efficacy for cervical ripening. [Not by prescription.] ▶? ♀?▶– $

FENUGREEK (*Trigonelle foenum-graecum*) Efficacy unclear for diabetes or hyperlipidemia. [Not by prescription.] ▶? ♀–▶– $$

FEVERFEW (*Chrysanthemum parthenium, MIG-99, Migra-Lief, MigraSpray, Tanacetum parthenium L*) <u>Prevention of migraine</u> (possibly effective): 50 to 100 mg extract PO daily; 2 to 3 fresh leaves PO with or after meals daily; 50 to 125 mg freeze-dried leaf PO daily. May take 1 to 2 months to be effective. Inadequate data to evaluate efficacy for acute migraine. [Not by prescription.] ▶? ♀–▶– $

FLAVOCOXID (*Limbrel, UP446*) OA (efficacy unclear): 250 to 500 mg PO two times per day. [Caps 250, 500 mg. Marketed as medical food by prescription only (not all medical foods require a prescription).] ▶L ♀–▶– $$$

GARCINIA (*Garcinia cambogia, Citri Lean*) Appears ineffective for wt loss. [Not by prescription.] ▶? ♀–▶– $

GARLIC SUPPLEMENTS (*Allium sativum, Kwai, Kyolic*) Ineffective for hyperlipidemia. Small reductions in BP, but efficacy in HTN unclear. Does not appear effective for diabetes. Significantly decreases saquinavir levels. May increase bleeding risk with warfarin with/without increase in INR. [Not by prescription.] ▶LK ♀–▶– $

GINGER (*Zingiber officinale*) <u>Prevention of motion sickness</u> (efficacy unclear): 500 to 1000 mg powdered rhizome PO single dose 1 h before exposure. <u>Acute chemotherapy-induced nausea</u> (possibly effective adjunct to standard antiemetics): 250 to 500 mg PO two times per day for 6 days, starting 3 days before chemo. Does not appear effective for post-op N/V. American College of Obstetrics and Gynecology considers ginger 250 mg PO four times per day a nonpharmacologic option for N/V of pregnancy. Some experts advise pregnant women to limit dose to usual dietary amount (no more than 1 g/day). Some European countries advise pregnant women to avoid ginger supplements because it is cytotoxic in vitro. [Not by prescription.] ▶bile ♀? ▶? $

GINKGO BILOBA (*EGb 761, Ginkgold, Ginkoba*) Dementia (efficacy unclear): 40 mg PO three times per day of standardized extract containing 24% ginkgo flavone glycosides and 6% terpene lactones. The American Psychiatric Association and others find evidence too weak to recommend for Alzheimer's or other dementias. Does not prevent dementia in elderly or improve memory in people with normal cognitive function. Does not appear effective for intermittent claudication or prevention of acute altitude sickness. Possible risk of stroke. [Not by prescription.] ▶K ♀– ▶– $

GINSENG-AMERICAN (*Panax quinquefolius L., Cold-fX*) Reduction of postprandial glucose in type 2 diabetes (possibly effective): 3 g PO taken with or up to 2 h before meal. Cold-fX (1 cap PO two times per day) may modestly reduce the frequency of colds/flu; approved in Canada for adults and children 12 yo and older. [Not by prescription.] ▶K ♀– ▶– $

GINSENG-ASIAN (*Panax ginseng, Ginsana, G115, Korean red ginseng*) Promoted to improve vitality and well-being: 200 mg PO daily. Ginsana: 2 caps PO daily or 1 cap PO two times per day. Preliminary evidence of efficacy for erectile dysfunction. Efficacy unclear for improving physical or psychomotor performance, diabetes, herpes simplex infections, cognitive, or immune function. American College of Obstetrics and Gynecologists and North American Menopause Society recommend against use for postmenopausal hot flashes. [Not by prescription.] ▶? ♀– ▶– $

GINSENG-SIBERIAN (*Eleutherococcus senticosus, Ci-wu-jia*) Does not appear effective for improving athletic endurance or chronic fatigue syndrome. May interfere with some digoxin assays. [Not by prescription.] ▶? ♀– ▶– $

GLUCOSAMINE (*Cosamin DS, Dona*) OA: Glucosamine HCl 500 mg PO three times per day or glucosamine sulfate (Dona $$) 1500 mg PO once daily. Appears ineffective overall for OA pain, but glucosamine plus chondroitin may improve pain in moderate to severe knee OA. [Not by prescription.] ▶L ♀– ▶– $

GOLDENSEAL (*Hydrastis canadensis*) Often used in attempts to achieve false-negative urine test for illicit drug use (efficacy unclear). Often combined with echinacea in cold remedies; but insufficient data to assess efficacy for common cold or URIs. [Not by prescription.] ▶? ♀– ▶– $

GRAPE SEED EXTRACT (*Vitis vinifera L., procyanidolic oligomers, PCO*) Small clinical trials suggest benefit in chronic venous insufficiency. No benefit in single study of seasonal allergic rhinitis. [Not by prescription.] ▶? ♀? ▶? $

GREEN TEA (*Camellia sinensis, Polyphenon E*) Efficacy unclear for cancer prevention, wt loss, hypercholesterolemia. Large doses might decrease INR with warfarin due to vitamin K content. Contains caffeine. [Not by prescription. Green tea extract available in caps standardized to polyphenol content.] ▶LK ♀+ in moderate amount in food, – in supplements ▶+ in moderate amount in food, – in supplements $

GUARANA (*Paullinia cupana*) Marketed as a source of caffeine in wt-loss dietary supplements. [Not by prescription.] ▶? ♀+ in food, – in supplements ▶+ in food, – in supplements $

GUGGULIPID (*Commiphora mukul extract, guggul*) Does not appear effective for hyperlipidemia. [Not by prescription.] ▶? ♀− ▶− $$

HAWTHORN (*Crataegus laevigata, monogyna, oxyacantha, standardized extract WS 1442 − Crataegutt novo, HeartCare*) Mild heart failure (possibly effective): 80 mg PO two times per day to 160 mg PO three times per day of standardized extract (19% oligomeric procyanidins; WS 1442; HeartCare 80 mg tabs). [Not by prescription.] ▶? ♀− ▶− $

HONEY (*Medihoney*) Topical for burn/wound (including diabetic foot, stasis leg ulcers, pressure ulcers, 1st and 2nd degree partial thickness burns): Apply Medihoney for 12 to 24 h/day. Oral for nocturnal cough due to upper respiratory tract infection in children (efficacy unclear): Give PO within 30 min before sleep. Dose is ½ tsp for 2 to 5 yo, 1 tsp for 6 to 11 yo, 2 tsp for 12 to 18 yo. Do not feed honey to children younger than 1 yo due to risk of infant botulism. [Mostly not by prescription. Medihoney is FDA approved.] ▶? ♀+ ▶+ $ for oral $$$ for Medihoney

HORSE CHESTNUT SEED EXTRACT (*Aesculus hippocastanum, buckeye, HCE50, Venastat*) Chronic venous insufficiency (effective): 1 cap Venastat (16% aescin standardized extract) PO two times per day with water before meals. Am College of Cardiology found evidence insufficient to recommend for peripheral arterial disease. [Not by prescription.] ▶? ♀− ▶− $

LICORICE (*Cankermelt, Glycyrrhiza glabra, Glycyrrhiza uralensis*) Insufficient data to assess efficacy for postmenopausal vasomotor symptoms. Chronic high doses can cause pseudo-primary aldosteronism (with HTN, edema, hypokalemia). Cankermelt (dissolving oral patch; efficacy unclear for aphthous ulcers): Apply patch to ulcer for 16 h/day until healed. [Not by prescription.] ▶Bile ♀− ▶− $

MELATONIN (*N-acetyl-5-methoxytryptamine*) To reduce jet lag after flights over more than 5 time zones (effective): 0.5 to 5 mg PO at bedtime for 3 to 6 nights starting on day of arrival. [Not by prescription.] ▶L ♀− ▶− $

METHYLSULFONYLMETHANE (*MSM, dimethyl sulfone, crystalline DMSO2*) Insufficient data to assess efficacy of oral and topical MSM for arthritis pain. [Not by prescription.] ▶? ♀− ▶− $

MILK THISTLE (*Silybum marianum, Legalon, silymarin, Thisyin*) Hepatic cirrhosis (efficacy unclear): 100 to 200 mg PO three times per day of standardized extract with 70 to 80% silymarin. [Not by prescription.] ▶LK ♀− ▶− $

NETTLE ROOT (*stinging nettle, Urtica dioica radix*) Efficacy unclear for treatment of BPH or OA. [Not by prescription.] ▶? ♀− ▶− $

NONI (*Morinda citrifolia*) Promoted for many medical disorders; but insufficient data to assess efficacy. Potassium content comparable to orange juice; hyperkalemia reported in chronic renal failure. Case reports of hepatotoxicity. [Not by prescription.] ▶? ♀− ▶− $$$

PEPPERMINT OIL (*Mentha x piperita oil*) Irritable bowel syndrome (possibly effective): 0.2 to 0.4 mL enteric-coated caps PO three times per day. Peds, 8 yo or older: 0.1 to 0.2 mL enteric-coated caps PO three times per day. Take before meals. [Not by prescription.] ▶LK ♀+ in food, ? in supplements ▶+ in food, ? in supplements $

POLICOSANOL (*CholeRx, Cholestin*) Ineffective for hyperlipidemia. [Not by prescription.] ▶? ♀– ▶– $

PROBIOTICS (*Acidophilus, Align, Bifantis, Bifidobacteria, Lactobacillus, Bacid, Culturelle, Florastor, IntestiFlora, LiveBac, Power-Dophilus, Primadophilus, Probiotica, Saccharomyces boulardii, VSL#3*) Prevention of antibiotic-associated diarrhea (effective): Florastor (Saccharomyces boulardii) 2 caps PO two times per day for adults; 1 cap PO two times per day for peds. Culturelle (Lactobacillus GG) 1 cap PO once daily or two times per day for peds. Give 2 h before/after antibiotic. IDSA recommends against probiotics to prevent C. difficile–associated diarrhea; safety and efficacy is unclear. Peds rotavirus gastroenteritis (effective): Lactobacillus GG at least 10 billion cells/day PO started early in illness. Ulcerative colitis or pouchitis: VSL#3 1 to 8 packets/day or 4 to 32 caps/day for adults; peds dose based on wt and number of bowel movements. Irritable bowel syndrome: VSL#3 either ½ to 1 packet PO daily or 2 to 4 caps PO daily to relieve gas/bloating. Align: 1 cap PO once daily to relieve abdominal pain/bloating. [Not by prescription.] Culturelle contains Lactobacillus GG 10 billion cells/cap. Florastor contains Saccharomyces boulardii 5 billion cells/250 mg cap. VSL#3 (nonprescription medical food) contains 450 billion cells/packet, 225 billion cells/2 caps (Bifidobacterium breve, longum, infantis; Lactobacillus acidophilus, plantarum, casei, bulgaricus; Streptococcus thermophilus). Align contains Bifidobacterium infantis 35624, 1 billion cells/cap.] ▶? ♀+ ▶+ $

PYCNOGENOL (*French maritime pine tree bark*) Promoted for many medical disorders; but efficacy unclear for chronic venous insufficiency, HTN, sperm dysfunction, melasma, OA, diabetes, and ADHD. [Not by prescription.] ▶L ♀? ▶? $

PYGEUM AFRICANUM (*African plum tree*) BPH (may have modest efficacy): 50 to 100 mg PO two times per day or 100 mg PO daily of standardized extract containing 14% triterpenes. [Not by prescription.] ▶? ♀– ▶– $

RED CLOVER (*red clover isoflavone extract, Trifolium pratense, trefoil, Promensil, Rimostil, Trinovin*) Postmenopausal vasomotor symptoms (conflicting evidence; does not appear effective overall, but may have modest benefit for severe symptoms): Promensil 1 tab PO daily to two times per day with meals. [Not by prescription.] Isoflavone content (genistein, daidzein, biochanin, formononetin) is 40 mg/tab in Promensil and Trinovin, 57 mg/tab in Rimostil.] ▶Gut, L, K ♀– ▶– $$

RED YEAST RICE (*Monascus purpureus, Xuezhikang, Zhibituo, Hypocol*) Hyperlipidemia: Usual dose is 1200 mg PO two times per day. Efficacy depends on whether formulation contains lovastatin or other statins. In the United States, red yeast rice should not contain more than trace amounts of statins, but some products contain up to 10 mg lovastatin per cap. Some clinicians consider red yeast rice an alternative for patients who develop myalgia with prescription statins. Can cause myopathy. Some formulations may contain citrinin, a potential nephrotoxin. [Not by prescription. Xuezhikang marketed in Asia, Norway (HypoCol).] ▶L ♀– ▶– $$

S-ADENOSYLMETHIONINE (*SAM-e, sammy*) Mild to moderate <u>depression</u> (effective): 800 to 1600 mg/day PO in divided doses with meals. Efficacy unclear for OA. [Not by prescription.] ▶L ♀? ▶? $$$

SAINT JOHN'S WORT (*Hypericum perforatum, Kira, LI-160*) Mild to moderate depression (effective): 300 mg PO three times per day of standardized extract (0.3% hypericin). Does not appear effective for ADHD. May decrease efficacy of other drugs (eg, ritonavir, oral contraceptives) by inducing liver metabolism. May cause serotonin syndrome with SSRIs, MAOIs. [Not by prescription.] ▶L ♀− ▶− $

SAW PALMETTO (*Serenoa repens*) <u>BPH</u> (does not appear effective): 160 mg PO two times per day or 320 mg PO daily of standardized liposterolic extract. Take with food. [Not by prescription.] ▶? ♀− ▶− $

SHARK CARTILAGE (*BeneFin, Cartilade*) Appears ineffective for palliative care of advanced cancer. [Not by prescription.] ▶? ♀− ▶− $$$$$

SOY (*Genisoy, Healthy Woman, Novasoy, Phytosoya, Supro*) Soy protein or isoflavone supplements do not substantially reduce hyperlipidemia or BP. Postmenopausal vasomotor symptoms (modest benefit if any): 20 to 60 g/day soy protein PO (40 to 80 mg/day isoflavones). Conflicting clinical trials for postmenopausal bone loss. [Not by prescription.] ▶Gut, L, K ♀+ for food, ? for supplements ▶+ for food, ? for supplements $

STEVIA (*Stevia rebaudiana*) Leaves traditionally used as sweetener. Rebaudioside A (a component of stevia) is FDA approved as a general purpose sweetener. Unrefined stevia is available as dietary supplement in US, but not FDA approved as a sweetener. [Not by prescription. Rebaudioside A available as Rebiana, Truvia, PureVia.] ▶L ♀− ▶? $

TEA TREE OIL (*melaleuca oil, Melaleuca alternifolia*) Not for oral use; CNS toxicity reported. Efficacy unclear for topical treatment of onychomycosis, tinea pedis, acne vulgaris, dandruff, pediculosis. [Not by prescription.] ▶? ♀− ▶− $

VALERIAN (*Valeriana officinalis, Alluna*) <u>Insomnia</u> (possibly modestly effective; conflicting clinical trials): 400 to 900 mg of standardized extract PO 30 min before bedtime. Alluna: 2 tabs PO 1 h before bedtime. [Not by prescription.] ▶? ♀− ▶− $

WILD YAM (*Dioscorea villosa*) Ineffective as topical "natural progestin." Was used historically to synthesize progestins, cortisone, and androgens; it is not converted to them or dehydroepiandrosterone (DHEA) in the body. [Not by prescription.] ▶L ♀? ▶? $

WILLOW BARK EXTRACT (*Salix alba, Salicis cortex, salicin*) <u>OA, low-back pain</u> (possibly effective): 60 to 240 mg/day salicin PO divided two to three times per day. [Not by prescription. Some products standardized to 15% salicin content.] ▶K ♀− ▶− $

YOHIMBE (*Corynanthe yohimbe, Pausinystalia yohimbe*) Promoted for impotence and as aphrodisiac, but some products contain little yohimbine. FDA considers yohimbe bark in herbal remedies an unsafe herb. [Not by prescription.] ▶L ♀− ▶− $

IMMUNOLOGY

Immunizations

NOTE: *For vaccine info see CDC website (www.cdc.gov).*

AVIAN INFLUENZA VACCINE H5N1—INACTIVATED INJECTION 1 mL IM for 2 doses, separated by 21 to 35 days. ▶Immune system ♀C ▶? ?

BCG VACCINE (*Tice BCG, ✚ OncoTICE, Immucyst*) 0.2 to 0.3 mL percutaneously. ▶Immune system ♀C ▶? $$$$ ▸

COMVAX (haemophilus B vaccine + hepatitis B vaccine) Infants born of HBsAg (negative) mothers: 0.5 mL IM for 3 doses, given at 2, 4, and 12 to 15 months. ▶Immune system ♀C ▶? $$$

DIPHTHERIA, TETANUS, AND ACELLULAR PERTUSSIS VACCINE (*DTaP, Tdap, Tripedia, Infanrix, Daptacel, Boostrix, Adacel, ✚ Tripacel*) 0.5 mL IM. Do not use Boostrix or Adacel for primary childhood vaccination series. ▶Immune system ♀C ▶–$$

DIPHTHERIA—TETANUS TOXOID (*Td, DT, ✚ D2T5*) 0.5 mL IM. [Injection DT (pediatric: 6 weeks to 6 yo). Td (adult and children at least 7 yo).] ▶Immune system ♀C ▶? $

HAEMOPHILUS B VACCINE (*ActHIB, HibTITER, PedvaxHIB*) 0.5 mL IM. Dosing schedule varies depending on formulation used and age of child at first dose. ▶Immune system ♀C ▶? $$$

HEPATITIS A VACCINE (*Havrix, Vaqta, ✚ Avaxim, Epaxal*) Adult formulation 1 mL IM, repeat in 6 to 12 months. Peds: 0.5 mL IM for age 1 yo or older, repeat 6 to 18 months later. [Single-dose vial (specify pediatric or adult).] ♀C ▶+ $$$

HEPATITIS B VACCINE (*Engerix-B, Recombivax HB*) Adults: 1 mL IM, repeat 1 and 6 months later. Separate pediatric formulations and dosing. ♀C ▶+ $$$

HUMAN PAPILLOMAVIRUS RECOMBINANT VACCINE (*Gardasil*) 0.5 mL IM, then repeat 2 and 6 months later. Gardisil is indicated in females and males, Cervarix is only indicated in females. ♀B ▶? $$$$$

INFLUENZA VACCINE—INACTIVATED INJECTION (*Afluria, Fluarix, FluLaval, Fluzone, Fluvirin, ✚ Fluviral, Vaxigrip*) 0.5 mL IM or 0.1 mL intradermal (Fluzone Intradermal, age 18 to 64 yo only). FluLaval, Fluzone High-Dose, and Fluzone Intradermal not indicated if age younger than 18 yo, Fluarix not indicated if age younger than 3 yo. Fluvirin not indicated if age younger than 4 yo. Do not use Afluria in younger than 9 yo due to risk of febrile reactions. ▶Immune system ♀C ▶+ $

INFLUENZA VACCINE—LIVE INTRANASAL (*FluMist*) 1 dose (0.2 mL) intranasally. Use only if 2 to 49 yo. ▶Immune system ♀C ▶+ $

JAPANESE ENCEPHALITIS VACCINE (*JE-Vax*) 1 mL SC for 3 doses on day 0, 7, and 30. ♀C ▶? $$$$

MEASLES, MUMPS, AND RUBELLA VACCINE (*M-M-R II, ✚ Priorix*) 0.5 mL (1 vial) SC. ▶Immune system ♀C ▶+ $$$

MENINGOCOCCAL VACCINE (*Menomune-A/C/Y/W-135, Menactra, Menveo ✚ Menjugate*) 0.5 mL SC (Menomune) or IM (Menactra) at 11 to 12 yo. Repeat at 16 yo. ♀C ▶? $$$$

PEDIARIX (diphtheria tetanus and acellular pertussis vaccine + hepatitis B vaccine + polio vaccine) 0.5 mL IM at 2, 4, 6 mo. ▶Immune system ♀C ▶? $$$

PLAGUE VACCINE 1 mL IM 1st dose, then 0.2 mL IM 1 to 3 months after the 1st injection, then 0.2 mL IM 5 to 6 months later for age 18 to 61 yo. ▶Immune system ♀C ▶+ $

PNEUMOCOCCAL 23-VALENT VACCINE (*Pneumovax*, ✦ *Pneumo 23*) 0.5 mL IM or SC. ▶Immune system ♀C ▶+ $$

PNEUMOCOCCAL 13-VALENT CONJUGATE VACCINE (*Prevnar 13*) 0.5 mL IM for 3 doses at age 2 to 6 mo, followed by a 4th dose at 12 to 15 mo. Do not use after 6th birthday. ♀C ▶? $$$

POLIO VACCINE (*IPOL*) 0.5 mL IM or SC. ♀C ▶? $$

PROQUAD (measles mumps and rubella vaccine + varicella vaccine, MMRV) 0.5 mL (1 vial) SC for age 12 mo to 12 yo. ▶Immune system ♀C ▶? $$$$

RABIES VACCINE (*RabAvert, Imovax Rabies, BioRab, Rabies Vaccine Adsorbed*) 1 mL IM in deltoid region on day 0, 3, 7, 14, 28. ♀C ▶? $$$$$

ROTAVIRUS VACCINE (*RotaTeq, Rotarix*) RotaTeq: First dose (2 mL PO) between 6 to 12 weeks of age, and then 2nd and 3rd doses at 4 to 10 week intervals thereafter (last dose no later than 32 weeks). Rotarix: First dose (1 mL) at 6 weeks of age, and 2nd dose (1 mL) at least 4 weeks later, and last dose prior to 24 weeks of age. [Trade only: Oral susp 2 mL (RotaTeq), 1 mL (Rotarix).] ▶? $$$$$

TETANUS TOXOID 0.5 mL IM or SC. ▶Immune system ♀C ▶+ $$

TRIHIBIT (haemophilus B vaccine + diphtheria tetanus and acellular pertussis vaccine) Use for 4th dose only, age 15 to 18 mo: 0.5 mL IM. ▶Immune system ♀C ▶− $$$

TWINRIX (hepatitis A vaccine + hepatitis B vaccine) Adults: 1 mL IM in deltoid, repeat 1 and 6 months later. Accelerated dosing schedule: 0, 7, 21, and 30 days and booster dose at 12 months. ▶Immune system ♀C ▶? $$$$

TYPHOID VACCINE—INACTIVATED INJECTION (*Typhim Vi*, ✦ *Typherix*) 0.5 mL IM single dose. May revaccinate q 2 to 5 years if high risk. ▶Immune system ♀C ▶? $$

TYPHOID VACCINE—LIVE ORAL (*Vivotif Berna*) 1 cap every other day for 4 doses. May revaccinate q 2 to 5 years if high risk. [Trade only: Caps.] ▶Immune system ♀C ▶? $$

VARICELLA VACCINE (*Varivax*, ✦ *Varilrix*) Children 1 to 12 yo: 0.5 mL SC. Repeat dose at ages 4 to 6 yo. Age 13 yo or older: 0.5 mL SC, repeat 4 to 8 weeks later. ♀C ▶+ $$$$

YELLOW FEVER VACCINE (*YF-Vax*) 0.5 mL SC. ♀C ▶+ $$$

ZOSTER VACCINE—LIVE (*Zostavax*) 0.65 mL SC single dose for age 50 yo or older. ▶Immune system ♀C ▶? $$$$

Immunoglobulins

ANTIVENIN—CROTALIDAE IMMUNE FAB OVINE POLYVALENT (*CroFab*) Rattlesnake envenomation: 4 to 6 vials IV infusion over 60 min, within 6 h of bite if possible. Administer 4 to 6 additional vials if no initial control of envenomation

(cont.)

CHILDHOOD IMMUNIZATION SCHEDULE*

Age	Birth	1	2	4	6	12	15	18	2	4–6	11–12
						Months			**Years**		
Hepatitis B	HB	HB				HB					
Rotavirus			Rota	Rota	Rota#						
DTP			DTaP	DTaP	DTaP		DTaP			DTaP	DTaP***
H influenza b			Hib	Hib	Hib	Hib					
Pneumococci**			PCV	PCV	PCV	PCV					
Polio			IPV	IPV		IPV				IPV#	
Influenza						Influenza (yearly)†					
MMR						MMR				MMR	
Varicella						Varicella				Vari	
Hepatitis A§						Hep A x 2§					
Papillomavirus¶											HPV x 3¶
Meningococcal˚											MCV˚

*2011 schedule from the CDC, ACIP, AAP, & AAFP, see CDC website (www.cdc.gov/vaccines/recs/schedules/default.htm).

**Administer 1 dose Prevnar 13 to all healthy children 24 to 59 months having an incomplete schedule.

***When immunizing adolescents 10 yo or older, consider DTaP if patient has never received a pertussis booster (Boostrix if 10 yo or older, Adacel if 11 to 64 yo).

#If using Rotarix at 2 and 4 months, dose at 6 months is not indicated. Max age for final dose is 8 mo.

Last IPV on or after 4th birthday, and at least 6 months since last dose. If 4 doses given before 4th birthday, give 5th dose at ages 4 to 6 yo.

†For healthy patients age 2 yo or greater can use intranasal form. If age less than 9 yo and receiving for first time, administer 2 doses 4 or more weeks apart for injected form and 6 or more weeks apart for intranasal form. FluLaval not indicated for younger than 18 yo. Use Afluria only if 9 yo or older due to risk of febrile reaction

§Two doses at least 6 months apart.

¶Second and third doses 2 and 6 months after first dose. Also approved (Gardasil) for males 9 to 18 yo to reduce risk of genital warts.

˚Vaccinate all children at 11 to 12 yo, booster at 16 yo. Give one dose between 13 yo and 18 yo, if previously unvaccinated. For children 2 to 10 yo at high risk for meningococcal disease, vaccinate with meningococcal polysaccharide vaccine (Menactra). Revaccinate after 3 years (first dose was at 2 to 6 yo) for children who remain at high risk or after 5 years (first dose was a 7 yo or older).

---

syndrome, then 2 vials q 6 h for up to 18 h (3 doses) after initial control has been established. ▶? ♀C ▷? $$$$$

BOTULISM IMMUNE GLOBULIN (*BabyBIG*) Infant botulism: 1 mL/kg (50 mg/kg) IV for age younger than 1 yo. ▶L ♀? ▷? $$$$$

HEPATITIS B IMMUNE GLOBULIN (*H-BIG, HyperHep B, HepaGam B, NABI-HB*) 0.06 mL/kg IM within 24 h of needlestick, ocular, or mucosal exposure, repeat in 1 month. ▶L ♀C ▷? $$$

IMMUNE GLOBULIN—INTRAMUSCULAR (*Baygam, ✦Gamastan*) Hepatitis A prophylaxis: 0.02 to 0.06 mL/kg IM depending on length of travel to endemic area. Measles (within 6 days postexposure): 0.2 to 0.25 mL/kg IM. ▶L ♀C ▷? $$$$ ■

IMMUNE GLOBULIN—INTRAVENOUS (*Carimune, Flebogamma, Gammagard, Gammaplex, Gamunex, Octagam, Privigen*) IV dosage varies by indication and product. ▶L ♀C ▷? $$$$$ ■

IMMUNE GLOBULIN—SUBCUTANEOUS (*Vivaglobulin, Hizentra*) 100 to 200 mg/kg SC weekly. ▶L ♀C ▷? $$$$$ ■

LYMPHOCYTE IMMUNE GLOBULIN (*Atgam*) Specialized dosing. ▶L ♀C ▷? $$$$$

RABIES IMMUNE GLOBULIN HUMAN (*Imogam Rabies-HT, HyperRAB S/D*) 20 units/kg, as much as possible infiltrated around bite, the rest IM. ▶L ♀C ▶? $$$$$

RSV IMMUNE GLOBULIN (*RespiGam*) IV infusion for RSV. ▶Plasma ♀C ▶? $$$$$

TETANUS IMMUNE GLOBULIN (*BayTet, ♦Hypertet S/D*) <u>Prophylaxis:</u> 250 units IM. ▶L ♀C ▶? $$$$

VARICELLA-ZOSTER IMMUNE GLOBULIN (*VariZIG, VZIG*) Specialized dosing. ▶L ♀C ▶? $$$$$

Immunosuppression

BASILIXIMAB (*Simulect*) Specialized dosing for <u>organ transplantation.</u> ▶Plasma ♀B ▶? $$$$$ ■

BELATACEPT (*Nulojix*) Specialized dosing for <u>organ transplantation.</u> [injection.] ▶serum– ♀C ▶– $$$$$ ■

CYCLOSPORINE (*Sandimmune, Neoral, Gengraf*) Specialized dosing for <u>organ transplantation, RA</u>, and <u>psoriasis.</u> [Generic/Trade: Microemulsion Caps 25, 100 mg. Generic/Trade: Caps (Sandimmune) 25, 100 mg. Soln (Sandimmune) 100 mg/mL. Microemulsion soln (Neoral, Gengraf) 100 mg/mL.] ▶L ♀C ▶– $$$$$ ■

DACLIZUMAB (*Zenapax*) Specialized dosing for <u>organ transplantation.</u> ▶L ♀C ▶? $$$$$ ■

MYCOPHENOLATE MOFETIL (*Cellcept, Myfortic*) Specialized dosing for <u>organ transplantation.</u> [Generic/Trade: Caps 250 mg. Tabs 500 mg. Trade only (CellCept): Susp 200 mg/mL. Trade only (Myfortic): Tabs, extended-release: 180, 360 mg.] ▶? ♀D ▶? $$$$$ ■

SIROLIMUS (*Rapamune*) Specialized dosing for <u>organ transplantation.</u> [Trade only: Soln 1 mg/mL (60 mL). Tabs 1, 2 mg.] ▶L ♀C ▶– $$$$$ ■

TACROLIMUS (*Prograf, FK 506*) Specialized dosing for <u>organ transplantation.</u> [Generic/Trade: Caps 0.5, 1, 5 mg.] ▶L ♀C ▶– $$$$$ ■

Other

HYMENOPTERA VENOM Specialized desensitization dosing protocol. ▶Serum ♀C ▶? $$$$

TUBERCULIN PPD (*Aplisol, Tubersol, Mantoux, PPD*) 5 tuberculin units (0.1 mL) intradermally, read 48 to 72 h later. ▶L ♀C ▶+ $

TETANUS WOUND CARE (www.cdc.gov)		
	Unknown or less than 3 prior tetanus immunizations	3 or more prior tetanus immunizations
Non-tetanus–prone wound (eg, clean and minor)	Td (DT age younger than 7 yo)	Td if more than 10 years since last dose
Tetanus prone wound (eg, dirt, contamination, punctures, crush components)	Td (DT age younger than 7 yo), tetanus immune globulin 250 units IM at site other than Td	Td if more than 5 years since last dose

If patient age 10 yo or older has never received a pertussis booster consider DTaP (*Boostrix* if 10 yo or younger, *Adacel* if 11–64 yo).

NEUROLOGY

Alzheimer's Disease—Cholinesterase Inhibitors

DONEPEZIL (*Aricept*) Start 5 mg PO at bedtime. May increase to 10 mg PO at bedtime in 4 to 6 weeks. Max 10 mg/day for mild to moderate disease. For moderate to severe disease (MMSE 10 or less); may increase after 3 months to 23 mg/day. [Generic/Trade: Tabs 5, 10 mg, Orally disintegrating tabs 5, 10 mg. Trade only: Tab 23 mg.] ▶LK ♀C ▶? $$$$

GALANTAMINE (*Razadyne, Razadyne ER, ✦Reminyl*) Extended-release: Start 8 mg PO q am with food; increase to 16 mg after 4 weeks. May increase to 24 mg after another 4 weeks. Immediate-release: Start 4 mg PO two times per day with food; increase to 8 mg two times per day after 4 weeks. May increase to 12 mg two times per day after another 4 weeks. [Generic/Trade: Tabs 4, 8, 12 mg. Extended-release caps 8, 16, 24 mg. Oral soln 4 mg/mL. Prior to April 2005 was called Reminyl in the US.] ▶LK ♀B ▶? $$$$

RIVASTIGMINE (*Exelon, Exelon Patch*) <u>Alzheimer's disease:</u> Start 1.5 mg PO two times per day with food. Increase to 3 mg two times per day after 2 weeks. Max 12 mg/day. Patch: Start 4.6 mg/24 h once daily; may increase after 1 month or more to max 9.5 mg/24 h. Rotate sites. <u>Dementia in Parkinson's disease:</u> Start 1.5 mg PO two times per day with food. Increase by 3 mg/day at intervals greater than 4 weeks to max 12 mg/day. Patch: Use dosing for Alzheimer's disease. [Trade only: Caps 1.5, 3, 4.5, 6 mg. Oral soln 2 mg/mL (120 mL). Transdermal patch: 4.6 mg/24 h (9 mg/patch), 9.5 mg/24 h (18 mg/patch).] ▶K ♀B ▶? $$$$$

Alzheimer's Disease—NMDA Receptor Antagonists

MEMANTINE (*Namenda, Namenda XR, ✦Ebixa*) Start 5 mg PO daily. Increase by 5 mg/day at weekly intervals to max 20 mg/day. Doses greater than 5 mg/day should be divided two times per day. Extended-release: start 7 mg once daily. Increase at weekly intervals to target dose of 28 mg/day. Reduce to 14 mg/day in renal impairment. [Trade only: Tabs 5, 10 mg. Oral soln 2 mg/mL. Extended-release caps 7, 14, 21, 28 mg.] ▶KL ♀B ▶? $$$$

Anticonvulsants

CARBAMAZEPINE (*Tegretol, Tegretol XR, Carbatrol, Epitol, Equetro*) <u>Epilepsy:</u> 200 to 400 mg PO divided into two to four doses per day. Extended-release: 200 mg PO two times per day. Age younger than 6 yo: 10 to 20 mg/kg/day PO divided into two to four doses per day. Age 6 to 12 yo: 100 mg PO two times per day or 50 mg PO four times per day (susp); increase by 100 mg/day at weekly intervals divided three to four doses per day (immediate-release), two times per day (extended-release), or four times per day (susp). <u>Bipolar disorder, acute manic/mixed episodes</u> (Equetro): Start 200 mg PO two times per day; increase by 200 mg/day to max 1600 mg/day. <u>Trigeminal neuralgia:</u> Start 100 mg PO two timer per day (regular and XR tabs) or 50 mg PO four times per day (susp). May increase by 200 mg/

(cont.)

day to pain relief or max 1200 mg/day. Aplastic anemia, agranulocytosis, many drug interactions. [Generic/Trade: Tabs 200 mg, Chewable tabs 100 mg. Susp 100 mg/5 mL. Extended-release tabs (Tegretol XR) 100, 200, 400 mg. Generic only: Tabs 100, 300, 400 mg, Chewable tabs 200 mg. Trade only: Extended-release caps (Carbatrol and Equetro): 100, 200, 300 mg.] ▶LK ♀D ▶+ $$ ■

CLOBAZAM (♣ *Frisium*) Canada only. Adults: Start 5 to 15 mg PO daily. Increase prn to max 80 mg/day. Children younger than 2 yo: 0.5 to 1 mg/kg PO daily. Children age 2 to 16 yo: Start 5 mg PO daily. May increase prn to max 40 mg/day. [Generic/Trade: Tabs 10 mg.] ▶L ♀X (first trimester) D (second/third trimesters) ▶- $

ETHOSUXIMIDE (*Zarontin*) Absence seizures, age 3 to 6 yo: Start 250 mg PO daily (or divided two times per day). Age older than 6 yo: Start 500 mg PO daily (or divided two times per day). Max 1.5 g/day. [Generic/Trade: Caps 250 mg. Syrup 250 mg/5 mL.] ▶LK ♀C ▶+ $$$$

FELBAMATE (*Felbatol*) Start 400 mg PO three times per day. Max 3600 mg/day. Peds: Start 15 mg/kg/day PO divided three to four times per day. Max 45 mg/kg/day. Aplastic anemia, hepatotoxicity. Not first line. Requires written informed consent. [Trade only: Tabs 400, 600 mg. Susp 600 mg/5 mL.] ▶KL ♀C ▶- $$$$$ ■

FOSPHENYTOIN (*Cerebyx*) Load: 15 to 20 mg "phenytoin equivalents" (PE) per kg IM/IV no faster than 150 PE mg/min. Maintenance: 4 to 6 PE/kg/day. ▶L ♀D ▶+ $$$$$

GABAPENTIN (*Neurontin, Horizant, Gralise*) Partial seizures, adjunctive therapy: Start 300 mg PO at bedtime. Increase gradually to 300 to 600 mg PO three times per day. Max 3600 mg/day divided three times per day. Postherpetic neuralgia, immediate-release tabs: Start 300 mg PO on day 1; increase to 300 mg two times per day on day 2, and to 300 mg three times per day on day 3. Max 1800 mg/day divided three times per day. Postherpetic neuralgia (Gralise): start 300 mg PO once daily with evening meal. Increase to 600 mg on day 2, 900 mg on days 3 to 6, 1200 mg on days 7 to 10, 1500 mg on days 11 to 14, and 1800 mg on day 15. Max 1800 mg/day. Partial seizures, initial monotherapy: Titrate as above. Usual effective dose is 900 to 1800 mg/day. Restless legs syndrome (Horizant): 600 mg PO once daily around 5 pm taken with food. [Generic only: Tabs 100, 300, 400 mg. Generic/Trade: Caps 100, 300, 400 mg. Tabs scored 600, 800 mg. Soln 50 mg/mL. Trade only: Tabs, extended release 600 mg (gabapentin enacarbil, Horizant). Trade only (Gralise): Tabs 300, 600 mg.] ▶K ♀C ▶? $$$$

LACOSAMIDE (*Vimpat*) Partial onset seizures, adjunctive (17 yo and older): Start 50 mg PO/IV two times per day. Increase by 50 mg two times per day to recommended dose of 100 to 200 mg two times per day. Max 600 mg/day or 300 mg/day in mild/mod hepatic or severe renal impairment. [Trade only: Tabs 50, 100, 150, 200 mg.] ▶KL ♀C ▶? $$$$$

LAMOTRIGINE (*Lamictal, Lamictal CD, Lamictal ODT*) Partial seizures, Lennox-Gastaut syndrome, or generalized tonic-clonic seizures adjunctive therapy with a single enzyme-inducing anticonvulsant. Age 2 to 12 yo: dosing is based on wt and concomitant meds (see prescribing information). Age older than 12 yo: 50 mg PO daily for 2 weeks, then 50 mg two times per day for 2 weeks, then gradually increase to 150 to 250 mg PO two times per day.

(cont.)

Conversion to monotherapy (age 16 yo or older): See prescribing information. Drug interaction with valproate (see prescribing information for adjusted dosing guidelines). Potentially life-threatening rashes reported in 0.3% of adults and 0.8% of children; discontinue at first sign of rash. [Generic/Trade: Tabs, 25, 100, 150, 200 mg. Trade only: Chewable dispersible tabs (Lamictal CD) 2, 5, 25 mg. Trade only: Orally disintegrating tabs (Lamictal ODT) 25, 50, 100, 200 mg. Chewable dispersible tabs (Lamictal CD) 2 mg may not be available in all pharmacies; obtain through manufacturer representative, or by calling 888-825-5249.] ▶LK ♀C (see notes) ▶– $$$$ ■

LEVETIRACETAM *(Keppra, Keppra XR)* <u>Partial seizures, juvenile myoclonic epilepsy (JME), or primary generalized tonic-clonic seizures (GTC), adjunctive:</u> Start 500 mg PO/IV two times per day (Keppra) or 1000 mg/day (Keppra XR, partial seizures only); increase by 1000 mg/day q 2 weeks prn to max 3000 mg/day (partial seizures) or to target dose of 3000 mg/day (JME or GTC). IV route not approved for GTC or if age less than 16 yo. [Generic/Trade: Tabs 250, 500, 750, 1000 mg, Oral soln 100 mg/mL. Trade only: Tabs extended-release 500, 750 mg.] ▶K ♀C ▶? $$$$$

OXCARBAZEPINE *(Trileptal)* Start 300 mg PO two times per day. Titrate to 1200 mg/day (adjunctive) or 1200 to 2400 mg/day (monotherapy). Peds 2 to 16 yo: Start 8 to 10 mg/kg/day divided two times per day. Life-threatening rashes and hypersensitivity reactions. [Generic/Trade: Tabs (scored) 150, 300, 600 mg. Trade only: Oral susp 300 mg/5 mL.] ▶LK ♀C ▶– $$$$$

PHENOBARBITAL *(Luminal)* Load: 20 mg/kg IV at rate no faster than 60 mg/min. Maintenance: 100 to 300 mg/day PO given once daily or divided two times per day. Peds 3 to 5 mg/kg/day PO divided two to three times per day. Many drug interactions. [Generic only: Tabs 15, 16.2, 30, 32.4, 60, 100 mg. Elixir 20 mg/5 mL.] ▶L ♀D ▶–©IV $

PHENYTOIN *(Dilantin, Phenytek)* <u>Status epilepticus:</u> Load 15 to 20 mg/kg IV no faster than 50 mg/min, then 100 mg IV/PO q 6 to 8 h. <u>Epilepsy:</u> Oral load: 400 mg PO initially, then 300 mg in 2 h and 4 h. Maintenance: 5 mg/kg (or 300 mg PO) given once daily (extended-release) or divided three times per day (susp and chew tabs) and titrated to a therapeutic level. Limit dose increases to 10% or less due to saturable metabolism. [Generic/Trade: Extended-release caps 30, 100 mg (Dilantin). Susp 125 mg/5 mL. Trade only: Extended-release caps 200, 300 mg (Phenytek). Chewable tabs 50 mg (Dilantin Infatabs). Generic only: Extended-release caps 200, 300 mg.] ▶I ♀D ▶+ $$

PREGABALIN *(Lyrica)* <u>Painful diabetic peripheral neuropathy:</u> Start 50 mg PO three times per day; may increase within 1 week to max 100 mg PO three times per day. <u>Postherpetic neuralgia:</u> Start 150 mg/day PO divided two to three times per day. May increase within 1 week to 300 mg/day divided two to three times per day; max 600 mg/day. <u>Partial seizures (adjunctive):</u> Start 150 mg/day PO divided two to three times per day; increase prn to max 600 mg/day divided two to three times per day. <u>Fibromyalgia:</u> Start 75 mg PO two times per day; may increase to 150 mg two times per day within 1 week; max 225 mg two times per day. [Trade only: Caps 25, 50, 75, 100, 150, 200, 225, 300 mg. Oral soln 20 mg/mL (480 mL).] ▶K ♀C ▶?©V $$$$$

PRIMIDONE *(Mysoline)* Start 100 to 125 mg PO at bedtime. Increase over 10 days to 250 mg three to four times per day. Max 2 g/day. Metabolized to phenobarbital. Essential tremor (unapproved): up to 750 mg/day. [Generic/Trade: Tabs 50, 250 mg.] ▶LK ♀D ▶– $$$$

RUFINAMIDE *(Banzel)* Start 400 to 800 mg/day PO divided two times per day. Increase by 400 to 800 mg/day q 2 days to max 3200 mg/day. [Trade only: Tabs 200, 400 mg.] ▶K ♀C ▶? $$$$$

TIAGABINE *(Gabitril)* Start 4 mg PO daily. Increase by 4 to 8 mg/day at weekly intervals prn to max 32 mg/day (age 12 to 18 yo) or max 56 mg/day (age older than 18 yo) divided two to four times per day. Avoid off-label use. [Trade only: Tabs 2, 4, 12, 16 mg.] ▶L ♀C ▶? $$$$$

TOPIRAMATE *(Topamax)* Partial seizures or primary generalized tonic-clonic seizures, monotherapy: Start 25 mg PO two times per day (week 1), 50 mg two times per day (week 2), 75 mg two times per day (week 3), 100 mg two times per day (week 4), 150 mg two times per day(week 5), then 200 mg two times per day as tolerated. Partial seizures, primary generalized tonic-clonic seizures or Lennox-Gastaut syndrome, adjunctive therapy: Start 25 to 50 mg PO at bedtime. Increase weekly by 25 to 50 mg per day to usual effective dose of 200 mg PO two times per day. Doses greater than 400 mg per day not shown to be more effective. Migraine prophylaxis: Start 25 mg PO at bedtime (week 1), then 25 mg two times per day (week 2), then 25 mg q am and 50 mg q pm (week 3), then 50 mg two times per day (week 4 and thereafter). Bipolar disorder (unapproved): Start 25 to 50 mg per day PO. Titrate prn to max 400 mg per day divided two times per day. [Trade: Tabs 25, 50, 100, 200 mg. Sprinkle Caps 15, 25 mg.] ▶K ♀D ▶? $$$$$

VALPROIC ACID *(Depakene, Depakote, Depakote ER, Depacon, Stavzor, divalproex, sodium valproate, ✦Immunoprin, Oprisine)* Epilepsy: 10 to 15 mg/kg/day PO/IV divided two to four times per day (standard-release, delayed-release, or IV) or given once daily (Depakote ER). Titrate to max 60 mg/kg/day. Use rate no faster than 20 mg/min when given IV. Migraine prophylaxis: Start 250 mg PO two times per day (Depakote or Stavzor) or 500 mg PO daily (Depakote ER) for 1 week, then increase to max 1000 mg/day PO divided two times per day (Depakote or Stavzor) or given once daily (Depakote ER). Hepatotoxicity, drug interactions, reduce dose in elderly. [Generic/Trade: Immediate-release caps 250 mg (Depakene), syrup (Depakene, valproic acid) 250 mg/5 mL. Delayed-release tabs (Depakote) 125, 250, 500 mg, extended-release tabs (Depakote ER) 250, 500 mg, delayed-release sprinkle caps (Depakote) 125 mg. Trade only (Stavzor): Delayed-release caps 125, 250, 500 mg.] ▶L ♀D ▶+ $$$$

ZONISAMIDE *(Zonegran)* Start 100 mg PO daily. Titrate q 2 weeks to 200 to 400 mg/day given once daily or divided two times per day. Max 600 mg/day. Drug interactions. Contraindicated in sulfa allergy. [Generic/Trade: Caps 25, 50, 100 mg.] ▶LK ♀C ▶? $$$$

Migraine Therapy—Triptans (5-HT1 Receptor Agonists)

NOTE: *May cause vasospasm. Avoid in ischemic or vasospastic heart disease, cerebrovascular syndromes, peripheral arterial disease, uncontrolled HTN, and*

(cont.)

hemiplegic or basilar migraine. Do not use within 24 h of ergots or other triptans. Risk of serotonin syndrome if used with SSRIs or MAOIs.

ALMOTRIPTAN (*Axert*) 6.25 to 12.5 mg PO. May repeat in 2 h prn. Max 25 mg/day. Avoid MAOIs. [Trade only: Tabs 6.25, 12.5 mg.] ▶LK ♀C ▶? $$

ELETRIPTAN (*Relpax*) 20 to 40 mg PO. May repeat in 2 h prn. Max 40 mg/dose or 80 mg/day. Drug interactions. Avoid MAOIs. [Trade only: Tabs 20, 40 mg.] ▶LK ♀C ▶? $$$$

FROVATRIPTAN (*Frova*) 2.5 mg PO. May repeat in 2 h prn. Max 7.5 mg/24 h. [Trade only: Tabs 2.5 mg.] ▶LK ♀C ▶? $$

NARATRIPTAN (*Amerge*) 1 to 2.5 mg PO. May repeat in 4 h prn. Max 5 mg/24 h. [Generic/Trade: Tabs 1, 2.5 mg.] ▶KL ♀C ▶? $$$

RIZATRIPTAN (*Maxalt, Maxalt MLT*) 5 to 10 mg PO. May repeat in 2 h prn. Max 30 mg/24 h. MLT form dissolves on tongue without liquids. Avoid MAOIs. [Trade only: Tabs 5, 10 mg. Orally disintegrating tabs (MLT) 5, 10 mg.] ▶LK ♀C ▶? $$

SUMATRIPTAN (*Imitrex, Alsuma*) 4 to 6 mg SC. May repeat in 1 h prn. Max 12 mg/ 24 h. Tabs: 25 to 100 mg PO (50 mg most common). May repeat q 2 h prn with 25 to 100 mg doses. Max 200 mg/24 h. Intranasal spray: 5 to 20 mg q 2 h. Max 40 mg/24 h. Avoid MAOIs. [Injection (STATdose System) 4, 6 mg prefilled cartridges.] ▶LK ♀C ▶+ $$$$

TREXIMET (sumatriptan + naproxen) 1 tab PO at onset; may repeat in 2 h. Max 2 tabs/24 h. [Trade only: Tabs 85 mg sumatriptan + 500 mg naproxen sodium.] ▶LK ♀C ▶– $$

ZOLMITRIPTAN (*Zomig, Zomig ZMT*) 1.25 to 2.5 mg PO q 2 h. Max 10 mg/24 h. Orally disintegrating tabs (ZMT) 2.5 mg PO. May repeat in 2 h prn. Max 10 mg/24 h. Nasal spray: 5 mg (1 spray) in 1 nostril. May repeat in 2 h. Max 10 mg/24 h. [Trade only: Tabs 2.5, 5 mg. Orally disintegrating tabs (ZMT) 2.5, 5 mg. Nasal spray 5 mg/spray.] ▶L ♀C ▶? $$

Migraine Therapy—Other

CAFERGOT (ergotamine + caffeine) 2 tabs PO at onset, then 1 tab q 30 min prn. Max 6 tabs/attack or 10/week. Drug interactions. Fibrotic complications. [Trade only: Tabs 1/100 mg ergotamine/caffeine.] ▶L ♀X ▶– $

DIHYDROERGOTAMINE (*D.H.E. 45, Migranal*) Soln (DHE 45) 1 mg IV/IM/SC. May repeat in 1 h prn. Max 2 mg (IV) or 3 mg (IM/SC) per day. Nasal spray (Migranal): 1 spray in each nostril. May repeat in 15 min prn. Max 6 sprays/24 h or 8 sprays/week. Drug interactions. Fibrotic complications. [Trade only: Nasal spray 0.5 mg/spray (Migranal). Self-injecting soln (D.H.E 45): 1 mg/mL.] ▶L ♀X ▶– $$ ■

FLUNARIZINE (*❋Sibelium*) Canada only. 10 mg PO at bedtime. [Generic/Trade: Caps 5 mg.] ▶L ♀C ▶– $$

MIDRIN (isometheptene + dichloralphenazone + acetaminophen, Amidrine, Durdrin, Migquin, Migratine, Migrazone, Va-Zone) Tension and vascular headache treatment: 1 to 2 caps PO q 4 h. Max 8 caps/day. Migraine treatment: 2 caps PO single dose, then 1 cap q 1 h prn to max 5 caps within 12 h. [Generic only: Caps (isometheptene/dichloralphenazone/acetaminophen) 65/100/325 mg.] ▶L ♀? ▶?©IV $

Multiple sclerosis

DALFAMPRIDINE (*Ampyra*) 10 mg PO two times per day. Contraindicated in seizure disorders or moderate to severe renal impairment. [Trade: Extended-release tabs 10 mg.] ▶K - ♀C ▶?

FINGOLIMOD (*Gilenya*) Multiple sclerosis: 0.5 mg PO two times per day. [Trade only: Caps 0.5 mg.] ▶L - ♀C ▶?

GLATIRAMER (*Copaxone*) Multiple sclerosis: 20 mg SC daily. [Trade only: Injection 20 mg single-dose vial.] ▶Serum ♀B ▶? $$$$$

INTERFERON BETA-1A (*Avonex, Rebif*) Multiple sclerosis: Avonex 30 mcg (6 million units) IM q week. Rebif start 8.8 mcg SC 3 times a week; titrate over 4 weeks to maintenance dose of 44 mcg 3 times a week. Suicidality, hepatotoxicity, blood dyscrasias. Follow LFTs and CBC. [Trade only (Avonex): Injection 30 mcg single-dose vial with or without albumin. Prefilled syringe 30 mcg. Trade only (Rebif): Starter kit 20 mcg prefilled syringe. Prefilled syringe 22, 44 mcg.] ▶L ♀C ▶? $$$$$

INTERFERON BETA-1B (*Betaseron*) Multiple sclerosis: Start 0.0625 mg SC every other day; titrate over 6 weeks to 0.25 mg (8 million units) SC every other day. Suicidality, hepatotoxicity. Follow LFTs. [Trade only: Injection 0.3 mg (9.6 million units) single-dose vial.] ▶L ♀C ▶? $$$$$

Myasthenia Gravis

EDROPHONIUM (*Tensilon, Enlon*) Evaluation for myasthenia gravis (diagnostic purposes only): 2 mg IV over 15 to 30 sec (test dose) while on cardiac monitor, then 8 mg IV after 45 sec. Atropine should be readily available in case of cholinergic reaction. Duration of effect is 5 to 10 min. [10 mg/mL MDV vial.] ▶Plasma ♀C ▶? $

NEOSTIGMINE (*Prostigmin*) 15 to 375 mg/day PO in divided doses, or 0.5 mg IM/SC. [Trade only: Tabs 15 mg.] ▶L ♀C ▶? $$$$

PYRIDOSTIGMINE (*Mestinon, Mestinon Timespan, Regonol*) Myasthenia gravis: 60 to 200 mg PO three times per day (standard-release) or 180 mg PO daily or divided two times per day (extended-release). [Generic/Trade: Tabs 60 mg. Trade only: Extended-release tabs 180 mg. Syrup 60 mg/ 5 mL.] ▶Plasma, K ♀C ▶+ $$

Parkinsonian Agents—Anticholinergics

BENZTROPINE MESYLATE (*Cogentin*) Parkinsonism: 0.5 to 2 mg IM/PO/IV given once daily or divided two times per day. Drug-induced extrapyramidal disorders: 1 to 4 mg PO/IM/IV given once daily or divided two times per day. [Generic only: Tabs 0.5, 1, 2 mg.] ▶LK ♀C ▶? $

BIPERIDEN (*Akineton*) 2 mg PO three to four times per day, max 16 mg/day. [Trade only: Tabs 2 mg.] ▶LK ♀C ▶? $$$

TRIHEXYPHENIDYL (*Artane*) Start 1 mg PO daily. Gradually increase to 6 to 10 mg/day divided three times per day. Max 15 mg/day. [Generic only: Tabs 2, 5 mg. Elixir 2 mg/5 mL.] ▶LK ♀C ▶? $

Parkinsonian Agents—COMT Inhibitors

ENTACAPONE (*Comtan*) Start 200 mg PO with each dose of carbidopa/levodopa. Max 8 tabs (1600 mg)/day. [Trade only: Tabs 200 mg.] ▶L ♀C ▶? $$$$$

Parkinsonian Agents—Dopaminergic Agents and Combinations

APOMORPHINE (*Apokyn*) Start 0.2 mL SC prn. May increase in 0.1 mL increments every few days. Monitor for orthostatic hypotension after initial dose and with dose escalation. Max 0.6 mL/dose or 2 mL/day. Potent emetic, pretreat with trimethobenzamide 300 mg PO three times per day starting 3 days prior to use and continue for at least 6 weeks. Contains sulfites. [Trade only: Cartridges (for injector pen, 10 mg/mL) 3 mL. Ampules (10 mg/mL) 2 mL.] ▶L ♀C ▶? $$$$$

CARBIDOPA/LEVODOPA (*Sinemet, Sinemet CR, Parcopa*) Start 1 tab (25/100) PO three times per day. Increase q 1 to 4 days prn. Sustained-release: Start 1 tab (50/200) PO two times per day; increase q 3 days prn. [Generic/Trade: Tabs (carbidopa/levodopa) 10/100, 25/100, 25/250 mg. Tabs, sustained-release (Sinemet CR, carbidopa-levodopa ER) 25/100, 50/200 mg. Trade only: Orally disintegrating tab (Parcopa) 10/100, 25/100, 25/250 mg.] ▶L ♀C ▶– $$$$

PRAMIPEXOLE (*Mirapex, Mirapex ER*) Parkinson's disease: Start 0.125 mg PO three times per day. Gradually increase to 0.5 to 1.5 mg PO three times per day. Extended-release: Start 0.375 mg PO daily. May increase after 5 to 7 days to 0.75 mg daily, then by 0.75 mg/day increments q 5 to 7 days to max 4.5 mg/day. Restless leg syndrome: Start 0.125 mg PO 2 to 3 h prior to bedtime. May increase q 4 to 7 days to max 0.5 mg/dose. [Generic/Trade: Tabs 0.125, 0.25, 0.5, 0.75, 1, 1.5 mg. Trade only: Tabs extended-release 0.375, 0.75, 1.5, 3, 4.5 mg.] ▶K ♀C ▶? $$$$$

ROPINIROLE (*Requip, Requip XL*) Parkinson's disease: Start 0.25 mg PO three times per day, then gradually increase over 4 weeks to 1 mg PO three times per day. Max 24 mg/day. Extended-release: Start 2 mg PO daily for 1 to 2 weeks, then gradually increase by 2 mg daily at weekly or longer intervals. Max 24 mg/day. Restless legs syndrome: Start 0.25 mg PO 1 to 3 h before bedtime for 2 days, then increase to 0.5 mg/day on days 3 to 7. Increase by 0.5 mg/day at weekly intervals prn to max 4 mg/day given 1 to 3 h before bedtime. [Generic/Trade: Tabs, immediate-release 0.25, 0.5, 1, 2, 3, 4, 5 mg. Trade only: Tabs, extended-release (Requip XL) 2, 3, 4, 6, 8, 12 mg.] ▶L ♀C ▶? $$$$$

STALEVO (carbidopa + levodopa + entacapone) Parkinson's disease (conversion from carbidopa/levodopa with or without entacapone): Start Stalevo tab that contains the same amount of carbidopa/levodopa as the patient was previously taking then titrate to desired response. May need to reduce levodopa dose if not already taking entacapone. [Trade only: Tabs (carbidopa/levodopa/entacapone): Stalevo 50 (12.5/50/200 mg), Stalevo 75 (18.75/75/200 mg), Stalevo 100 (25/100/200 mg), Stalevo

125 (31.25/125/200 mg), Stalevo 150 (37.5/150/200 mg), Stalevo 200 (50/200/200 mg).] ▶L ♀C ▶− $$$$$

Parkinsonian Agents—Monoamine Oxidase Inhibitors (MAOIs)

RASAGILINE (*Azilect*) Parkinson's disease, monotherapy: 1 mg PO q am. Parkinson's disease, adjunctive: 0.5 mg PO q am. Max 1 mg/day. Requires an MAOI diet. [Trade only: Tabs 0.5, 1 mg.] ▶L ♀C ▶? $$$$$
SELEGILINE (*Eldepryl, Zelapar*) Parkinson's disease: 5 mg PO q am and at noon, max 10 mg/day. Zelapar ODT: 1.25 to 2.5 mg q am, max 2.5 mg/day. [Generic/Trade: Caps 5 mg. Tabs 5 mg. Trade only: Oral disintegrating tabs (Zelapar ODT) 1.25 mg.] ▶LK ♀C ▶? $$$$

Dermatomes

MOTOR FUNCTION BY NERVE ROOTS

Level	Motor Function
C3/C4/C5	Diaphragm
C5/C6	Deltoid/biceps
C7/C8	Triceps
C8/T1	Finger flexion/intrinsics
T1–T12	Intercostal/abd muscles
L2/L3	Hip flexion
L2/L3/L4	Hip adduction/quads
L4/L5	Ankle dorsiflexion
S1/S2	Ankle plantarflexion
S2/S3/S4	Rectal tone

LUMBOSACRAL NERVE ROOT COM-PRESSIONs	Root	Motor	Sensory	Reflex
	L4	quadriceps	medial foot	knee-jerk
	L5	dorsiflexors	dorsum of foot	medial hamstring
	S1	plantarflexors	lateral foot	ankle-jerk

GLASGOW COMA SCALE

Eye Opening	Verbal Activity	Motor Activity
4. Spontaneous	5. Oriented	6. Obeys commands
3. To command	4. Confused	5. Localizes pain
2. To pain	3. Inappropriate	4. Withdraws to pain
1. None	2. Incomprehensible	3. Flexion to pain
	1. None	2. Extension to pain
		1. None

Other Agents

MANNITOL (*Osmitrol, Resectisol*) Intracranial HTN: 0.25 to 2 g/kg IV over 30 to 60 min. ▶K ♀C ▶? $$

MILNACIPRAN (*Savella*) Day 1: 12.5 mg PO once. Days 2 to 3: 12.5 mg two times per day. Days 4 to 7: 25 mg two times per day, then 50 mg two times per day thereafter. Max 200 mg/day. [Trade only: Tabs 12.5, 25, 50, 100 mg.] ▶KL ♀C ▶? $$$$

NIMODIPINE (*Nimotop*) Subarachnoid hemorrhage: 60 mg PO q 4 h for 21 days. [Generic only: Caps 30 mg.] ▶L ♀C ▶– $$$$$

OXYBATE (*Xyrem, GHB*, gamma hydroxybutyrate) Cataplexy or excessive daytime sleepiness in narcolepsy: 2.25 g PO at bedtime. Repeat in 2.5 to 4 h. May increase by 1.5 g/day at 2 week intervals to max ½ g/day. From a centralized pharmacy. [Trade only: Soln 180 mL (500 mg/mL) supplied with measuring device and child-proof dosing cups.] ▶L ♀B ▶?©III $$$$$ ■

RILUZOLE (*Rilutek*) ALS: 50 mg PO q 12 h. Monitor LFTs. [Trade only: Tabs 50 mg.] ▶LK ♀C ▶– $$$$$

TETRABENAZINE (*Xenazine,* ✦ *Nitoman*) Chorea associated with Huntington's disease: Start 12.5 mg PO q am. Increase after 1 week to 12.5 mg PO two time per day. May increase by 12.5 mg/day weekly. Doses greater than 37.5 to 50 mg/day should be divided and given three times per day. For doses greater than 50 mg/day, genotype for CYP2D6, titrate by 12.5 mg/day weekly and divide in doses three times per day to max 37.5 mg/dose and 100 mg/day (extensive/intermediate metabolizers) or 25 mg/dose and 50 mg/day (poor metabolizers). Associated with suicidality and orthostatic hypotension. [Trade only: Tabs 12.5, 25 mg.] ▶L ♀C ▶? ? $$$$$ ■

OB/GYN

Contraceptives—Other

LEVONORGESTREL (*Next Choice*) Emergency contraception: 1 tab PO ASAP but within 72 h of intercourse. 2nd tab 12 h later. [OTC Trade only: Kit contains 2 tabs 0.75 mg.] ▶L ♀X ▶– $$

LEVONORGESTREL 1S (*Plan B One-Step*) Emergency contraception: 1 tab PO ASAP but within 72 h of intercourse. [OTC Trade only: Tabs 1.5 mg.] ▶L ♀X ▶– $$

NUVARING (ethinyl estradiol vaginal ring + etonogestrel) Contraception: 1 ring intravaginally for 3 weeks each month. [Trade only: Flexible intravaginal ring, 15 mcg ethinyl estradiol/0.120 mg etonogestrel/day in 1, 3 rings/box.] ▶L ♀X ▶– $$$ ■

ORTHO EVRA (norelgestromin + ethinyl estradiol transdermal, ✦ *Evra*) Contraception: 1 patch q week for 3 weeks, then 1 week patch-free. [Trade only: Transdermal patch: 150 mcg norelgestromin/20 mcg ethinyl estradiol/day in 1, 3 patches/box.] ▶L ♀X ▶– $$$ ■

ULIPRISTAL ACETATE (*Ella*) Emergency contraception: 1 tab PO ASAP within 5 days of intercourse. [Trade only: Tabs 30 mg.] ▶L ♀X ▶?

Estrogens

NOTE: *See also Hormone Combinations. Unopposed estrogens increase the risk of endometrial cancer in postmenopausal women.*

ESTERIFIED ESTROGENS (*Menest*) 0.3 to 1.25 mg PO daily. [Trade only: Tabs 0.3, 0.625, 1.25, 2.5 mg.] ▶L ♀X ▶– $$ ■

ESTRADIOL (*Estrace, Gynodiol*) 1 to 2 mg PO daily. [Generic/Trade: Tabs, micronized 0.5, 1, 2 mg, scored. Trade only: 1.5 mg (Gynodiol).] ▶L ♀X ▶– $ ■

ESTRADIOL ACETATE (*Femtrace*) 0.45 to 1.8 mg PO daily. [Trade only: Tabs, 0.45, 0.9, 1.8 mg.] ▶L ♀X ▶– $$ ■

ESTRADIOL ACETATE VAGINAL RING (*Femring*) Insert and replace after 90 days. [Trade only: 0.05 mg/day and 0.1 mg/day.] ▶L ♀X ▶– $$$ ■

ESTRADIOL CYPIONATE (*Depo-Estradiol*) 1 to 5 mg IM q 3 to 4 weeks. ▶L ♀X ▶– $ ■

ESTRADIOL GEL (*Divigel, Estrogel, Elestrin*) Thinly apply contents of 1 complete pump depression to one entire arm (Estrogel) or upper arm (Elestrin) or contents of 1 foil packet (Divigel) to one upper thigh. [Trade only: Gel 0.06% in nonaerosol, metered-dose pump with #64 or #32 1.25 g doses (Estrogel), #100 0.87 g doses (Elestrin). Gel 0.1% in single-dose foil packets of 0.25, 0.5, 1.0 g, carton of 30 (Divigel).] ▶L ♀X ▶– $$$ ■

ESTRADIOL TOPICAL EMULSION (*Estrasorb*) Rub in contents of 1 pouch each to left and right legs (spread over thighs and calves) q am. Daily dose is equivalent to two 1.74 g pouches. [Trade only: Topical emulsion, 56 pouches/carton.] ▶L ♀X ▶– $$ ■

ESTRADIOL TRANSDERMAL PATCH (*Alora, Climara, Esclim, Estraderm, FemPatch, Menostar, Vivelle, Vivelle Dot, ✦ Estradot, Oesclim*) Apply 1 patch weekly (Climara, FemPatch, Estradiol, Menostar) or two times per week (Esclim, Estraderm, Vivelle, Vivelle Dot, Alora). [Generic/Trade: Transdermal patches doses in mg/day: Climara (once a week) 0.025, 0.0375, 0.05, 0.06, 0.075, 0.1. Trade only: FemPatch (once a week) 0.025. Esclim (two times per week) 0.025, 0.0375, 0.05, 0.075, 0.1. Vivelle, Vivelle Dot (two times a week) 0.025, 0.0375, 0.05, 0.075, 0.1. Estraderm (two times per week) 0.05, 0.1. Alora (two times a week) 0.025, 0.05, 0.075, 0.1.] ▶L ♀X ▶– $$ ■

ESTRADIOL TRANSDERMAL SPRAY (*Evamist*) 1 to 3 sprays daily to forearm. [Trade only: Spray: 1.53 mg estradiol per 90 mcL spray, 56 sprays per metered-dose pump.] ▶L ♀X ▶– $$$ ■

ESTRADIOL VAGINAL RING (*Estring*) Insert and replace after 90 days. [Trade only: 2 mg ring single pack.] ▶L ♀X ▶– $$$ ■

ESTRADIOL VAGINAL TAB (*Vagifem*) 1 tab vaginally daily for 2 weeks, then 1 tab vaginally two times a week. [Trade only: Vaginal tab: 10 mcg or 25 mcg in disposable single-use applicators, 8, 18/pack.] ▶L ♀X ▶– $$$ ■

ESTRADIOL VALERATE (*Delestrogen*) 10 to 20 mg IM q 4 weeks. ▶L ♀X ▶– $$ ■

ESTROGEN VAGINAL CREAM (*Premarin, Estrace*) <u>Menopausal atrophic vaginitis:</u> Premarin: 0.5 to 2 g daily. Estrace: 2 to 4 g daily for 2 weeks, then reduce. <u>Moderate</u>

(cont.)

to severe menopausal dyspareunia: Premarin: 0.5 g daily, then reduce to two times per week. [Trade only: Premarin: 0.625 mg conjugated estrogens/g in 42.5 g with or without calibrated applicator. Estrace: 0.1 mg estradiol/g in 42.5 g with calibrated applicator. Generic only: Cream 0.625 mg synthetic conjugated estrogens/g in 30 g with calibrated applicator.] ▶L ♀X ▶? $$$$ ■

ESTROGENS CONJUGATED (*Premarin, C.E.S., Congest*) 0.3 to 1.25 mg PO daily. <u>Abnormal uterine bleeding:</u> 25 mg IV/IM. Repeat in 6 to 12 h if needed. [Trade only: Tabs 0.3, 0.45, 0.625, 0.9, 1.25 mg.] ▶L ♀X ▶– $$$ ■

ESTROGENS SYNTHETIC CONJUGATED A (*Cenestin*) 0.3 to 1.25 mg PO daily. [Trade only: Tabs 0.3, 0.45, 0.625, 0.9, 1.25 mg.] ▶L ♀X ▶– $$$ ■

ESTROGENS SYNTHETIC CONJUGATED B (*Enjuvia*) 0.3 to 1.25 mg PO daily. [Trade only: Tabs 0.3, 0.45, 0.625, 0.9, 1.25 mg.] ▶L ♀X ▶– $$ ■

ESTROPIPATE (*Ogen, Ortho-Est*) 0.75 to 6 mg PO daily. [Generic/Trade: Tabs 0.75, 1.5, 3, 6 mg of estropipate.] ▶L ♀X ▶– $ ■

Hormone Combinations

NOTE: See also Estrogens.

ACTIVELLA (estradiol + norethindrone) 1 tab PO daily. [Trade only: Tabs 1/0.5 mg and 0.5/0.1 mg estradiol/norethindrone acetate in calendar dial pack dispenser.] ▶L ♀X ▶– $$$ ■

ANGELIQ (estradiol + drospirenone) 1 tab PO daily. [Trade only: Tabs 1 mg estradiol/0.5 mg drospirenone.] ▶L ♀X ▶– $$$ ■

CLIMARA PRO (estradiol + levonorgestrel) 1 patch weekly. [Trade only: Transdermal 0.045/0.015 estradiol/levonorgestrel in mg/day, 4 patches/box.] ▶L ♀X ▶– $$$ ■

COMBIPATCH (estradiol + norethindrone, ✦Estalis) 1 patch two times per week. [Trade only: Transdermal patch 0.05 estradiol/0.14 norethindrone and 0.05 estradiol/0.25 norethindrone in mg/day, 8 patches/box.] ▶L ♀X ▶– $$$ ■

EEMT D.S. (esterified estrogens + methyltestosterone) 1 tab PO daily. [Generic only: Tabs 1.25 mg esterified estrogens/2.5 mg methyltestosterone.] ▶L ♀X ▶– $$$$ ■

EEMT H.S. (esterified estrogens + methyltestosterone) 1 tab PO daily. [Generic only: Tabs 0.625 mg esterified estrogens/1.25 mg methyltestosterone.] ▶L ♀X ▶– $$$ ■

FEMHRT (ethinyl estradiol + norethindrone) 1 tab PO daily. [Trade only: Tabs 5/1, 2.5/0.5 mcg ethinyl estradiol/mg norethindrone, 28/blister card.] ▶L ♀X ▶– $$$ ■

PREFEST (estradiol + norgestimate) 1 pink tab PO daily for 3 days followed by 1 white tab PO daily for 3 days, sequentially throughout the month. [Trade only: Tabs in 30 days blister packs 1 mg estradiol (15 pink), 1 mg estradiol/0.09 mg norgestimate (15 white).] ▶L ♀X ▶– $$$ ■

PREMPHASE (estrogens conjugated + medroxyprogesterone) 1 tab PO daily. [Trade only: Tabs in 28 days EZ-Dial dispensers: 0.625 mg conjugated estrogens (14), 0.625 mg/5 mg conjugated estrogens/medroxyprogesterone (14).] ▶L ♀X ▶– $$$ ■

EMERGENCY CONTRACEPTION Emergency contraception within 72 h of unprotected sex. Progestin-only methods (causes less nausea and may be more effective. Available OTC for age at least 17 yo): *Plan B One-Step* (levonorgestrel 1.5 mg tab): take one pill. *Next Choice* (levonorgestrel 0.75 mg): take one tab ASAP and 2nd dose 12 h later. Progestin and estrogen method: Dose is defined as 2 pills of Ogestrel, 4 pills of Cryselle, Enpresse*, Jolessa, Levora, Lo/Ovral, Low Ogestrel, Nordette, Portia, Quasense, Seasonale, Seasonique, Solia, or Trivora*, or 5 pills of Aviane, Lessina, LoSeasonique, Lutera, or Sronyx: Take first dose ASAP and 2nd dose 12 h later. If vomiting occurs within 1 h of taking dose, consider repeating that dose with an antiemetic 1 h prior.

Emergency contraception within 120 h of unprotected sex. *Ella* (ulipristal 50mg): take 1 pill. More info at: www.not-2-late.com.

*Use 0.125 mg levonorgestrel/30 mcg ethinyl estradiol tab.

PREMPRO (**estrogens conjugated + medroxyprogesterone**, *◆ Premplus*) 1 tab PO daily. [Trade only: Tabs in 28-day EZ-Dial dispensers: 0.625 mg/5 mg, 0.625 mg/2.5 mg, 0.45 mg/1.5 mg (Prempro low dose), or 0.3 mg/1.5 mg conjugated estrogens/medroxyprogesterone.] ▶L ♀X ▶– $$$ ■

Labor Induction / Cervical Ripening

DINOPROSTONE (**PGE2, Prepidil, Cervidil, Prostin E2**) Cervical ripening: 1 syringe of gel placed directly into the cervical os for cervical ripening or 1 insert in the posterior fornix of the vagina. [Trade only: Gel (Prepidil) 0.5 mg/3 g syringe. Vaginal insert (Cervidil) 10 mg. Vaginal supps (Prostin E2) 20 mg.] ▶Lung ♀C ▶? $$$$$ ■

MISOPROSTOL- OB (**PGE1, Cytotec**) Cervical ripening: 25 mcg intravaginally q 3 to 6 h (or 50 mcg q 6 h). First trimester pregnancy failure: 800 mcg intravaginally, repeat on day 3 if expulsion incomplete. [Generic/Trade: Oral tabs 100, 200 mcg.] ▶LK ♀X ▶– $$$$ ■

OXYTOCIN (**Pitocin**) Labor induction: 10 units in 1000 mL NS (10 milliunits/mL), start at 6 to 12 mL/h (1 to 2 milliunits/min). Postpartum bleeding: 10 units IM or 10 to 40 units in 1000 mL NS IV, infuse 20 to 40 milliunits/min. ▶LK ♀? ▶– $ ■

Ovulation Stimulants

CLOMIPHENE (**Clomid, Serophene**) Specialized dosing for ovulation induction. [Generic/Trade: Tabs 50 mg, scored.] ▶L ♀D ▶? $$$$$

Progestins

MAKENA (**hydroxyprogesterone caproate**) [Trade only. 5mL MDV (250mg/ml) hydroxyprogesterone caproate in castor oil solution.] ▶L + glucuronidation ♀B ▶? $$$$$

MEDROXYPROGESTERONE (**Provera**) 10 mg PO daily for last 10 to 12 days of month, or 2.5 to 5 mg PO daily. Secondary amenorrhea, abnormal uterine

(cont.)

ORAL CONTRACEPTIVES* ►L CX Monophasic	Estrogen (mcg)	Progestin (mg)
Necon 1/50, Norinyl 1+50	50 mestranol	1 norethindrone
Ovcon-50	50 ethinyl estradiol	1 norethindrone
Demulen 1/50, Zovia 1/50E		1 ethynodiol
Ogestrel		0.5 norgestrel
Necon 1/35, Norinyl 1+35, Nortrel 1/35, Ortho-Novum 1/35		1 norethindrone
Brevicon, Modicon, Necon 0.5/35, Nortrel 0.5/35	35 ethinyl estradiol	0.5 norethindrone
Balziva, Femcon Fe, Ovcon-35, Zenchent, Zeosa		0.4 norethindrone
Previfem		0.18 norgestimate
MonoNessa, Ortho-Cyclen, Sprintec-28		0.25 norgestimate
Demulen 1/35, Kelnor 1/35, Zovia 1/35E		1 ethynodiol
Junel 1.5/30, Junel 1.5/30 Fe, Loestrin 21 1.5/30, Loestrin Fe 1.5/30, Microgestin Fe 1.5/30		1.5 norethindrone
Cryselle, Lo/Ovral, Low-Ogestrel	30 ethinyl estradiol	0.3 norgestrel
Apri, Desogen, Ortho-Cept, Reclipsen		0.15 desogestrel
Levora, Nordette, Portia, Solia		0.15 levonorgestrel
Ocella, Safyral, Yasmin, Zarah		3 drospirenone
Generess Fe	25 ethinyl estradiol	0.8 norethindrone
Junel 1/20, Junel Fe 1/20, Loestrin 21 1/20, Loestrin Fe 1/20, Loestrin 24 Fe, Microgestin Fe 1/20		1 norethindrone
Aviane, Lessina, Lutera, Sronyx	20 ethinyl estradiol	0.1 levonorgestrel
Amethyst†, Lybrel†		0.09 levonorgestrel
Gianvi, Yaz		3 drospirenone
Beyaz		2 drospirenone
Azurette, Kariva, Mircette	20/10 ethinyl estradiol	0.15 desogestrel
Progestin-only		
Camila, Errin, Jolivette, Micronor, Nor-Q.D., Nora-BE	none	0.35 norethindrone
Biphasic (estrogen and progestin contents vary)		
Necon 10/11	35 ethinyl estradiol	0.5/1 norethindrone
Triphasic (estrogen and progestin contents vary)		
Caziant, Cesia, Cyclessa, Velivet	25 ethinyl estradiol	0.100/0.125/0.150 desogestrel
Ortho-Novum 7/7/7, Necon 7/7/7, Nortrel 7/7/7	35 ethinyl estradiol	0.5/0.75/1 norethindrone
Aranelle, Leena, Tri-Norinyl		0.5/1/0.5 norethindrone
Enpresse, Trivora-28	30/40/30 ethinyl estradiol	0.5/0.75/0.125 levonorgestrel
Ortho Tri-Cyclen, Tri-Nessa, Tri-Previfem, Tri-Sprintec	35 ethinyl estradiol	0.0.18/0.215/0.25 norgestimate
Ortho Tri-Cyclen Lo	25 ethinyl estradiol	norgestimate
Estrostep Fe, Tilia Fe, Tri-Legest, Tri-Legest Fe	20/30/35 ethinyl estradiol	1 norethindrone
Four-phasic (estrogen and progestin contents vary)		
Natazia	3mg/2mg estradiol valerate	2/3/0 dienogest
Extended Cycle††		
Jolessa, Quasense, Seasonale	30 ethinyl estradiol	0.15 levonorgestrel
Amethia, Seasonique	30/10 ethinyl estradiol	0.15 levonorgestrel
LoSeasonique	20 ethinyl estradiol	0.1 levonorgestrel

*All: Not recommended in smokers. Increase risk of thromboembolism, CVA, MI, hepatic neoplasia, and gallbladder disease. Nausea, breast tenderness, and breakthrough bleeding are common transient side effects. Effectiveness reduced by hepatic enzyme-inducing drugs such as certain anticonvulsants and barbiturates, rifampin, rifabutin, griseofulvin, and protease inhibitors. Coadministration with St. John's wort may decrease efficacy. Vomiting or diarrhea may also increase the risk of contraceptive failure. Consider an additional form of birth control in above circumstances. See product insert for instructions on missing doses. Most available in 21 and 28 day packs. **Progestin only:** Must be taken at the same time every day. Because much of the literature regarding OC adverse effects pertains mainly to estrogen/progestin combinations, the extent to which progestin-only contraceptives cause these effects is unclear. No significant interaction has been found with broad-spectrum antibiotics. The effect of St. John's wort is unclear. No placebo days, start new pack immediately after finishing current one. Available in 28-day packs. Readers may find the following website useful: www.managingcontraception.com. † Approved for continuous use without a "pill-free" period. †† 84 active pills and 7 placebo pills.

bleeding: 5 to 10 mg PO daily for 5 to 10 days. <u>Endometrial hyperplasia</u>: 10 to 30 mg PO daily. [Generic/Trade: Tabs 2.5, 5, 10 mg, scored.] ▶L ♀X ▶+ $

MEDROXYPROGESTERONE-INJECTABLE (*Depo-Provera, depo-subQ provera 104*) <u>Contraception/Endometriosis</u>: 150 mg IM in deltoid or gluteus maximus or 104 mg SC in anterior thigh or abdomen q 13 weeks. ▶L ♀X ▶+ $ ■

MEGESTROL (*Megace, Megace ES*) <u>Endometrial hyperplasia</u>: 40 to 160 mg PO daily for 3 to 4 months. <u>AIDS anorexia</u>: 800 mg (20 mL) susp PO daily or 625 mg (5 mL) ES daily. [Generic/Trade: Tabs 20, 40 mg. Susp 40 mg/mL in 240 mL. Trade only: Megace ES susp 125 mg/mL (150 mL).] ▶L ♀D ▶? $$$$$

NORETHINDRONE (*Aygestin, Micronor, Nor-Q.D., Camila, Errin, Jolivette, Nora-BE*) <u>Amenorrhea, abnormal uterine bleeding</u>: 2.5 to 10 mg PO daily for 5 to 10 days during the 2nd half of the menstrual cycle. <u>Endometriosis</u>: 5 mg PO daily for 2 weeks. Increase by 2.5 mg q 2 weeks to 15 mg. [Generic/Trade: Tabs scored 5 mg. Trade only: 0.35 mg tabs.] ▶L ♀D/X ▶See notes $ ■

PROGESTERONE GEL (*Crinone, Prochieve*) <u>Secondary amenorrhea</u>: 45 mg (4%) intravaginally every other day up to 6 doses. If no response, use 90 mg (8%) every other day up to 6 doses. Infertility: Special dosing. [Trade only: 4%, 8% single-use, prefilled applicators.] ▶Plasma ♀− ▶? $$$

PROGESTERONE MICRONIZED (*Prometrium*) 200 mg PO at bedtime 10 to 12 days per month or 100 mg at bedtime daily. <u>Secondary amenorrhea</u>: 400 mg PO at bedtime for 10 days. Contraindicated in peanut allergy. [Trade only: Caps 100, 200 mg.] ▶L ♀B ▶+ $$ ■

PROGESTERONE VAGINAL INSERT (*Endometrin*) Infertility: Special dosing. [Trade only: 100 mg vaginal insert.] ▶Plasma ♀− ▶? $$$$

Selective Estrogen Receptor Modulators

RALOXIFENE (*Evista*) <u>Osteoporosis prevention/treatment, breast cancer prevention</u>: 60 mg PO daily. [Trade only: Tabs 60 mg.] ▶L ♀X ▶− $$$$ ■

TAMOXIFEN (*Nolvadex, Soltamox, Tamone, ✦Tamofen*) <u>Breast cancer prevention</u>: 20 mg PO daily for 5 years. <u>Breast cancer</u>: 10 to 20 mg PO two times per day. [Generic/Trade: Tabs 10, 20 mg. Trade only (Soltamox): Sugar-free soln 10 mg/5 mL (150 mL).] ▶L ♀D ▶− $$ ■

Uterotonics

CARBOPROST (*Hemabate, 15-methyl-prostaglandin F2 alpha*) <u>Refractory postpartum uterine bleeding</u>: 250 mcg deep IM. ▶LK ♀C ▶? $$$

METHYLERGONOVINE (*Methergine*) <u>Refractory postpartum uterine bleeding</u>: 0.2 mg IM/PO three to four times per day prn. [Trade only: Tabs 0.2 mg.] ▶LK ♀C ▶? $$

Vaginitis Preparations

NOTE: *See also STD/vaginitis table in antimicrobial section.*

DRUGS GENERALLY ACCEPTED AS SAFE IN PREGNANCY (selected)

Analgesics: acetaminophen, codeine*, meperidine*, methadone*, oxycodone*.
Antimicrobials: azithromycin, cephalosporins, clotrimazole, erythromycins (not estolate), metronidazole, penicillins, permethrin, nitrofurantoin***, nystatin. Antivirals: acyclovir, famciclovir, valacyclovir. CV: hydralazine*, labetalol, methyldopa, nifedipine. Derm: benzoyl peroxide, clindamycin, erythromycin. Endo: insulin, levothyroxine, liothyronine. ENT: chlorpheniramine, diphenhydramine, dextromethorphan, guaifenesin, nasal steroids, nasal cromolyn. GI: antacids*, bisacodyl, cimetidine, docusate, doxylamine, famotidine, lactulose, loperamide, meclizine, metoclopramide, nizatidine, ondansetron, psyllium, ranitidine, simethicone, trimethobenzamide. Heme: Heparin, low molecular wt heparins. Psych: bupropion, buspirone, desipramine, doxepin. Pulmonary: beclomethasone, budesonide, cromolyn, montelukast, nedocromil, prednisone**, short-acting inhaled beta-2 agonists, theophylline. *Except if used long-term or in high dose at term. **Except I[st] trimester. ***Contraindicated at term and during labor and delivery.

BORIC ACID <u>Resistant vulvovaginal candidiasis</u>: 1 vaginal suppository at bedtime for 2 weeks. [No commercial preparation; must be compounded by pharmacist. Vaginal supps 600 mg in gelatin caps.] ▶Not absorbed ♀? ▶− $

BUTOCONAZOLE (*Gynazole, Mycelex-3*) <u>Vulvovaginal candidiasis</u>: Mycelex 3: 1 applicatorful at bedtime for 3 to 6 days. Gynazole-1: 1 applicatorful intravaginally once at bedtime. [OTC: Trade only (Mycelex 3): 2% vaginal cream in 5 g prefilled applicators (3s), 20 g tube with applicators. Rx: Trade only (Gynazole-1): 2% vaginal cream in 5 g prefilled applicator.] ▶LK ♀C ▶? $(OTC), $$$(Rx)

CLINDAMYCIN-VAGINAL (*Cleocin, Clindesse, ✦ Dalacin*) <u>Bacterial vaginosis</u>: Cleocin: 1 applicatorful cream at bedtime for 7 days or 1 vaginal suppository at bedtime for 3 days. Clindesse: 1 applicatorful once. [Generic/Trade: 2% vaginal cream in 40 g tube with 7 disposable applicators (Cleocin). Vag suppository (Cleocin Ovules) 100 mg (3) with applicator. 2% vaginal cream in a single-dose prefilled applicator (Clindesse).] ▶L ♀− ▶+ $$

CLOTRIMAZOLE-VAGINAL (*Mycelex 7, Gyne-Lotrimin, ✦ Canesten, Clotrimaderm*) <u>Vulvovaginal candidiasis</u>: 1 applicatorful 1% cream at bedtime for 7 days. 1 applicatorful 2% cream at bedtime for 3 days. 1 vaginal suppository 100 mg at bedtime for 7 days. 200 mg suppository at bedtime for 3 days. [OTC Generic/Trade: 1% vaginal cream with applicator (some prefilled). 2% vaginal cream with applicator and 1% topical cream in some combination packs. OTC Trade only (Gyne-Lotrimin): Vaginal suppository 100 mg (7), 200 mg (3) with applicators.] ▶LK ♀B ▶? $

METRONIDAZOLE-VAGINAL (*MetroGel-Vaginal, Vandazole*) <u>Bacterial vaginosis</u>: 1 applicatorful at bedtime or two times per day for 5 days. [Generic/Trade: 0.75% gel in 70 g tube with applicator.] ▶LK ♀B ▶? $$

MICONAZOLE (*Monistat, Femizol-M, M-Zole, Micozole, Monazole*) <u>Vulvovaginal candidiasis</u>: 1 applicatorful at bedtime for 3 (4%) or 7 (2%) days. 100 mg vaginal suppository at bedtime for 7 days. 400 mg vaginal suppository at bedtime for 3 days. 1200 mg vaginal suppository once. [OTC Generic/Trade: 2% vaginal cream in 45 g with 1 applicator or 7 disposable applicators. Vaginal suppository 100 mg

(cont.)

(7) OTC Trade only: 400 mg (3), 1200 mg (1) with applicator. Generic/Trade: 4% vaginal cream in 25 g tubes or 3 prefilled applicators. Some in combination packs with 2% miconazole cream for external use.] ▶LK ♀+ ▶? $

NYSTATIN-VAGINAL (*Mycostatin*, ✦ *Nilstat*, *Nyaderm*) Vulvovaginal candidiasis: 1 vaginal tab at bedtime for 14 days. [Generic only: Vaginal tabs 100,000 units in 15s with applicator.] ▶Not metabolized ♀A ▶? $$

TERCONAZOLE (*Terazol*) Vulvovaginal candidiasis: 1 applicatorful of 0.4% cream at bedtime for 7 days, or 1 applicatorful of 0.8% cream at bedtime for 3 days, or 80 mg vaginal suppository at bedtime for 3 days. [All forms supplied with applicators: Generic/Trade: Vaginal cream 0.4% (Terazol 7) in 45 g tube, 0.8% (Terazol 3) in 20 g tube. Vaginal suppository (Terazol 3) 80 mg (#3).] ▶LK ♀C ▶– $$

TIOCONAZOLE (*Monistat 1-Day*, *Vagistat-1*) Vulvovaginal candidiasis: 1 applicatorful of 6.5% ointment intravaginally at bedtime single-dose. [OTC Trade only: Vaginal ointment: 6.5% (300 mg) in 4.6 g prefilled single-dose applicator.] ▶Not absorbed ♀C ▶– $$

Other OB/GYN Agents

DANAZOL (*Danocrine*, ✦ *Cyclomen*) Endometriosis: Start 400 mg PO two times per day, then titrate downward to maintain amenorrhea for 3 to 6 months. Fibrocystic breast disease: 100 to 200 mg PO two times per day for 4 to 6 months. [Generic only: Caps 50, 100, 200 mg.] ▶L ♀X ▶– $$$$$ ■

MIFEPRISTONE (*Mifeprex*, *RU-486*) Termination of pregnancy, up to 49 days: 600 mg PO followed by 400 mcg misoprostol on day 3, if abortion not confirmed. [Trade only: Tabs 200 mg.] ▶L ♀X ▶? $$$$$ ■

PREMESIS-RX (pyridoxine + folic acid + cyanocobalamin + calcium carbonate) Pregnancy-induced nausea: 1 tab PO daily. [Trade only: Tabs 75 mg vitamin B6 (pyridoxine), sustained-release, 12 mcg vitamin B12 (cyanocobalamin), 1 mg folic acid, and 200 mg calcium carbonate.] ▶L ♀A ▶+ $$

RHO IMMUNE GLOBULIN (*HyperRHO S/D*, *MICRhoGAM*, *RhoGAM*, *Rhophylac*, *WinRho SDF*) Prevention of hemolytic disease of the newborn if mother RH– and baby is or might be RH+: 300 mcg vial IM to mother at 28 weeks gestation followed by a second dose within 72 h of delivery. Microdose (50 mcg, MICRhoGAM) is appropriate if spontaneous abortion less than 12 weeks gestation. ▶L ♀C ▶? $$$$$

ONCOLOGY

ALKYLATING AGENTS altretamine (*Hexalen*), bendamustine (*Treanda*), busulfan (*Myleran*, *Busulfex*), carmustine (*BCNU*, *BiCNU*, *Gliadel*), chlorambucil (*Leukeran*), cyclophosphamide (*Cytoxan*, *Neosar*), dacarbazine (*DTIC-Dome*), ifosfamide (*Ifex*), lomustine (*CeeNu*, *CCNU*), mechlorethamine (*Mustargen*), melphalan (*Alkeran*), procarbazine (*Matulane*), streptozocin (*Zanosar*),

(cont.)

temozolomide (*Temodar*, ✦*Temodal*), thiotepa (*Thioplex*). **ANTIBIOTICS:** bleomycin (*Blenoxane*), dactinomycin (*Cosmegen*), daunorubicin *(Cerubidine)*, doxorubicin liposomal (*Doxil*, ✦*Caelyx, Myocet*), doxorubicin non-liposomal (*Adriamycin, Rubex*), epirubicin (*Ellence*, ✦*Pharmorubicin*), idarubicin (*Idamycin*), mitomycin (*Mutamycin, Mitomycin-C*), mitoxantrone (*Novantrone*), valrubicin (*Valstar*, ✦*Valtaxin*). **ANTIMETABOLITES:** azacitidine (*Vidaza*), capecitabine (*Xeloda*), cladribine (*Leustatin, chlorodeoxyadenosine*), clofarabine (*Clolar*), cytarabine (*Cytosar, AraC*), cytarabine liposomal (*Depo-Cyt*),decitabine (*Dacogen*), floxuridine (*FUDR*), fludarabine (*Fludara*), fluorouracil (*Adrucil, 5-FU*), gemcitabine (*Gemzar*), hydroxyurea (*Hydrea, Droxia*), mercaptopurine (*6-MP, Purinethol*), methotrexate (*Rheumatrex, Trexall*), nelarabine (*Arranon*), pemetrexed (*Alimta*), pentostatin (*Nipent*), Pralatrexate (*Folotyn*), thioguanine (*Tabloid*, ✦*Lanvis*). **CYTOPROTECTIVE AGENTS:** amifostine (*Ethyol*), dexrazoxane (*Zinecard, Totect*), leucovorin (folinic acid), levoleucovorin (Fusilev), mesna (*Mesnex*, ✦*Uromitexan*), palifermin (*Kepivance*). **HORMONES:** anastrozole (*Arimidex*), bicalutamide (*Casodex*), cyproterone, (*Androcur, Androcur Depot*), degarelix (*Firmagon*), estramustine (*Emcyt*), exemestane (*Aromasin*), flutamide (*Eulexin*, ✦*Euflex*), fulvestrant (*Faslodex*), goserelin (*Zoladex*), histrelin (*Vantas, Supprelin LA*), letrozole (*Femara*), leuprolide (*Eligard, Lupron, Lupron Depot, Lupron Depot-Ped*), nilutamide (*Nilandron*), raloxifene (*Evista*), tamoxifen (Nolvadex), toremifene (*Fareston*), triptorelin (*Trelstar Depot*). **IMMUNOMODULATORS:** aldesleukin (*Proleukin, interleukin-2*), alemtuzumab (*Campath*, ✦*MabCampath*), BCG (*Bacillus of Calmette & Guerin, Pacis, TheraCys, Tice BCG*, ✦*OncoTICE*, ✦*Immucyst*), bevacizumab (*Avastin*), cetuximab (*Erbitux*), denileukin (*Ontak*), everolimus (*Afinitor*), ibritumomab (*Zevalin*), interferon alfa-2b (*Intron-A*), lenalidomide (*Revlimid*), ofatumumab (*Arzerra*), panitumumab (*Vectibix*), rituximab (*Rituxan*), temsirolimus (*Torisel*), thalidomide (*Thalomid*), tositumomab (*Bexxar*), trastuzumab (*Herceptin*). **MITOTIC INHIBITORS:** Cabazitaxel (*Jevtana*), Docetaxel (*Taxotere*), eribulin (*Halaven*), ixabepilone (*Ixempra*), paclitaxel (*Taxol, Abraxane, Onxol*), vinblastine (*Velban, VLB*), vincristine (*Oncovin, Vincasar, VCR*), vinorelbine (*Navelbine*). **PLATINUM-CONTAINING AGENTS:** carboplatin (*Paraplatin*), cisplatin (*Platinol-AQ*), oxaliplatin (*Eloxatin*). **RADIOPHARMACEUTICALS:** samarium 153 (*Quadramet*), strontium-89 (*Metastron*). **TOPOISOMERASE INHIBITORS:** etoposide (*VP-16, Etopophos, Toposar, VePesid*), irinotecan (*Camptosar*), teniposide (*Vumon, VM-26*), topotecan (*Hycamtin*). **MISCELLANEOUS:** arsenic trioxide (*Trisenox*), asparaginase (*Elspar*, ✦*Kidrolase*), bexarotene (*Targretin*), bortezomib (*Velcade*), dasatinib (*Sprycel*), erlotinib (*Tarceva*) gefitinib (*Iressa*), imatinib (*Gleevec*), lapatinib (*Tykerb*), mitotane (*Lysodren*), nilotinib (*Tasigna*), pazopanib (*Votrient*), pegaspargase (*Oncaspar*), porfimer (*Photofrin*), rasburicase (*Elitek*), romidepsin (*Istodax*), sorafenib (*Nexavar*), sunitinib (*Sutent*), tretinoin (*Vesanoid*), vorinostat (*Zolinza*).

OPHTHALMOLOGY

NOTE: *Most eye medications can be administered 1 gtt at a time despite common manufacturer recommendations of 1 to 2 gtts concurrently. Even a single gtt is typically more than the eye can hold, and thus a second gtt is wasteful and increases the possibility of systemic toxicity. If 2 gtts of the medication are desired, separate single gtt by at least 5 min.*

Antiallergy—Decongestants & Combinations

NAPHAZOLINE (*Albalon, All Clear, AK-Con, Naphcon, Clear Eyes*) 1 to 2 gtts in each affected eye four times per day for up to 3 days. [OTC Generic/Trade: Soln 0.012, 0.025% (15, 30 mL). Rx Generic/Trade: 0.1% (15 mL).] ▶? ♀C ▶? $

NAPHCON-A (naphazoline + pheniramine, *Visine-A*) 1 gtt in each affected eye four times per day prn for up to 3 days. [OTC Trade only: Soln 0.025% + 0.3% (15 mL).] ▶L ♀C ▶? $

VASOCON-A (naphazoline + antazoline) 1 gtt in each affected eye four times per day prn for up to 3 days. [OTC Trade only: Soln 0.05% + 0.5% (15 mL).] ▶L ♀C ▶? $

Antiallergy—Dual Antihistamine & Mast Cell Stabilizer

AZELASTINE—OPHTHALMIC (*Optivar*) 1 gtt in each affected eye two times per day. [Trade only: Soln 0.05% (6 mL).] ▶L ♀C ▶? $$$

EPINASTINE (*Elestat*) 1 gtt in each affected eye two times per day. [Trade only: Soln 0.05% (5 mL).] ▶K ♀C ▶? $$$$

KETOTIFEN-OPHTHALMIC (*Alaway, Zaditor*) 1 gtt in each affected eye q 8 to 12 h. [OTC Generic/Trade: Soln 0.025% (5 mL).] ▶Minimal absorption ♀C ▶? $

OLOPATADINE (*Pataday, Patanol*) 1 gtt of 0.1% soln in each affected eye two times per day (Patanol) or 1 gtt of 0.2% soln in each affected eye daily (Pataday). [Trade only: Soln 0.1% (5 mL, Patanol), 0.2% (2.5 mL, Pataday).] ▶K ♀C ▶? $$$$

Antiallergy—Pure Antihistamines

ALCAFTADINE (*Lastacaft*) <u>Allergic conjunctivitis:</u> 1 gtt into each eye once daily. [Trade: Soln 0.25% 3 mL.] ▶minimal absorption – ♀B ▶? $$$

BEPOTASTINE (*Bepreve*) 1 gtt in each affected eye two times per day [Trade only: Soln 1.5% (2.5, 5, 10 mL)] ▶L (but minimal absorption) – ♀C ▶? $$$

EMEDASTINE (*Emadine*) 1 gtt in each affected eye daily to four times per day. [Trade only: Soln 0.05% (5 mL).] ▶L ♀B ▶? $$$

LEVOCABASTINE—OPHTHALMIC (*Livostin*) 1 gtt in each affected eye one to four times per day for 2 weeks. [Trade only: Susp 0.05% (5, 10 mL).] ▶Minimal absorption ♀C ▶? $$$

Antiallergy—Pure Mast Cell Stabilizers

CROMOLYN—OPHTHALMIC (*Crolom, Opticrom*) 1 to 2 gtts in each affected eye four to six times per day. [Generic/Trade: Soln 4% (10 mL).] ▶L ♀B ▶? $$

LODOXAMIDE (*Alomide*) 1 to 2 gtts in each affected eye four times per day. [Trade only: Soln 0.1% (10 mL).] ▶K ♀B ▶? $$$

NEDOCROMIL—OPHTHALMIC (*Alocril*) 1 to 2 gtts in each affected eye two times per day. [Trade only: Soln 2% (5 mL).] ▶L ♀B ▶? $$$

PEMIROLAST (*Alamast*) 1 to 2 gtts in each affected eye four times per day. [Trade only: Soln 0.1% (10 mL).] ▶? ♀C ▶? $$$

Antibacterials—Aminoglycosides

GENTAMICIN—OPHTHALMIC (*Garamycin, Genoptic, Gentak, ✦ Diogent*) 1 to 2 gtts in each affected eye q 2 to 4 h; ½ inch ribbon of ointment two to three times per day. [Generic/Trade: Soln 0.3% (5, 15 mL) Ointment 0.3% (3.5 g tube).] ▶K ♀C ▶? $

TOBRAMYCIN—OPHTHALMIC (*Tobrex*) 1 to 2 gtts in each affected eye q 1 to 4 h or ½ inch ribbon of ointment q 3 to 4 h or two or three times per day. [Generic/Trade: Soln 0.3% (5 mL). Trade only: Ointment 0.3% (3.5 g tube).] ▶K ♀B ▶– $

Antibacterials—Fluoroquinolones

BESIFLOXACIN (*Besivance*) 1 gtt in each affected eye three times per day for 7 days. [Trade: Soln 0.6% (5 mL).] ▶LK ♀C ▶? ?

CIPROFLOXACIN—OPHTHALMIC (*Ciloxan*) 1 to 2 gtts in each affected eye q 1 to 6 h or ½ inch ribbon ointment two to three times per day. [Generic/Trade: Soln 0.3% (2.5, 5, 10 mL). Trade only: Ointment 0.3% (3.5 g tube).] ▶LK ♀C ▶? $$

GATIFLOXACIN—OPHTHALMIC (*Zymaxid*) 1 to 2 gtts in each affected eye q 2 h while awake (up to 8 times per day) on day 1 and 2, then 1 to 2 gtts q 4 h (up to four times per day) on days 3 to 7. [Trade only: Soln 0.3% (5 mL).] ▶K ♀C ▶? $$$

LEVOFLOXACIN—OPHTHALMIC (*Iquix, Quixin*) Quixin: 1 to 2 gtts in each affected eye q 2 h while awake (up to 8 times per day) on days 1 and 2, then 1 to 2 gtts q 4 h (up to four times per day) on days 3 to 7. Iquix: 1 to 2 gtts q 30 min to 2 h while awake and q 4 to 6 h overnight on days 1 to 3, then 1 to 2 gtts q 1 to 4 h while awake on day 4 to completion of therapy. [Trade only: Soln 0.5% (Quixin, 5 mL), 1.5% (Iquix, 5 mL).] ▶KL ♀C ▶? $$$

MOXIFLOXACIN—OPHTHALMIC (*Vigamox, Moxeza*) 1 gtt in each affected eye three times per day for 7 days (Vigamox) or 1 gtt in each affected eye two times per day for 7 days (Moxeza). [Trade only: Soln 0.5% (3 mL, Vigamox, 4 mL, Moxeza).] ▶LK ♀C ▶? $$$

OFLOXACIN—OPHTHALMIC (*Ocuflox*) 1 to 2 gtts in each affected eye q 1 to 6 h for 7 to 10 days. [Generic/Trade: Soln 0.3% (5, 10 mL).] ▶LK ♀C ▶? $$

Antibacterials—Other

AZITHROMYCIN—OPHTHALMIC (*Azasite*) 1 gtt in each affected eye two times per day for 2 days, then 1 gtt once daily for 5 more days. [Trade only: Soln 1% (2.5 mL).] ▶L ♀B ▶? $$$

BACITRACIN—OPHTHALMIC (*AK Tracin*) Apply ¼ to ½ inch ribbon of ointment in each affected eye q 3 to 4 h or two to four times per day for 7 to 10 days. [Generic/Trade: Ointment 500 units/g (3.5 g tube).] ▶Minimal absorption ♀C ▶? $

ERYTHROMYCIN—OPHTHALMIC (*Ilotycin, AK-Mycin*) ½ inch ribbon of ointment in each affected eye q 3 to 4 h or two to six times per day. [Generic only: Ointment 0.5% (1, 3.5 g tube).] ▶L ♀B ▶+ $

NEOSPORIN OINTMENT—OPHTHALMIC (neomycin + bacitracin + polymyxin) ½ inch ribbon of ointment in each affected eye q 3 to 4 h for 7 to 10 days or ½ inch ribbon two to three times per day for mild to moderate infection. [Generic only: Ointment. (3.5 g tube).] ▶K ♀C ▶? $$

NEOSPORIN SOLUTION—OPHTHALMIC (neomycin + polymyxin + gramicidin) 1 to 2 gtts in each affected eye q 4 to 6 h for 7 to 10 days. [Generic/Trade: Soln (10 mL).] ▶KL ♀C ▶? $$

POLYSPORIN—OPHTHALMIC (polymyxin + bacitracin) ½ inch ribbon of ointment in each affected eye q 3 to 4 h for 7 to 10 days or ½ inch ribbon two to three times per day for mild to moderate infection. [Generic only: Ointment (3.5 g tube).] ▶K ♀C ▶? $$

POLYTRIM—OPHTHALMIC (polymyxin + trimethoprim) 1 to 2 gtts in each affected eye q 4 to 6 h (up to 6 gtts per day) for 7 to 10 days. [Generic/Trade: Soln (10 mL).] ▶KL ♀C ▶? $

SULFACETAMIDE—OPHTHALMIC (*Bleph-10, Sulf-10*) 1 to 2 gtts in each affected eye q 2 to 6 h for 7 to 10 days or ½ inch ribbon of ointment q 3 to 8 h for 7 to 10 days. [Generic/Trade: Soln 10% (15 mL), Ointment 10% (3.5 g tube). Generic only: Soln 30% (15 mL).] ▶K ♀C ▶– $

Antiviral Agents

GANCICLOVIR (*Zirgan*) <u>Herpetic keratitis</u>: 1 gtt five times per day (approximately q 3 h) until ulcer heals, then 1 gtt 3 times/day for 7 days. [Trade only: Gel 0.15% (5g).] ▶Minimal absorption ♀C ▶? $$$$

TRIFLURIDINE (*Viroptic*) <u>Herpetic keratitis</u>: 1 gtt q 2 to 4 h for 7 to 14 days, max 9 gtts per day and max of 21 days of therapy. [Generic/Trade Soln 1% (7.5 mL).] ▶Minimal absorption ♀C ▶– $$$

Corticosteroid & Antibacterial Combinations

NOTE: *Recommend that only ophthalmologists or optometrists prescribe due to infection, cataract, corneal/scleral perforation, and glaucoma risk from prolonged use. Monitor intraocular pressure.*

BLEPHAMIDE (prednisolone—ophthalmic + sulfacetamide) 1 to 2 gtts in each affected eye q 1 to 8 h or ½ inch ribbon to lower conjunctival sac 3 to 4 times per day and 1 to 2 times at bedtime. [Generic/Trade: Soln/Susp (5, 10 mL), Trade only: Ointment (3.5 g tube).] ▶KL ♀C ▶? $

CORTISPORIN-OPHTHALMIC (neomycin + polymyxin + hydrocortisone—ophthalmic) 1 to 2 gtts or ½ inch ribbon of ointment in each affected eye q 3 to 4 h or more frequently prn. [Generic only: Susp (7.5 mL), Ointment (3.5 g tube).] ▶LK ♀C ▶? $

FML-S LIQUIFILM (prednisolone—ophthalmic + sulfacetamide) 1 to 2 gtts in each affected eye q 1 to 8 h or ½ inch ribbon of ointment one to four times per day. [Trade only: Susp (10 mL).] ▶KL ♀C ▶? $$

MAXITROL (dexamethasone—ophthalmic + neomycin + polymyxin) Small amount (about ½ inch) ointment in affected eye 3 to 4 times per day or at bedtime as an adjunct with gtts. 1 to 2 susp gtts into affected eye q 3 to 4 h; in severe disease, gtts may be used hourly and tapered to discontinuation. [Generic/Trade: Susp (5 mL), Ointment (3.5 g tube).] ▶KL ♀C ▶? $$

PRED G (prednisolone—ophthalmic + gentamicin) 1 to 2 gtts in each affected eye q 1 to 8 h daily to four times per day or ½ inch ribbon of ointment two to four times per day. [Trade only: Susp (2, 5, 10 mL), Ointment (3.5 g tube).] ▶KL ♀C ▶? $$

TOBRADEX (tobramycin + dexamethasone—ophthalmic) 1 to 2 gtts in each affected eye q 2 to 6 h or ½ inch ribbon of ointment two to four times per day. [Trade only (tobramycin 0.3%/dexamethasone 0.1%): Susp (2.5, 5, 10 mL), Ointment (3.5 g tube).] ▶L ♀C ▶? $$$

TOBRADEX ST (tobramycin + dexamethasone—ophthalmic) 1 gtt in each affected eye q 2 to 6 h. [Trade only: Tobramycin 0.3%/dexamethasone 0.05%: Susp (2.5, 5, 10 mL).] ▶L ♀C ▶? $$$

VASOCIDIN (prednisolone—ophthalmic + sulfacetamide) 1 to 2 gtts in each affected eye q 1 to 8 h or ½ inch ribbon of ointment one to four times per day. [Generic only: Soln (5, 10 mL).] ▶KL ♀C ▶? $

ZYLET (loteprednol + tobramycin) 1 to 2 gtts in each affected eye q 1 to 2 h for 1 to 2 days then 1 to 2 gtts q 4 to 6 h. [Trade only: Susp 0.5% loteprednol + 0.3% tobramycin (2.5, 5, 10 mL).] ▶LK ♀C ▶? $$$

Corticosteroids

NOTE: *Recommend that only ophthalmologists or optometrists prescribe due to infection, cataract, corneal/scleral perforation, and glaucoma risk. Monitor intraocular pressure. Gradually taper when discontinuing.*

DIFLUPREDNATE (*Durezol*) 1 gtt into affected eye four times per day, beginning 24 h after surgery for 2 weeks, then 1 gtt into affected eye two times per day for 1 week, then taper based on response. [Trade only: Ophthalmic emulsion 0.05% (2.5, 5 mL).] ▶Not absorbed ♀C ▶? $$$$

FLUOROMETHOLONE (*FML, FML Forte, Flarex*) 1 to 2 gtts in each affected eye q 1 to 12 h or ½ inch ribbon of ointment q 4 to 24 h. [Trade only: Susp 0.1% (5, 10, 15 mL), 0.25% (2, 5, 10, 15 mL), Ointment 0.1% (3.5 g tube).] ▶L ♀C ▶? $$

LOTEPREDNOL (*Alrex, Lotemax*) 1 to 2 gtts in each affected eye four times per day. [Trade only: Susp 0.2% (Alrex 5, 10 mL), 0.5% (Lotemax 2.5, 5, 10, 15 mL).] ▶L ♀C ▶? $$$

PREDNISOLONE—OPHTHALMIC (*Pred Forte, Pred Mild, Inflamase Forte, Econopred Plus, ♦Diopred*) Soln: 1 to 2 gtts in each affected eye (up to q 1 h during day and q 2 h at night); when response observed, then 1 gtt in each affected eye q 4 h, then 1 gtt three to four times per day. Susp: 1 to 2 gtts in each affected eye two to four times per day. [Generic/Trade: Soln, Susp 1% (5, 10, 15 mL). Trade only (Pred Mild): Susp 0.12% (5, 10 mL), Susp (Pred Forte) 1% (1 mL).] ▶L ♀C ▶? $$

RIMEXOLONE (*Vexol*) 1 to 2 gtts in each affected eye q 1 to 6 h. [Trade only: Susp 1% (5, 10 mL).] ▶L ♀C ▶? $$

Glaucoma Agents—Beta-Blockers

NOTE: *Use caution in cardiac conditions and asthma.*

BETAXOLOL—OPHTHALMIC (*Betoptic, Betoptic S*) 1 to 2 gtts in each affected eye two times per day. [Trade only: Susp 0.25% (5, 10, 15 mL). Generic only: Soln 0.5% (5, 10, 15 mL).] ▶LK ♀C ▶? $$

CARTEOLOL—OPHTHALMIC (*Ocupress*) 1 gtt in each affected eye two times per day. [Generic only: Soln 1% (5, 10, 15 mL).] ▶KL ♀C ▶? $

LEVOBUNOLOL (*Betagan*) 1 to 2 gtts in each affected eye one to two times per day. [Generic/Trade: Soln 0.25% (5, 10 mL), 0.5% (5, 10, 15 mL. Trade only: Soln 0.25% 2 mL).] ▶? ♀C ▶– $$

METIPRANOLOL (*Optipranolol*) 1 gtt in each affected eye two times per day. [Generic/Trade: Soln 0.3% (5, 10 mL).] ▶? ♀C ▶? $

TIMOLOL—OPHTHALMIC (*Betimol, Timoptic, Timoptic XE, Istalol, Timoptic Ocudose*) 1 gtt in each affected eye two times per day. Timoptic XE, Istalol: 1 gtt in each affected eye daily. [Generic/Trade: Soln 0.25, 0.5% (5, 10, 15 mL), Preservative-free soln (Timoptic Ocudose) 0.25% (0.2 mL), Gel-forming soln (Timoptic XE) 0.25, 0.5% (2.5, 5 mL).] ▶LK ♀C ▶+ $$

Glaucoma Agents—Carbonic Anhydrase Inhibitors

NOTE: *Sulfonamide derivatives; verify absence of sulfa allergy before prescribing.*

BRINZOLAMIDE (*Azopt*) 1 gtt in each affected eye three times per day. [Trade only: Susp 1% (5, 10, 15 mL).] ▶LK ♀C ▶? $$$

DORZOLAMIDE (*Trusopt*) 1 gtt in each affected eye three times per day. [Generic/Trade: Soln 2% (5, 10 mL).] ▶KL ♀C ▶– $$$

METHAZOLAMIDE (*Neptazane*) 25 to 50 mg PO daily (up to three times per day). [Generic only: Tabs 25, 50 mg.] ▶LK ♀C ▶? $$

Glaucoma Agents—Combinations and Other

COMBIGAN (brimonidine + timolol) 1 gtt in each affected eye q 12 h. [Trade only: Soln brimonidine 0.2% + timolol 0.5% (5, 10 mL).] ▶LK ♀C ▶– $$$

COSOPT (dorzolamide + timolol) 1 gtt in each affected eye two times per day. [Generic/Trade: Soln dorzolamide 2% + timolol 0.5% (5, 10 mL).] ▶LK ♀D ▶– $$$

Glaucoma Agents—Miotics

PILOCARPINE—OPHTHALMIC (*Pilopine HS, Isopto Carpine, ✦Akarpine*) 1 gtt in each affected eye up to four times per day or ½ inch ribbon of gel bedtime. [Generic only: Soln 0.5% (15 mL), 1% (2 mL), 2% (2 mL), 3% (15 mL), 4% (2 mL), 6% (15 mL). Generic/Trade: Soln 1% (15 mL), 2% (15 mL), 4% (15 mL). Trade only (Pilopine HS): Gel 4% (4 g tube).] ▶Plasma ♀C ▶ $

Glaucoma Agents—Prostaglandin Analogs

BIMATOPROST (*Lumigan, Latisse*) 1 gtt to eyelashes (Latisse) or each affected eye (Lumigan) at bedtime. [Trade only: Soln 0.01%, 0.03% (Lumigan, 2.5, 5, 7.5 mL), (Latisse, 3 mL with 60 sterile, disposable applicators).] ▶LK ♀C ▶? $$$

LATANOPROST (*Xalatan*) 1 gtt in each affected eye at bedtime. [Trade only: Soln 0.005% (2.5 mL).] ▶LK ♀C ▶? $$$

TRAVOPROST (*Travatan, Travatan Z*) 1 gtt in each affected eye at bedtime. [Trade only: Soln (Travatan), benzalkonium chloride-free (Travatan Z) 0.004% (2.5, 5 mL).] ▶L ♀C ▶? $$$

Glaucoma Agents—Sympathomimetics

BRIMONIDINE (*Alphagan P, ✦Alphagan*) 1 gtt in each affected eye three times per day. [Trade only: Soln 0.1% (5, 10, 15 mL). Generic/Trade: Soln 0.15% (5, 10, 15 mL). Generic only: Soln 0.2% (5, 10, 15 mL).] ▶L ♀B ▶? $$

Mydriatics & Cycloplegics

ATROPINE—OPHTHALMIC (*Isopto Atropine, Atropine Care*) 1 to 2 gtts in each affected eye before procedure or daily to four times per day or ⅓ to ¼ inch ointment before procedure or one to three times per day. Cycloplegia may last up to 5 to 10 days and mydriasis may last up to 7 to 14 days. [Generic/Trade: Soln 1% (2, 5, 15 mL). Generic only: Ointment 1% (3.5 g tube)] ▶I ♀C ▶+ $

CYCLOPENTOLATE (*AK-Pentolate, Cyclogyl, Pentolair*) 1 to 2 gtts in each affected eye for 1 to 2 doses before procedure. Cycloplegia may last 6 to 24 h; mydriasis may last 1 day. [Generic/Trade: Soln 1% (2, 15 mL). Trade only (Cyclogyl): 0.5% (15 mL), 1% (5 mL) and 2% (2, 5, 15 mL).] ▶? ♀C ▶? $

HOMATROPINE (*Isopto Homatropine*) 1 to 2 gtts in each affected eye before procedure or two to three times per day. Cycloplegia and mydriasis lasts 1 to 3 days. [Trade only: Soln 2% (5 mL), 5% (15 mL). Generic/Trade: Soln 5% (5 mL).] ▶? ♀C ▶? $

PHENYLEPHRINE—OPHTHALMIC (*AK-Dilate, Altafrin, Mydfrin, Refresh*) 1 to 2 gtts in each affected eye before procedure or three to four times per day. No cycloplegia; mydriasis may last up to 5 h. [Rx Generic/Trade: Soln 2.5% (2, 3, 5, 15 mL), 10% (5 mL). OTC Trade only (Altafrin and Refresh): Soln 0.12% (15 mL).] ▶Plasma, L ♀C ▶? $

TROPICAMIDE (*Mydriacyl, Tropicacyl*) 1 to 2 gtts in each affected eye before procedure. Mydriasis may last 6 h. [Generic/Trade: Soln 0.5% (15 mL), 1% (3, 15 mL). Generic only: Soln 1% (2 mL).] ▶? ♀? ▶? $

Non-Steroidal Anti-Inflammatories

BROMFENAC—OPHTHALMIC (*Bromday*) 1 gtt in each affected eye once daily beginning 1 day prior to surgery and continuing for 14 days after surgery. [Trade only: Soln 0.09% (1.7 mL).] ▶Minimal absorption ♀C, D (3rd trimester) ▶? $$$$$

DICLOFENAC—OPHTHALMIC (*Voltaren, ✦ Voltaren Ophtha*) 1 gtt in each affected eye four times per day. [Generic/Trade: Soln 0.1% (2.5, 5 mL).] ▶L ♀B, D (3rd trimester) ▶? $$$

KETOROLAC—OPHTHALMIC (*Acular, Acular LS*) 1 gtt in each affected eye four times per day. [Generic/Trade: Soln (Acular LS) 0.4%. Trade only: Acular 0.5% (3, 5, 10 mL), preservative-free Acular 0.5% unit dose (0.4 mL).] ▶L ♀C ▶? $$$$

NEPAFENAC (*Nevanac*) 1 gtt in each affected eye three times per day for 2 weeks. [Trade only: Susp 0.1% (3 mL).] ▶Minimal absorption ♀C ▶? $$$

Other Ophthalmologic Agents

ARTIFICIAL TEARS (*Tears Naturale, Hypotears, Refresh Tears, GenTeal, Systane*) 1 to 2 gtts in each eye three to four times per day prn. [OTC Generic/Trade: Soln (15, 30 mL, among others).] ▶Minimal absorption ♀A ▶+ $

CYCLOSPORINE—OPHTHALMIC (*Restasis*) 1 gtt in each eye q 12 h. [Trade only: Emulsion 0.05% (0.4 mL single-use vials).] ▶Minimal absorption ♀C ▶? $$$$

HYDROXYPROPYL CELLULOSE (*Lacrisert*) Moderate to severe dry eyes: 1 insert in each eye daily. Some patients may require twice daily use. [Trade only: Ocular insert 5 mg.] ▶Minimal absorption ♀+ ▶+ $$$

LIDOCAINE—OPHTHALMIC (*Akten*) Do not prescribe for unsupervised or prolonged use. Corneal toxicity and ocular infections may occur with repeated use. 2 gtts before procedure, repeat prn. [Generic only: Gel 3.5% (5 mL).] ▶L ♀B ▶? ?

PETROLATUM (*Lacrilube, Dry Eyes, Refresh PM, ✦ Duolube*) Apply ¼ to ½ inch ointment to inside of lower lid prn. [OTC Trade only: Ointment (3.5, 7 g) tube.] ▶Minimal absorption ♀A ▶+ $

PROPARACAINE (*Ophthaine, Ophthetic, ✦ Alcaine*) Do not prescribe for unsupervised or prolonged use. Corneal toxicity and ocular infections may occur with repeated use. 1 to 2 gtts into affected eye before procedure. [Generic/Trade: Soln 0.5% (15 mL).] ▶L ♀C ▶? $

TETRACAINE—OPHTHALMIC (*Pontocaine*) Do not prescribe for unsupervised or prolonged use. Corneal toxicity and ocular infections may occur with repeated use. 1 to 2 gtts or ½ to 1 inch ribbon of ointment in each affected eye before procedure. [Generic only: Soln 0.5% (15 mL), unit-dose vials (0.7, 2 mL).] ▶Plasma ♀C ▶? $

PSYCHIATRY

Antidepressants—Heterocyclic Compounds

AMITRIPTYLINE *(Elavil)* <u>Depression</u>: Start 25 to 100 mg PO at bedtime; gradually increase to usual effective dose of 50 to 300 mg/day. Primarily inhibits serotonin reuptake. Demethylated to nortriptyline, which primarily inhibits norepinephrine reuptake. Suicidality. [Generic: Tabs 10, 25, 50, 75, 100, 150 mg. Elavil brand name no longer available; has been retained in this entry for name recognition purposes only.] ▶L ♀D ▶– $$

CLOMIPRAMINE *(Anafranil)* <u>OCD</u>: Start 25 mg PO at bedtime; gradually increase to usual effective dose of 150 to 250 mg/day. Max 250 mg/day. Primarily inhibits serotonin reuptake. Suicidality. [Generic/Trade: Caps 25, 50, 75 mg.] ▶L ♀C ▶+ $$$

DESIPRAMINE *(Norpramin)* <u>Depression</u>: Start 25 to 100 mg PO given once daily or in divided doses. Gradually increase to usual effective dose of 100 to 200 mg/day, max 300 mg/day. Primarily inhibits norepinephrine reuptake. Suicidality. [Generic/Trade: Tabs 10, 25, 50, 75, 100, 150 mg.] ▶L ♀C ▶+ $$

DOXEPIN *(Sinequan, Silenor)* <u>Depression</u>: Start 75 mg PO at bedtime. Gradually increase to usual effective dose of 75 to 150 mg/day, max 300 mg/day. Primarily inhibits norepinephrine reuptake. <u>Insomnia</u> (Silenor): 6 mg PO 30 min before bedtime, 3 mg in age 65 yo or older. Suicidality. [Generic/Trade: Caps 10, 25, 50, 75, 100, 150 mg. Oral concentrate 10 mg/mL.] ▶L ♀C ▶– $$

IMIPRAMINE *(Tofranil, Tofranil PM)* <u>Depression</u>: Start 75 to 100 mg PO at bedtime or in divided doses; gradually increase to max 300 mg/day. <u>Enuresis</u>: 25 to 75 mg PO at bedtime. Suicidality. [Generic/Trade: Tabs 10, 25, 50 mg. Caps 75, 100, 125, 150 mg (as pamoate salt).] ▶L ♀D ▶– $$$

NORTRIPTYLINE *(Aventyl, Pamelor)* <u>Depression</u>: Start 25 mg PO given once daily or divided two to four times per day. Usual effective dose is 75 to 100 mg/day, max 150 mg/day. Primarily inhibits norepinephrine reuptake. Suicidality. [Generic/Trade: Caps 10, 25, 50, 75 mg. Oral soln 10 mg/5 mL.] ▶L ♀D ▶+ $$$

PROTRIPTYLINE *(Vivactil)* <u>Depression</u>: 15 to 40 mg/day PO divided three to four times per day. Max 60 mg/day. Suicidality. [Trade only: Tabs 5, 10 mg.] ▶L ♀C ▶+ $$$$

VILAZODONE *(Viibryd)* <u>Depression</u>: Start 10 mg PO once daily. Max 40 mg/day. [Trade only: Tabs 10, 20, and 40 mg.] Give this medication with food. ▶L – ♀C ▶?

Antidepressants—Monoamine Oxidase Inhibitors (MAOIs)

NOTE: *Must be on tyramine-free diet throughout treatment and for 2 weeks after discontinuation. Numerous drug interactions; risk of hypertensive crisis*

(cont.)

and serotonin syndrome with many medications, including OTC. Allow at least 2 weeks wash-out when converting from an MAOI to an SSRI (6 weeks after fluoxetine), TCA, or other antidepressant.

ISOCARBOXAZID (*Marplan*) <u>Depression</u>: Start 10 mg PO two times per day; increase by 10 mg q 2 to 4 days. Usual effective dose is 20 to 40 mg/day. MAOI diet. Suicidality. [Trade only: Tabs 10 mg.] ▶L ♀C ▶? $$$

PHENELZINE (*Nardil*) <u>Depression</u>: Start 15 mg PO three times per day. Usual effective dose is 60 to 90 mg/day in divided doses. MAOI diet. Suicidality. [Trade only: Tabs 15 mg.] ▶L ♀C ▶? $$$

SELEGILINE—TRANSDERMAL (*Emsam*) <u>Depression</u>: Start 6 mg/24 h patch, change daily. Max 12 mg/24 h. MAOI diet for doses 9 mg/day or higher. Suicidality. [Trade only: Transdermal patch 6 mg/day, 9 mg/24 h, 12 mg/24 h.] ▶L ♀C ▶ $$$$$

TRANYLCYPROMINE (*Parnate*) <u>Depression</u>: Start 10 mg PO q am; increase by 10 mg/day at 1- to 3- week intervals to usual effective dose of 10 to 40 mg/day divided two times per day. MAOI diet. Suicidality. [Generic/Trade: Tabs 10 mg.] ▶L ♀C ▶– $$

Antidepressants—Selective Serotonin Reuptake Inhibitors (SSRIs)

CITALOPRAM (*Celexa*) <u>Depression</u>: Start 20 mg PO daily; usual effective dose is 20 to 40 mg/day, max 60 mg/day. Suicidality. [Generic/Trade: Tabs 10, 20, 40 mg. Oral soln 10 mg/5 mL. Generic only: Oral disintegrating tab 10, 20, 40 mg.] ▶LK ♀C but - in third trimester ▶ $$$

ESCITALOPRAM (*Lexapro*, ✦*Cipralex*) <u>Depression-generalized anxiety disorder</u>, adults, and age 12 yo or older: Start 10 mg PO daily; max 20 mg/day. Suicidality. [Generic/Trade: Tabs 5, 10, 20 mg. Trade only: Oral soln 1 mg/mL.] ▶LK ♀C but - in 3rd trimester ▶– $$$

FLUOXETINE (*Prozac, Prozac Weekly, Sarafem*) <u>Depression, OCD</u>: Start 20 mg PO q am; usual effective dose is 20 to 40 mg/day, max 80 mg/day. <u>Depression</u>, maintenance: 20 to 40 mg/day (standard-release) or 90 mg PO once a week (Prozac Weekly) starting 7 days after last standard-release dose. <u>Bulimia</u>: 60 mg PO daily; may need to titrate slowly, over several days. <u>Panic disorder</u>: Start 10 mg PO q am; titrate to 20 mg/day after 1 week, max 60 mg/day. <u>Premenstrual dysphoric disorder</u> (Sarafem): 20 mg PO daily, given either throughout the menstrual cycle or for 14 days prior to menses; max 80 mg/day. Doses greater than 20 mg/day can be divided two times per day (in morning and at noon). <u>Bipolar depression</u>, olanzapine + fluoxetine: Start 5 mg olanzapine + 20 mg fluoxetine daily in the evening. Increase to usual range of 5 to 12.5 mg olanzapine plus 20 to 50 mg fluoxetine as tolerated. <u>Treatment-resistant depression</u>, olanzapine + fluoxetine: Start 5 mg olanzapine + 20 mg fluoxetine daily in the evening. Increase to usual range of 5 to 20 mg olanzapine plus 20 to 50 mg fluoxetine as tolerated. Suicidality, many drug interactions. [Generic/Trade: Tabs 10 mg. Caps 10, 20, 40 mg. Oral soln 20 mg/5 mL. Caps (Sarafem) 10, 20 mg. Trade only: Tabs (Sarafem) 10, 15, 20 mg. Caps delayed-release (Prozac Weekly) 90 mg. Generic only: Tabs 20, 40 mg.] ▶L ♀C but - in 3rd trimester ▶– $$$

FLUVOXAMINE (*Luvox, Luvox CR*) <u>OCD</u>: Start 50 mg PO at bedtime; usual effective dose is 100 to 300 mg/day divided two times per day, max 300 mg/day. <u>OCD and social anxiety disorder</u> (CR): Start 100 mg PO at bedtime; increase by 50 mg/day q week prn to max 300 mg/day. <u>OCD</u> (children age 8 yo or older): Start 25 mg PO at bedtime; usual effective dose is 50 to 200 mg/day divided two times per day, max 200 mg/day. Do not use with thioridazine, pimozide, alosetron, cisapride, tizanidine, tryptophan, or MAOIs; use caution with benzodiazepines, TCAs, theophylline, and warfarin. Suicidality. [Generic/Trade: Tabs 25, 50, 100 mg. Trade only: Caps extended-release 100, 150 mg.] ▶L ♀C but - in third trimester ▶– $$$$

PAROXETINE (*Paxil, Paxil CR, Pexeva*) <u>Depression</u>: Start 20 mg PO q am, max 50 mg/day. <u>Depression, controlled-release</u>: Start 25 mg PO q am, max 62.5 mg/day. <u>OCD</u>: Start 10 to 20 mg PO q am, max 60 mg/day. <u>Social anxiety disorder</u>: Start 10 to 20 mg PO q am, max 60 mg/day. <u>Social anxiety disorder, controlled-release</u>: Start 12.5 mg PO q am, max 37.5 mg/day. <u>Generalized anxiety disorder</u>: Start 20 mg PO q am, max 50 mg/day. <u>Panic disorder</u>: Start 10 mg PO q am, increase by 10 mg/day at intervals of 1 week or more to usual effective dose of 10 to 60 mg/day; max 60 mg/day. <u>Panic disorder, controlled-release</u>: Start 12.5 mg PO q am, max 75 mg/day. <u>Post-traumatic stress disorder</u>: Start 20 mg PO q am, max 50 mg/day. <u>Premenstrual dysphoric disorder</u> (PMDD), continuous dosing: Start 12.5 mg PO q am (controlled-release); may increase dose after 1 week to max 25 mg q am. <u>PMDD</u>, intermittent dosing (given for 2 weeks prior to menses): 12.5 mg PO q am (controlled-release), max 25 mg/day. Suicidality, many drug interactions. [Generic/Trade: Tabs 10, 20, 30, 40 mg. Oral susp 10 mg/5 ml. Controlled-release tabs 12.5, 25 mg. Trade only: (Paxil CR) 37.5 mg.] ▶LK ♀D ▶? $$$

SERTRALINE (*Zoloft*) <u>Depression, OCD</u>: Start 50 mg PO daily; usual effective dose is 50 to 200 mg/day, max 200 mg/day. <u>Panic disorder, post-traumatic stress disorder, social anxiety disorder</u>: Start 25 mg PO daily, max 200 mg/day. <u>PMDD</u>, continuous dosing: Start 50 mg PO daily, max 150 mg/day. <u>PMDD</u>, intermittent dosing (given for 14 days prior to menses): Start 50 mg PO daily for 3 days, then increase to 100 mg/day. Suicidality. [Generic/Trade: Tabs 25, 50, 100 mg. Oral concentrate 20 mg/mL (60 mL).] ▶LK ♀C but–in third trimester ▶+ $$$

Antidepressants—Serotonin-Norepinephrine Reuptake Inhibitors (SNRIs)

DESVENLAFAXINE (*Pristiq*) 50 mg PO daily. Max 400 mg/day. [Trade only: Tabs extended-release 50, 100 mg.] ▶LK ♀C ▶? $$$$

DULOXETINE (*Cymbalta*) <u>Depression</u>: 20 mg PO two times per day; max 60 mg/day given once daily or divided two times per day. <u>Generalized anxiety disorder</u>: Start 30 to 60 mg PO daily, max 120 mg/day. <u>Diabetic peripheral neuropathic pain</u>: 60 mg PO daily. <u>Fibromyalgia</u>: Start 30 to 60 mg PO daily, max 60 mg/day. Suicidality, hepatotoxicity, many drug interactions. [Trade only: Caps 20, 30, 60 mg.] ▶L ♀C ▶? $$$$

VENLAFAXINE (*Effexor, Effexor XR*) <u>Depression/anxiety</u>: Start 37.5 to 75 mg PO daily (Effexor XR) or 75 mg/day divided two to three times per day (Effexor).

(cont.)

Usual effective dose is 150 to 225 mg/day, max 225 mg/day (Effexor XR) or 375 mg/day (Effexor). Generalized anxiety disorder: Start 37.5 to 75 mg PO daily (Effexor XR), max 225 mg/day. Social anxiety disorder: 75 mg PO daily (Effexor XR). Panic disorder: Start 37.5 mg PO daily (Effexor XR), may titrate by 75 mg/day at weekly intervals to max 225 mg/day. Suicidality, seizures, HTN. [Generic/Trade: Caps extended-release 37.5, 75, 150 mg. Tabs 25, 37.5, 50, 75, 100 mg. Generic only: Tabs extended-release 37.5, 75, 150, 225 mg.] ▶LK ♀C but–in 3rd trimester ▶? $$$$

Antidepressants—Other

BUPROPION (*Wellbutrin, Wellbutrin SR, Wellbutrin XL, Aplenzin, Zyban, Buproban*) Depression: Start 100 mg PO two times per day (immediate-release tabs); can increase to 100 mg three times per day after 4 to 7 days. Usual effective dose is 300 to 450 mg/day, max 150 mg/dose and 450 mg/day. Sustained-release: Start 150 mg PO q am; may increase to 150 mg two times per day after 4 to 7 days, max 400 mg/day. Give last dose no later than 5 pm. Extended-release: Start 150 mg PO q am; may increase to 300 mg q am after 4 days, max 450 mg q morning. Extended-release (Aplenzin): Start 174 mg PO q am; increase to target dose of 348 mg/day after 4 days or more. May increase to max dose of 522 mg/day after 4 weeks or more. Seasonal affective disorder: Start 150 mg of extended-release PO q am in autumn; can increase to 300 mg q am after 1 week, max 300 mg/day. In the spring, decrease to 150 mg/day for 2 weeks and then discontinue. Smoking cessation (Zyban, Buproban): Start 150 mg PO q am for 3 days, then increase to 150 mg PO two times per day for 7 to 12 weeks. Max 150 mg PO two times per day. Give last dose no later than 5 pm. Seizures, suicidality. [Generic/Trade (for depression, bupropion HCl): Tabs 75, 100 mg. Sustained-release tabs 100, 150, 200 mg. Extended-release tabs 150, 300 mg (Wellbutrin XL). Generic/Trade (Smoking cessation): Sustained-release tabs 150 mg (Zyban, Buproban). Trade only: Extended-release (Aplenzin, bupropion hydrobromide) tabs 174, 348, 522 mg.] ▶LK ♀C ▶– $$$$
MIRTAZAPINE (*Remeron, Remeron SolTab*) Start 15 mg PO at bedtime. Usual effective dose is 15 to 45 mg/day. Agranulocytosis in 0.1% of patients. Suicidality. [Generic/Trade: Tabs 15, 30, 45 mg. Tabs orally disintegrating (SolTab) 15, 30, 45 mg. Generic only: Tabs 7.5 mg.] ▶LK ♀C ▶? $$
TRAZODONE (*Desyrel, Oleptro*) Depression: Start 50 to 150 mg/day PO in divided doses; usual effective dose is 400 to 600 mg/day. Extended-release: Start 150 mg PO at bedtime. May increase by 75 mg/day q 3 days to max 375 mg/day. Insomnia: 50 to 150 mg PO at bedtime. [Trade only: Extended release tabs (Oleptro) 150, 300 mg. Generic only: Tabs 50, 100, 150, 300 mg.] ▶L ♀C ▶– $

Antimanic (Bipolar) Agents

LAMOTRIGINE (*Lamictal, Lamictal CD, Lamictal ODT, Lamictal XR*) Adults with bipolar disorder (maintenance): Start 25 mg PO daily, 50 mg PO daily if on enzyme-

(cont.)

inducing drugs, or 25 mg PO every other day if on valproate; titrate to 200 mg/day, 400 mg/day divided two times per day if on enzyme-inducing drugs, or 100 mg/day if on valproate. Potentially life-threatening rashes in 0.3% of adults and 0.8% of children; discontinue at first sign of rash. Drug interaction with valproic acid; see prescribing information for adjusted dosing guidelines. [Generic/Trade: Chewable dispersible tabs (Lamictal CD) 5, 25 mg. Tabs 25, 100, 150, 200 mg. Trade only: Orally disintegrating tabs (ODT) 25, 50, 100, 200 mg. Extended-release tabs (XR) 25, 50, 100, 200 mg.] ▶LK ♀C (see notes) ▶− $$$$

LITHIUM (*Eskalith, Eskalith CR, Lithobid, ✦ Lithane*) <u>Acute mania:</u> Start 300 to 600 mg PO two to three times per day; usual effective dose is 900 to 1800 mg/day. Steady state is achieved in 5 days. <u>Bipolar maintenance:</u> usually 900 to 1200 mg/day titrated to therapeutic trough level of 0.6 to 1.2 mEq/L. [Generic/Trade: Caps 300, extended-release tabs 300, 450 mg. Generic only: Caps 150, 600 mg, Tabs 300 mg, Syrup 300/5 mL.] ▶K ♀D ▶− $

TOPIRAMATE (*Topamax*) Bipolar disorder (unapproved): Start 25 to 50 mg/day PO. Titrate prn to max 400 mg/day divided two times per day. [Trade: Tabs 25, 50, 100, 200 mg. Sprinkle Caps 15, 25 mg.] ▶K ♀D ▶? $$$$$

VALPROIC ACID (*Depakote, Depakote ER, Stavzor, divalproex, ✦ Epival*) <u>Mania:</u> 250 mg PO three times per day (Depakote) or 25 mg/kg once daily (Depakote ER); max 60 mg/kg/day. Hepatotoxicity, drug interactions, reduce dose in the elderly. [Generic only: Syrup (Valproic acid) 250 mg/5 mL. Generic/Trade: Delayed-release tabs (Depakote) 125, 250, 500 mg. Extended-release tabs (Depakote ER) 250, 500 mg. Delayed-release sprinkle caps (Depakote) 125 mg. Trade only: Stavzor): Delayed-release caps 125, 250, 500 mg.] ▶L ♀D ▶+ $$$$

Antipsychotics—First Generation (Typical)

CHLORPROMAZINE (*Thorazine*) Start 10 to 50 mg PO/IM two to three times per day, usual dose 300 to 800 mg/day. [Generic only: Tabs 10, 25, 50, 100, 200 mg. Generic/Trade: Oral concentrate 30 mg/mL, 100 mg/mL. Trade only: Syrup 10 mg/5 mL, Supps 25, 100 mg.] ▶LK ♀C ▶− $$$

FLUPHENAZINE (*Prolixin, ✦ Modicate, Moditen*) 1.25 to 10 mg/day IM divided q 6 to 8 h. Start 0.5 to 10 mg/day PO divided q 6 to 8 h. Usual effective dose 1 to 20 mg/day. Depot (fluphenazine decanoate/enanthate): 12.5 to 25 mg IM/SC q 3 weeks is equivalent to 10 to 20 mg/day PO fluphenazine. [Generic/Trade: Tabs 1, 2.5, 5, 10 mg. Elixir 2.5 mg/5 mL. Oral concentrate 5 mg/mL.] ▶LK ♀C ▶? $$$

HALOPERIDOL (*Haldol*) 2 to 5 mg IM. Start 0.5 to 5 mg PO two to three times per day, usual effective dose 6 to 20 mg/day. Therapeutic range 2 to 15 nanogram/mL. Depot haloperidol (haloperidol decanoate): 100 to 200 mg IM q 4 weeks is equivalent to 10 mg/day oral haloperidol. [Generic only: Tabs 0.5, 1, 2, 5, 10, 20 mg. Oral concentrate 2 mg/mL.] ▶LK ♀C ▶− $$

PERPHENAZINE Start 4 to 8 mg PO three times per day or 8 to 16 mg PO two to four times per day (hospitalized patients), maximum 64 mg/day PO. Can give 5 to 10 mg IM q 6 h, maximum 30 mg/day IM. [Generic only: Tabs 2, 4, 8, 16 mg. Oral concentrate 16 mg/5 mL.] ▶LK ♀C ▶? $$$

PIMOZIDE (*Orap*) <u>Tourette syndrome</u>: Start 1 to 2 mg/day PO in divided doses, increase q 2 days to usual effective dose of 1 to 10 mg/day. [Trade only: Tabs 1, 2 mg.] ▶L ♀C ▶– $$$

THIORIDAZINE (*Mellaril*) Start 50 to 100 mg PO three times per day, usual dose 200 to 800 mg/day. Not 1st-line therapy. Causes QTc prolongation, torsades de pointes, and sudden death. Contraindicated with SSRIs, propranolol, pindolol. Monitor baseline ECG and potassium. Pigmentary retinopathy with doses greater than 800 mg/day. [Generic only: Tabs 10, 15, 25, 50, 100, 150, 200 mg. Oral concentrate 30, 100 mg/mL.] ▶LK ♀C ▶? $$

THIOTHIXENE (*Navane*) Start 2 mg PO three times per day. Usual effective dose is 20 to 30 mg/day, maximum 60 mg/day PO. [Generic/Trade: Caps 1, 2, 5, 10. Oral concentrate 5 mg/mL. Trade only: Caps 20 mg.] ▶LK ♀C ▶? $$$

TRIFLUOPERAZINE (*Stelazine*) Start 2 to 5 mg PO two times per day. Usual effective dose is 15 to 20 mg/day. [Generic/Trade: Tabs 1, 2, 5, 10 mg. Trade only: Oral concentrate 10 mg/mL.] ▶LK ♀C ▶– $$$

Antipsychotics—Second Generation (Atypical)

ARIPIPRAZOLE (*Abilify, Abilify Discmelt*) <u>Schizophrenia</u>: Start 10 to 15 mg PO daily. Max 30 mg daily. <u>Bipolar disorder</u>: Start 15 mg PO daily. Max 30 mg/day. <u>Agitation associated with schizophrenia or Bipolar disorder</u>: 9.75 mg IM recommended. May repeat in 2 h up to max 30 mg/day. <u>Depression, adjunctive therapy</u>: Start 2 to 5 mg PO daily. Max 15 mg/day. [Trade only: Tabs 2, 5, 10, 15, 20, 30 mg. Oral soln 1 mg/mL (150 mL). Orally disintegrating tabs (Discmelt) 10, 15, 20, 30 mg.] ▶L ♀C ▶? $$$$$

ASENAPINE (*Saphris*) <u>Schizophrenia</u>: Initial and maintenance 5 mg SL two times per day. Max 10 mg/day. <u>Bipolar disorder, acute manic or mixed episodes</u>: Start 5 mg sublingual two times per day (adjunctive) or 10 mg sublingual two times per day (monotherapy). Max 20 mg/day. [Trade: Sublingual tabs 5, 10 mg] ▶L ♀C ▶–

CLOZAPINE (*Clozaril, FazaClo ODT*) Start 12.5 mg PO one to two times per day. Usual effective dose is 300 to 450 mg/day divided two times per day, max 900 mg/day. Agranulocytosis 1 to 2%; check WBC and ANC weekly for 6 months, then q 2 weeks. Seizures, myocarditis, cardiopulmonary arrest. [Generic/Trade: Tabs 25, 100 mg. Generic only: Tabs 12.5, 50, 200 mg. Trade only: Orally disintegrating tab (Fazaclo ODT) 12.5, 25, 100 mg (scored).] ▶L ♀B ▶– $$$$$

ILOPERIDONE (*Fanapt*) Start 1 mg PO two times per day. Increase to 2 mg PO two times per day on day 2, then by 2 mg per dose each day to usual effective range of 6 to 12 mg PO two times per day. Max 24 mg/day. [Trade: Tabs 1, 2, 4, 6, 8, 10, 12 mg.] ▶L ♀C ▶– ?

LURASIDONE (*Latuda*) Start 40 mg PO daily, max 80 mg/day. Take with food. [Trade only: Tabs 40, 80 mg.] ▶K ♀B ▶?

OLANZAPINE (*Zyprexa, Zyprexa Zydis, Zyprexa Relprevv*) <u>Agitation in acute bipolar mania or schizophrenia</u>: Start 10 mg IM (2.5 to 5 mg in elderly or

(cont.)

debilitated patients); may repeat in 2 h to max 30 mg/day. Schizophrenia, oral therapy: Start 5 to 10 mg PO daily; usual effective dose is 10 to 15 mg/day. Schizophrenia, long-acting injection: dose based on prior oral dose and ranges from 150 mg to 300 mg deep IM (gluteal) q 2 weeks or 300 mg to 405 mg q 4 weeks. See prescribing information. Bipolar disorder, maintenance treatment or monotherapy for acute manic or mixed episodes: Start 10 to 15 mg PO daily. Increase by 5 mg/day at intervals after 24 h to usual effective dose of 5 to 20 mg/day, max 20 mg/day. Bipolar disorder, adjunctive for acute manic or mixed episodes: Start 10 mg PO daily; usual effective dose is 5 to 20 mg/day, max 20 mg/day. Bipolar depression, olanzapine + fluoxetine: Start 5 mg olanzapine + 20 mg fluoxetine daily in the evening. Increase to usual range of 5 to 12.5 mg olanzapine plus 20 to 50 mg fluoxetine as tolerated. Treatment-resistant depression, olanzapine + fluoxetine: Start 5 mg olanzapine + 20 mg fluoxetine daily in the evening. Increase to usual range of 5 to 20 mg olanzapine plus 20 to 50 mg fluoxetine as tolerated. [Trade only: Tabs 2.5, 5, 7.5, 10, 15, 20 mg. Tabs orally disintegrating (Zyprexa Zydis) 5, 10, 15, 20 mg. Long-acting injection (Zyprexa Relprevv) 210, 300, 405 mg/vial.] ▶L ♀C ▶ – $$$$$

PALIPERIDONE (*Invega, Invega Sustenna*) Schizophrenia and schizoaffective disorder (adjunctive and monotherapy): Start 6 mg PO q am. 3 mg/day may be sufficient in some. Max 12 mg/day. Extended-release injection: Start 234 mg IM (deltoid) and then 156 mg IM 1 week later. Recommended monthly dose 117 mg IM (deltoid or gluteal) or within range of 36 to 234 mg, based on response. [Trade only: Extended-release tabs 1.5, 3, 6, 9 mg.] ▶KL ♀C ▶ – $$$$$

QUETIAPINE (*Seroquel, Seroquel XR*) Schizophrenia: Start 25 mg PO two times per day (regular tabs); increase by 25 to 50 mg two to three times per day on days 2 and 3, and then to target dose of 300 to 400 mg/day divided two to three times per day on day 4. Usual effective dose is 150 to 750 mg/day, max 800 mg/day. Schizophrenia, extended-release: Start 300 mg PO daily in evening, increase by up to 300 mg/day at intervals of more than 1 day to usual effective range of 400 to 800 mg/day. Acute bipolar mania, monotherapy, or adjunctive: Start 50 mg PO two times per day on day 1, then increase to no higher than 100 mg two times per day on day 2, 150 mg two times per day on day 3, and 200 mg two times per day on day 4. May increase prn to 300 mg two times per day on day 5 and 400 mg two times per day thereafter. Usual effective dose is 400 to 800 mg/day. Acute bipolar mania, monotherapy or adjunctive, extended-release: Start 300 mg PO evening of day 1, 600 mg day 2, and 400 to 800 mg/day thereafter. Bipolar depression, regular- and extended-release: 50 mg PO at bedtime on day 1, 100 mg at bedtime day 2, 200 mg at bedtime day 3, and 300 mg at bedtime day 4. May increase prn to 400 mg at bedtime on day 5 and 600 mg at bedtime on day 8. Bipolar maintenance: Continue dose required to maintain remission. Major depressive disorder, adjunctive to antidepressants, extended-release: Start 50 mg evening of day 1, may increase to 150 mg on day 3. Max 300 mg/day. Eye exam for cataracts recommended q 6 months. [Trade only: Tabs 25, 50, 100, 200, 300, 400 mg. Extended-release tabs 50, 150, 200, 300, 400 mg.] ▶LK ♀C ▶ – $$$$$

ANTIPSYCHOTIC RELATIVE ADVERSE EFFECTS[a]

Genera-tion	Antipsychotic	Anticho-linergic	Sedation	Hypoten-sion	EPS	Weight Gain	Diabetes/ Hypergly-cemia	Dyslipi-demia
1st	chlorpromazine	+++	+++	++	++	++	?	?
1st	fluphenazine	++	+	+	++++	++	?	?
1st	haloperidol	+	+	+	++++	++	0	?
1st	loxapine	++	+	++	++	+	?	?
1st	molindone	++	++	+	++	+	?	?
1st	perphenazine	++	++	+	++	+	+/?	?
1st	pimozide	+	+	+	+++	?	?	?
1st	thioridazine	++++	+++	+++	+	+++	+/?	?
1st	thiothixene	+	++	++	+++	++	?	?
1st	trifluoperazine	++	+	+	+++	++	?	?
2nd	aripiprazole	++	+	0	0	0/+	0	0
2nd	asenapine	+	+	++	++	+	?	?
2nd	clozapine	++++	+++	+++	0	+++	+	+
2nd	iloperidone	++	+	+++	+	++	?	?
2nd	olanzapine	+++	++	+	0b	+++	++	++
2nd	paliperidone	+	+	++	++	++	?	?
2nd	risperidone	+	++	+	+b	++	++	++
2nd	quetiapine	+	+++	++	0	++	?	?
2nd	ziprasidone	+	+	0	0	0/+	0	0

[a]Risk of specific adverse effects is graded from 0 (absent) to ++++ (high). ? = Limited or inconsistent comparative data. [b]EPS (EPS) are dose-related and are more likely for risperidone >6-8 mg/day/olanzapine >20 mg/day. Akathisia risk remains unclear and may not be reflected in these ratings. There are limited comparative data for aripiprazole iloperidone, paliperidone, and asenapine relative to other second generation antipsychotics.

References: Goodman & Gilman 11e p461-500, Applied Therapeutics 8e p78, APA schizophrenia practice guideline, Psychiatry Q 2002; 73:297, Diabetes Care 2004;27:596, Pharmacotherapy. A Pathophysiologic Approach, 8th ed. pg 1158, 2011.

RISPERIDONE   (*Risperdal, Risperdal Consta*)   <u>Schizophrenia</u> (adults): Start 2 mg/day PO given once daily or divided two times per day (0.5 mg two times per day in the elderly, debilitated, or with hypotension, severe renal or hepatic disease); increase by 1 to 2 mg/day (no more than 0.5 mg two times per day in elderly and debilitated) at intervals of 24 h or more to usual effective dose of 4 to 8 mg/day given once daily or divided two times per day, max 16 mg/day. Long-acting injection (Consta): <u>Schizophrenia, Bipolar type 1</u> maintenance: Start 25 mg IM q 2 weeks while continuing oral dose for 3 weeks. May increase at 4-week intervals to max 50 mg q 2 weeks. <u>Schizophrenia</u> (13 to 17 yo): Start 0.5 mg PO daily; increase by 0.5 to 1 mg/day at intervals of 24 h or more to target dose of 3 mg/day. Max 6 mg/day. <u>Bipolar mania</u> (adults): Start 2 to

(cont.)

3 mg PO daily; may increase by 1 mg/day at 24 h intervals to max 6 mg/day. <u>Bipolar mania</u> (10 to 17 yo): Start 0.5 mg PO daily; increase by 0.5 to 1 mg/day at intervals of 24 h to recommended dose of 2.5 mg/day. Max 6 mg/day. <u>Autistic disorder irritability</u> (age 5 to 16 yo): Start 0.25 mg (for wt less than 20 kg) or 0.5 mg (wt 20 kg or greater) PO daily. May increase after 4 days to 0.5 mg/day (for wt less than 20 kg) or 1.0 mg/day (wt 20 kg or greater). Maintain at least 14 days. May then increase at 14 days intervals or more by increments of 0.25 mg/day (for wt less than 20 kg) or 0.5 mg/day (wt 20 kg or greater) to max 1.0 mg/day (for wt less than 20 kg), 2.5 mg/day (20 to 44 kg) or 3.0 mg/day (wt more than 45 kg). [Generic/Trade: Tabs 0.25, 0.5, 1, 2, 3, 4 mg. Oral soln 1 mg/mL (30 mL). Orally disintegrating tabs 0.5, 1, 2, 3, 4 mg. Generic only: Orally disintegrating tabs 0.25 mg.] ▶LK ♀C ▶– $$$$$

ZIPRASIDONE (*Geodon*) <u>Schizophrenia</u>: Start 20 mg PO two times per day with food; may adjust at more than 2-day intervals to max 80 mg PO two times per day. <u>Acute agitation</u>: 10 to 20 mg IM, max 40 mg/day. <u>Bipolar mania</u>: Start 40 mg PO two times per day with food; may increase to 60 to 80 mg two times per day on day 2. Usual effective dose is 40 to 80 mg two times per day. [Trade only: Caps 20, 40, 60, 80 mg, Susp 10 mg/mL.] ▶L ♀C ▶– $$$$$

Anxiolytics/Hypnotics—Benzodiazepines—Long Half-Life (25-100 h)

BROMAZEPAM (*✦Lectopam*) Canada only. 6 to 18 mg/day PO in divided doses. [Generic/Trade: Tabs 1.5, 3, 6 mg.] ▶L ♀D ▶– $

CHLORDIAZEPOXIDE (*Librium*) <u>Anxiety</u>: 5 to 25 mg PO or 25 to 50 mg IM/IV three to four times per day. <u>Acute alcohol withdrawal</u>: 50 to 100 mg PO/IM/IV, repeat q 3 to 4 h prn up to 300 mg/day. Half-life 5 to 30 h. [Generic/Trade: Caps 5, 10, 25 mg.] ▶LK ♀D ▶–©IV $$

CLONAZEPAM (*Klonopin, Klonopin Wafer, ✦Rivotril, Clonapam*) <u>Panic disorder</u>: Start 0.25 to 0.5 mg PO two to three times per day, max 4 mg/day. Half-life 18 to 50 h. <u>Epilepsy</u>: Start 0.5 mg PO three times per day. Max 20 mg/day. [Generic/Trade: Tabs 0.5, 1, 2 mg. Orally disintegrating tabs (approved for panic disorder only) 0.125, 0.25, 0.5, 1, 2 mg.] ▶LK ♀D ▶–©IV $$

CLORAZEPATE (*Tranxene, Tranxene SD*) Start 7.5 to 15 mg PO at bedtime or two to three times per day, usual effective dose is 15 to 60 mg/day. <u>Acute alcohol withdrawal</u>: 60 to 90 mg/day on 1st day divided two to three times per day, reduce dose to 7.5 to 15 mg/day over 5 days. [Generic/Trade: Tabs 3.75, 7.5, 15 mg. Trade only (Tranxene SD): Tabs extended-release 11.25, 22.5 mg.] ▶LK ♀D ▶–©IV $$

DIAZEPAM (*Valium, Diastat, Diastat AcuDial, ✦Diazemuls*) <u>Active seizures</u>: 5 to 10 mg IV q 10 to 15 min to max 30 mg, or 0.2 to 0.5 mg/kg rectal gel PR. <u>Skeletal muscle spasm, spasticity related to cerebral palsy, paraplegia, athetosis, "stiff man syndrome"</u>: 2 to 10 mg PO/PR three to four times per day. <u>Anxiety</u>: 2 to 10 mg PO two to four times per day. Half-life 20 to 80 h. <u>Alcohol withdrawal</u>: 10 mg PO three to four times per day for 24 h then 5 mg PO three to four times per day prn. [Generic/Trade: Tabs 2, 5, 10 mg. Generic only: Oral soln 5 mg/5 mL. Oral concentrate (Intensol) 5 mg/mL. Trade only: Rectal gel (Diastat) 2.5, 5, 10, 15, 20 mg. Rectal gel (Diastat AcuDial) 10, 20 mg.] ▶LK ♀D ▶–©IV $

FLURAZEPAM   (*Dalmane*) 15 to 30 mg PO at bedtime. Half-life 70 to 90 h. [Generic/Trade: Caps 15, 30 mg.] ▶LK ♀X ▶–◎IV $

Anxiolytics/Hypnotics—Benzodiazepines—Medium Half-Life (10 to 15 h)

ESTAZOLAM   (*ProSom*) 1 to 2 mg PO at bedtime. [Generic/Trade: Tabs 1, 2 mg.] ▶LK ♀X ▶–◎IV $$
LORAZEPAM   (*Ativan*) Anxiety: 0.5 to 2 mg IV/IM/PO q 6 to 8 h, max 10 mg/day. Half-life 10 to 20 h. Status epilepticus: Adult: 4 mg IV over 2 min; may repeat in 10 to 15 min. Status epilepticus: Peds: 0.05 to 0.1 mg/kg (max 4 mg) IV over 2 to 5 min; may repeat 0.05 mg/kg once in 10 to 15 min. [Generic/Trade: Tabs 0.5, 1, 2 mg. Generic only: Oral concentrate 2 mg/mL.] ▶LK ♀D ▶–◎IV $
TEMAZEPAM   (*Restoril*) 7.5 to 30 mg PO at bedtime. Half-life 8 to 25 h. [Generic/Trade: Caps 7.5, 15, 22.5, 30 mg.] ▶LK ♀X ▶–◎IV $

Anxiolytics/Hypnotics—Benzodiazepines—Short Half-Life (< 12 h)

NOTE: *To avoid withdrawal, gradually taper when discontinuing after prolonged use. Sedative-hypnotics have been associated with severe allergic reactions and complex sleep behaviors including sleep driving. Use caution and discuss with patients.*

ALPRAZOLAM   (*Xanax, Xanax XR, Niravam*) 0.25 to 0.5 mg PO two to three times per day. Half-life 12 h. Multiple drug interactions. [Generic/Trade: Tabs 0.25, 0.5, 1, 2 mg. Tabs extended-release 0.5, 1, 2, 3 mg. Orally disintegrating tab (Niravam) 0.25, 0.5, 1, 2 mg. Generic only: Oral concentrate (Intensol) 1 mg/mL.] ▶LK ♀D ▶–◎IV $
OXAZEPAM   (*Serax*) 10 to 30 mg PO three to four times per day. Half-life 8 h. [Generic/Trade: Caps 10, 15, 30 mg. Trade only: Tabs 15 mg.] ▶LK ♀D ▶–◎IV $$$
TRIAZOLAM   (*Halcion*) 0.125 to 0.5 mg PO at bedtime. 0.125 mg/day in elderly. Half-life 2 to 3 h. [Generic/Trade: Tabs 0.125, 0.25 mg.] ▶LK ♀X ▶–◎IV $

Anxiolytics/Hypnotics—Other

BUSPIRONE   (*BuSpar, Vanspar*) Anxiety: Start 15 mg "dividose" daily (7.5 mg PO two times per day), usual effective dose 30 mg/day. Max 60 mg/day. [Generic/Trade: Tabs 5, 10, Dividose Tabs 15, 30 mg (scored to be easily bisected or trisected). Generic only: Tabs 7.5 mg.] ▶K ♀B ▶– $$$
CHLORAL HYDRATE   (*Aquachloral Supprettes, Somnote*) 25 to 50 mg/kg/day up to 1000 mg PO/PR. Many physicians use higher than recommended doses in children (eg, 75 mg/kg). [Generic only: Syrup 500 mg/5 mL, rectal supps 500 mg. Trade only: Caps 500 mg. Rectal supps: 325, 650 mg.] ▶LK ♀C ▶+◎IV $
ESZOPICLONE   (*Lunesta*) 2 mg PO at bedtime prn. Max 3 mg. Elderly: 1 mg PO at bedtime prn, max 2 mg. [Trade only: Tabs 1, 2, 3 mg.] ▶L ♀C ▶?◎IV $$$$
RAMELTEON   (*Rozerem*) Insomnia: 8 mg PO at bedtime. [Trade only: Tabs 8 mg.] ▶L ♀C ▶? $$$$

ZALEPLON (*Sonata*) 5 to 10 mg PO at bedtime prn, max 20 mg. Do not use for benzodiazepine or alcohol withdrawal. [Generic/Trade: Caps 5, 10 mg.] ▶L ♀C ▶–©IV $$$$

ZOLPIDEM (*Ambien, Ambien CR, Zolpimist, Edluar*) Adult: Insomnia: Standard tabs: 10 mg PO at bedtime. For age older than 65 yo or debilitated: 5 mg PO at bedtime. Oral spray: 10 mg PO at bedtime. For age older than 65 yo or debilitated: 5 mg PO at bedtime. Control-release tabs: 12.5 mg PO at bedtime. For age older than 65 yo or debilitated: give 6.25 mg PO at bedtime. Do not use for benzodiazepine or alcohol withdrawal. [Generic/Trade: Tabs 5, 10 mg. Trade only: Controlled-release tabs 6.25, 12.5 mg, oral spray 5 mg/actuation (Zolpimist); sublingual tab 5, 10 mg (Edluar).] ▶L ♀C ▶+©IV $$$$

ZOPICLONE (*✛Imovane*) Canada only. Adults: 5 to 7.5 mg PO at bedtime. Reduce dose in elderly. [Generic/Trade: Tabs 5, 7.5 mg. Generic only: Tabs 3.75 mg.] ▶L ♀D ▶– $

Combination Drugs

SYMBYAX (olanzapine + fluoxetine) Bipolar type 1 with depression and treatment-resistant depression: Start 6/25 mg PO at bedtime. Max 18/75 mg/day. [Trade only: Caps (olanzapine/fluoxetine) 3/25, 6/25, 6/50, 12/25, 12/50 mg.] ▶LK ♀C ▶– $$$$$

Drug Dependence Therapy

ACAMPROSATE (*Campral*) Maintenance of abstinence from alcohol: 666 mg (2 tabs) PO three times per day. Start after alcohol withdrawal and when patient is abstinent. [Trade only: Tabs delayed-release 333 mg.] ▶K ♀C ▶? $$$$

DISULFIRAM (*Antabuse*) Sobriety: 125 to 500 mg PO daily. Patient must abstain from any alcohol for at least 12 h before using. Metronidazole and alcohol in any form (cough syrups, tonics, etc.) contraindicated. [Trade only: Tabs 250, 500 mg.] ▶L ♀C ▶? $$$

NALTREXONE (*ReVia, Depade, Vivitrol*) Alcohol/opioid dependence: 25 to 50 mg PO daily. Extended-release injectable susp: 380 mg IM q 4 weeks or monthly. Avoid if recent ingestion of opioids (past 7 to 10 days). Hepatotoxicity with higher than approved doses. [Generic/Trade: Tabs 50 mg. Trade only (Vivitrol): Extended-release injectable susp kits 380 mg.] ▶LK ♀C ▶? $$$$

NICOTINE GUM (*Nicorette, Nicorette DS*) Smoking cessation: Gradually taper: 1 piece q 1 to 2 h for 6 weeks, 1 piece q 2 to 4 h for 3 weeks, then 1 piece q 4 to 8 h for 3 weeks, max 30 pieces/day of 2 mg or 24 pieces/day of 4 mg. Use Nicorette DS 4 mg/piece in high cigarette use (more than 24 cigarettes/day). [OTC/Generic/Trade: Gum 2, 4 mg.] ▶LK ♀C ▶– $$$$

NICOTINE INHALATION SYSTEM (*Nicotrol Inhaler, ✛Nicorette inhaler*) 6 to 16 cartridges/day for 12 weeks. [Trade only: Oral inhaler 10 mg/cartridge (4 mg nicotine delivered), 42 cartridges/box.] ▶LK ♀D ▶– $$$$$

NICOTINE LOZENGE (*Commit, Nicorette*) Smoking cessation: In those who smoke within 30 min of waking use 4 mg lozenge; others use 2 mg. Take 1 to

(cont.)

2 lozenges q 1 to 2 h for 6 weeks, then q 2 to 4 h weeks 7 to 9, then q 4 to 8 h weeks 10 to 12. Length of therapy 12 weeks. [OTC Generic/Trade: Lozenge 2, 4 mg in 48, 72, 168 count packages.] ▶LK ♀D ▶– $$$$$

NICOTINE NASAL SPRAY (*Nicotrol NS*) Smoking cessation: 1 to 2 doses q 1 h, each dose is 2 sprays, 1 in each nostril (1 spray contains 0.5 mg nicotine). Minimum recommended: 8 doses/day, max 40 doses/day. [Trade only: Nasal soln 10 mg/mL (0.5 mg/inhalation); 10 mL bottles.] ▶LK ♀D ▶– $$$$$

NICOTINE PATCHES (*Habitrol, NicoDerm CQ, Nicotrol, ✦Prostep*) Smoking cessation: Start 1 patch (14 to 22 mg) daily, taper after 6 weeks. Ensure patient has stopped smoking. [OTC/Rx/Generic/Trade: Patches 11, 22 mg/24 h. 7, 14, 21 mg/24 h (Habitrol and NicoDerm). OTC/Trade: 15 mg/16 h (Nicotrol).] ▶LK ♀D ▶– $$$$

SUBOXONE (buprenorphine + naloxone) Treatment of opioid dependence: Maintenance: 16 mg SL daily. Can individualize to range of 4 to 24 mg SL daily. [Trade only: SL tabs and film 2/0.5 and 8/2 mg buprenorphine/naloxone.] ▶L ♀C ▶– ⊚III $$$$$

VARENICLINE (*Chantix, ✦Champix*) Smoking cessation: Start 0.5 mg PO daily for day 1 to 3, then 0.5 mg two times per day days 4 to 7, then 1 mg two times per day thereafter. Take after meals with full glass of water. Start 1 week prior to cessation and continue for 12 weeks. [Trade only: Tabs 0.5, 1 mg.] ▶K ♀C ▶? $$$$

Stimulants/ADHD/Anorexiants

ADDERALL (dextroamphetamine + amphetamine, *Adderall XR*) ADHD, standard-release tabs: Start 2.5 mg (3 to 5 yo) or 5 mg (age 6 yo or older) PO one to two times per day, increase by 2.5 to 5 mg q week, max 40 mg/day. ADHD, extended-release caps (Adderall XR): If age 6 to 12 yo, then start 5 to 10 mg PO daily to a max of 30 mg/day. If 13 to 17 yo, then start 10 mg PO daily to a max of 20 mg/day. If adult, then 20 mg PO daily. Narcolepsy, standard-release: Start 5 to 10 mg PO q am, increase by 5 to 10 mg q week, max 60 mg/day. Avoid evening doses. Monitor growth and use drug holidays when appropriate. [Generic/Trade: Tabs 5, 7.5, 10, 12.5, 15, 20, 30 mg. Trade only: Caps, extended-release (Adderall XR) 5, 10, 15, 20, 25, 30 mg.] ▶L ♀C ▶– ⊚II $$$$

ARMODAFINIL (*Nuvigil*) Obstructive sleep apnea/hypopnea syndrome and narcolepsy: 150 to 250 mg PO q am. Inconsistent evidence for improved efficacy of 250 mg/day dose. Shift work sleep disorder: 150 mg PO 1 h prior to start of shift. [Trade only: Tabs 50, 100, 150, 200, 250 mg.] ▶L ♀C ▶? ⊚IV $$$$$

ATOMOXETINE (*Strattera*) ADHD: All ages wt greater than 70 kg: Start 40 mg PO daily, then increase after more than 3 days to target of 80 mg/day divided one to two times per day. Max 100 mg/day. [Trade only: Caps 10, 18, 25, 40, 60, 80, 100 mg.] ▶K ♀C ▶? $$$$$

CAFFEINE (*NoDoz, Vivarin, Caffedrine, Stay Awake, Quick-Pep, Cafcit*) 100 to 200 mg PO q 3 to 4 h prn. [OTC Generic/Trade: Tabs/Caps 200 mg. Oral soln caffeine citrate (Cafcit) 20 mg/mL. OTC Trade only: Tabs extended-release 200 mg. Lozenges 75 mg.] ▶L ♀B/C ▶? $

DEXMETHYLPHENIDATE (*Focalin, Focalin XR*) <u>ADHD</u>, extended-release, not already on stimulants: Start 5 mg (children) or 10 mg (adults) PO q am. Max 30 mg/day (children) or 40 mg/day (Adults). Immediate-release, not already on stimulants: 2.5 mg PO two times per day. Max 20 mg/day. If taking racemic methylphenidate, use conversion of 2.5 mg for each 5 mg of methylphenidate. [Generic/Trade: Tabs, immediate-release 2.5, 5, 10 mg. Trade only: Extended-release caps (Focalin XR) 5, 10, 15, 20, 30 mg.] ▶LK ♀C ▶?©II $$$

DEXTROAMPHETAMINE (*Dexedrine, Dextrostat*) <u>Narcolepsy</u>: Age 6 to 12 yo: Start 5 mg PO q am, increase by 5 mg/day q week. Age older than 12 yo: Start 10 mg PO q am, increase by 10 mg/day q week. Usual dose range 5 to 60 mg/day in divided doses (tabs) or daily (extended-release). <u>ADHD</u>: 2.5 to 5 mg PO q am, usual max 40 mg/day. Avoid evening doses. Monitor growth and use drug holidays when appropriate. [Generic/Trade: Caps extended-release 5, 10, 15 mg. Generic only: Tabs 5, 10 mg. Oral soln 5 mg/5 mL.] ▶L ♀C ▶–©II $$$$

GUANFACINE (*Intuniv*) Start 1 mg PO q am. Increase by 1 mg/week to max 4 mg/day. [Trade only: Tabs 1, 2, 3, 4 mg.] ▶LK– ♀B ▶?

LISDEXAMFETAMINE (*Vyvanse*) <u>ADHD</u> adults and children ages 6 to 12 yo: Start 30 mg PO q am. May increase weekly by 10 to 20 mg/day to max 70 mg/day. Avoid evening doses. Monitor growth and use drug holidays when appropriate. [Trade: Caps 20, 30, 40, 50, 60, 70 mg.] ▶L ♀C ▶–©II $$$$

METHYLPHENIDATE (*Ritalin, Ritalin LA, Ritalin SR, Methylin, Methylin ER, Metadate ER, Metadate CD, Concerta, Daytrana, ✦ Biphentin*) <u>ADHD/Narcolepsy</u>: 5 to 10 mg PO two to three times per day or 20 mg PO q am (sustained and extended-release), max 60 mg/day. Or 18 to 36 mg PO q am (Concerta), max 72 mg/day. Avoid evening doses. Monitor growth and use drug holidays when appropriate. [Trade only: Tabs 5, 10, 20 mg (Ritalin, Methylin, Metadate). Tabs extended-release 10, 20 mg (Methylin ER, Metadate ER). Tabs extended-release 18, 27, 36, 54 mg (Concerta). Caps extended-release 10, 20, 30, 40, 50, 60 mg (Metadate CD) May be sprinkled on food. Tabs sustained-release 20 mg (Ritalin SR). Caps extended-release 10, 20, 30, 40 mg (Ritalin LA). Tabs chewable 2.5, 5, 10 mg (Methylin). Oral soln 5 mg/5 mL, 10 mg/5 mL (Methylin). Transdermal patch (Daytrana) 10 mg/9 h, 15 mg/9 h, 20 mg/9 h, 30 mg/9 h. Generic only: Tabs 5, 10, 20 mg, tabs extended-release 10, 20 mg, tabs sustained-release 20 mg.] ▶LK ♀C ▶?©II $$

BODY MASS INDEX*		Heights are in feet and inches; weights are in pounds					
BMI	*Class.*	4' 10"	5' 0"	5' 4"	5' 8"	6' 0"	6' 4"
<19	Underweight	<91	<97	<110	<125	<140	<156
19–24	Healthy Weight	91–119	97–127	110–144	125–163	140–183	156–204
25–29	Overweight	120–143	128–152	145–173	164–196	184–220	205–245
30–40	Obese	144–191	153–204	174–233	197–262	221–293	246–328
>40	Very Obese	>191	>204	>233	>262	>293	>328

*BMI = kg/m² = (wt in pounds)(703)/(height in inches)². Anorectants appropriate if BMI ≥30 with comorbidities ≥27); surgery an option if BMI >40 with comorbidities 35–40). www.nhlbi.nih.gov

MODAFINIL (*Provigil, ✦ Alertec*) <u>Narcolepsy and sleep apnea/hypopnea:</u> 200 mg PO q am. <u>Shift work sleep disorder:</u> 200 mg PO 1 h before shift. [Trade only: Tabs 100, 200 mg.] ▶L ♀C D?©IV $$$$$

PHENTERMINE (*Adipex-P, Ionamin, Pro-Fast*) 8 mg PO three times per day or 15 to 37.5 mg/day q am or 10 to 14 h before retiring. For short-term use. [Generic/Trade: Caps 15, 30, 37.5 mg. Tabs 37.5 mg. Trade only: Caps extended-release 15, 30 mg (Ionamin). Generic only (Pro-Fast): Caps 18.75 mg, Tabs 8 mg.] ▶KL ♀C D–©IV $$

SIBUTRAMINE (*Meridia*) Start 10 mg PO q am, max 15 mg/day. Monitor pulse and BP. [Trade only: Caps 5, 10, 15 mg.] ▶KL ♀C D–©IV $$$$

PULMONARY

Beta Agonists—Short-Acting

ALBUTEROL (*AccuNeb, Ventolin HFA, Proventil HFA, ProAir HFA, VoSpire ER, ✦ Airomir, Asmavent, salbutamol*) MDI: 2 puffs q 4 to 6 h prn. Soln: 0.5 mL of 0.5% soln (2.5 mg) nebulized three to four times per day. One 3 mL unit dose (0.083%) nebulized three to four times per day. Caps for inhalation: 200 to 400 mcg q 4 to 6 h. Tabs: 2 to 4 mg PO three times per day to four times per day or extended-release 4 to 8 mg PO q 12 h up to 16 mg PO q 12 h. Peds: 0.1 to 0.2 mg/kg/dose PO three times per day up to 4 mg three times per day for age 2 to 5 yo, 2 to 4 mg or extended-release 4 mg PO q 12 h for age 6 to 12 yo. <u>Prevention of exercise-induced bronchospasm:</u> MDI: 2 puffs 10 to 30 min before exercise. [Trade only: MDI 90 mcg/actuation, 200 metered doses/canister. "HFA" inhalers use hydrofluoroalkane propellant instead of CFCs but are otherwise equivalent. Generic/Trade: Soln for inhalation 0.021% (AccuNeb), 0.042% (AccuNeb), and 0.083% in 3 mL vials, 0.5% (5 mg/mL) in 20 mL with dropper. Tabs extended-release 4, 8 mg (VoSpire ER). Generic only: Syrup 2 mg/5 mL. Tabs immediate-release 2, 4 mg.] ▶L ♀C D? $$

LEVALBUTEROL (*Xopenex, Xopenex HFA*) MDI 2 puffs q 4 to 6 h prn. Nebulizer 0.63 to 1.25 mg q 6 to 8 h. Peds: 0.31 mg nebulized three times per day for age 6 to 11 yo. [Generic/Trade: Soln for inhalation 0.31, 0.63, 1.25 mg in 3 mL and 1.25 mg in 0.5 mL unit-dose vials. Trade only: HFA MDI 45 mcg/actuation, 15 g 200/canister. "HFA" inhalers use hydrofluoroalkane propellant.] ▶L ♀C D? $$$

PIRBUTEROL (*Maxair Autohaler*) MDI: 1 to 2 puffs q 4 to 6 h. [Trade only: MDI 200 mcg/actuation, 14 g 400/canister.] ▶L ♀C D? $$$$

Beta Agonists—Long-Acting

ARFORMOTEROL (*Brovana*) <u>COPD:</u> 15 mcg nebulized two times per day. [Trade only: Soln for inhalation 15 mcg in 2 mL vial.] ▶L ♀C D? $$$$$ ■

FORMOTEROL (*Foradil, Perforomist, ✦ Oxeze Turbuhaler*) 1 puff two times per day. Nebulized: 20 mcg q 12 h. Not for acute bronchospasm. Use

(cont.)

only in combination with corticosteroids. [Trade only: DPI 12 mcg, 12, 60 blisters/pack (Foradil). Soln for inhalation: 20 mcg in 2 mL vial (Perforomist). Canada only (Oxeze): DPI 6, 12 mcg 60 blisters/pack.] ▶L ♀C ▶? $$$ ■

SALMETEROL (*Serevent Diskus*) 1 puff two times per day. Not for acute bronchospasm. For asthma, use only in combination with corticosteroids. [Trade only: DPI (Diskus): 50 mcg, 60 blisters.] ▶L ♀C ▶? $$$$

Combinations

ADVAIR (fluticasone–inhaled + salmeterol, Advair HFA) <u>Asthma</u>: DPI: 1 puff two times per day (all strengths). MDI: 2 puffs two times per day (all strengths). <u>COPD</u>: DPI: 1 puff two times per day (250/50 only). [Trade only: DPI: 100/50, 250/50, 500/50 mcg fluticasone/salmeterol per actuation; 60 doses/DPI. Trade only (Advair HFA): MDI 45/21, 115/21, 230/21 mcg fluticasone/salmeterol per actuation; 120 doses/canister.] ▶L ♀C ▶? $$$$$ ■

COMBIVENT (albuterol + ipratropium) 2 puffs four times per day, max 12 puffs/day. Contraindicated in soy or peanut allergy. [Trade only: MDI: 90 mcg albuterol/18 mcg ipratropium per actuation, 200/canister.] ▶L ♀C ▶? $$$$

DULERA (mometasone - inhaled + formoterol, *Zenhale*) <u>Asthma</u>: 2 puffs two times per day (all strengths). [Trade only: MDI 100/5, 200/5 mcg mometasone/formoterol per actuation; 120 doses/canister.] ▶L ♀C ▶? $$$$$ ■

DUONEB (albuterol + ipratropium, *Combivent inhalation soln*) 1 unit dose four times per day. [Generic/Trade: Unit dose: 2.5 mg albuterol/0.5 mg ipratropium per 3 mL vial, premixed; 30, 60 vials/carton.] ▶L ♀C ▶? $$$$$

SYMBICORT (budesonide + formoterol) <u>Asthma</u>: 2 puffs two times per day (both strengths). <u>COPD</u>: 2 puffs two times per day (160/4.5). [Trade only: MDI: 80/4.5, 160/4.5 mcg budesonide/formoterol per actuation; 120 doses/canister.] ▶L ♀C ▶? $$$$ ■

Inhaled Steroids

NOTE: *See Endocrine-Corticosteroids when oral steroids necessary.*

BECLOMETHASONE—INHALED (*QVAR*) 1 to 4 puffs two times per day (40 mcg). 1 to 2 puffs two times per day (80 mcg). [Trade only: HFA MDI: 40, 80 mcg/actuation, 7.3 g 100 actuations/canister.] ▶L ♀C ▶? $$$

PREDICTED PEAK EXPIRATORY FLOW (liters/min) *Am Rev Resp Dis* 1963; 88:644

Age (yr)	Women *(height in inches)*					Men *(height in inches)*					Child *(height in inches)*	
	55″	60″	65″	70″	75″	60″	65″	70″	75″	80″		
20 yr	390	423	460	496	529	554	602	649	693	740	44″	160
30 yr	380	413	448	483	516	532	577	622	664	710	46″	187
40 yr	370	402	436	470	502	509	552	596	636	680	48″	214
50 yr	360	391	424	457	488	486	527	569	607	649	50″	240
60 yr	350	380	412	445	475	463	502	542	578	618	52″	267
70 yr	340	369	400	432	461	440	477	515	550	587	54″	293

INHALED STEROIDS: ESTIMATED COMPARATIVE DAILY DOSES*

ADULTS AND CHILDREN OLDER THAN 12 yo				
Drug	Form	Low Dose†	Medium Dose†	High Dose†
beclomethasone HFA MDI	40 mcg/puff	2–6	6–12	>12
	80 mcg/puff	1–3	3–6	>6
budesonide DPI	90 mcg/dose	2–6	6–13	>13
	180 mcg/dose	1–3	3–7	>7
budesonide	soln for nebs	-	-	-
flunisolide HFA MDI	80 mcg/puff	4	5–8	>8
fluticasone HFA MDI	44 mcg/puff	2–6	6–10	>10
	110 mcg/puff	1–2	2–4	>4
	220 mcg/puff	1	1–2	>2
fluticasone DPI	50 mcg/dose	2–6	6–10	>10
	100 mcg/dose	1–3	3–5	>5
	250 mcg/dose	1	2	>2
mometasone DPI	220 mcg/dose	1	2	>2

CHILDREN (age 5 to 11 yo)				
Drug	Form	Low Dose†	Medium Dose†	High Dose†
beclomethasone HFA MDI	40 mcg/puff	2–4	4–8	>8
	80 mcg/puff	1–2	2–4	>4
budesonide DPI	90 mcg/dose	2–4	4–9	>9
	180 mcg/dose	1–2	2–4	>4
budesonide	soln for nebs	0.5 mg 0.25–0.5 mg (0–4 yo)	1 mg >0.5–1 mg (0–4 yo)	2 mg >1 mg (0–4 yo)
flunisolide HFA MDI	80 mcg/puff	2	4	≥8
fluticasone HFA MDI (0–11 yo)	44 mcg/puff	2–4	4–8	>8
	110 mcg/puff	1–2	2–3	>4
	220 mcg/puff	n/a	1–2	>2
fluticasone DPI	50 mcg/dose	2–4	4–8	>8
	100 mcg/dose	1–2	2–4	>4
	250 mcg/dose	n/a	1	>1
mometasone DPI	220 mcg/dose	n/a	n/a	n/a

*HFA = Hydrofluoroalkane (propellant). MDI = metered dose inhaler. DPI = dry powder inhaler. Reference: http://www.nhlbi.nih.gov/guidelines/asthma/asthsumm.pdf
†Numbers in dosage columns are indicated as puffs/inhalations per day.

BUDESONIDE—INHALED (*Pulmicort Respules, Pulmicort Flexhaler*) 1 to 2 puffs daily up to 4 puffs two times per day. Respules: 0.5 to 1 mg daily or divided two times per day. [Trade only: DPI (Flexhaler) 90, 180 mcg powder/actuation 60, 120 doses respectively/canister. Respules 1 mg/2 mL unit dose. Generic/Trade: Respules 0.25, 0.5 mg/2 mL unit dose.] ▶L ♀B ▶? $$$$

CICLESONIDE—INHALED (*Alvesco*) 80 mcg/puff: 1 to 4 puffs two times per day. 160 mcg/puff: 1 to 2 puffs two times per day. [Trade only: 80 mcg/actuation, 60 per canister. 160 mcg/actuation, 60, 120 per canister.] ▶L ♀C ▶? $$$$

INHALER COLORS   (Body then cap—Generics may differ)

Advair:	purple	*Asmanex:*	white/pink	*Maxair*	
Advair HFA:	purple/light purple	*Atrovent HFA:*	clear/green	*Autohaler:*	white/white
				ProAir HFA:	red/white
Aerobid-M:	grey/green	*Combivent:*	clear/orange	*Proventil*	
Aerospan:	purple/grey			*HFA:*	yellow/orange
Alupent:	clear/blue	*Flovent HFA:*	orange/peach	*Pulmicort:*	white/brown
Alvesco				*QVAR 40 mcg:*	beige/grey
80 mcg:	brown/red	*Foradil:*	grey/beige	*QVAR 80 mcg:*	mauve/grey
Alvesco		*Intal:*	white/blue	*Serevent*	
160 mcg:	red/red	*Maxair:*	white/white	*Diskus:*	green
				Spiriva:	grey
				Ventolin HFA:	light blue/navy
				Xopenex HFA:	blue/red

FLUNISOLIDE—INHALED   (*AeroBid, AeroBid-M, Aerospan*) 2 to 4 puffs two times per day. [Trade only: MDI: 250 mcg/actuation, 100 metered doses/canister. AeroBid-M (AeroBid + menthol flavor). Aerospan HFA MDI: 80 mcg/actuation, 60, 120 metered doses/canister.] ▶L ♀C ▶? $$$

FLUTICASONE—INHALED   (*Flovent HFA, Flovent Diskus*) 2 to 4 puffs two times per day. [Trade only: HFA MDI: 44, 110, 220 mcg/actuation 120/canister. DPI (Diskus): 50, 100, 250 mcg/actuation delivering 44, 88, 220 mcg respectively.] ▶L ♀C ▶? $$$$

MOMETASONE—INHALED   (*Asmanex Twisthaler*) 1 to 2 puffs in the evening or 1 puff two times per day. If prior oral corticosteroid therapy: 2 puffs two times per day. [Trade only: DPI: 110 mcg/actuation with #30 dosage units, 220 mcg/actuation with #30, 60, 120 dosage units.] ▶L ♀C ▶? $$$$

TRIAMCINOLONE—INHALED   (*Azmacort*) 2 puffs three to four times per day or 4 puffs two times per day; max dose 16 puffs/day. [Trade only: MDI: 75 mcg/actuation, 240/canister. Built-in spacer.] ▶L ♀C ▶? $$$$

Leukotriene Inhibitors

MONTELUKAST   (*Singulair*) Adults: 10 mg PO daily. <u>Chronic asthma, allergic rhinitis</u>: give 5 mg PO daily for age 6 to 14 yo, give 4 mg (chew tab or oral granules) PO daily for age 2 to 5 yo. <u>Asthma</u> age 12 to 23 mo: 4 mg (oral granules) PO daily. <u>Allergic rhinitis</u> age 6 to 23 mo: 4 mg (oral granules) PO daily. <u>Prevention of exercise-induced bronchoconstriction</u>: 10 mg PO 2 h before exercise. [Trade only: Tabs 10 mg. Oral granules 4 mg packet, 30/box. Chewable tabs (cherry flavored) 4, 5 mg.] ▶L ♀B ▶? $$$$

ZAFIRLUKAST   (*Accolate*) 20 mg PO two times per day. Peds age 5 to 11 yo: 10 mg PO two times per day. Take at least 1 h before or 2 h after meals. Potentiates warfarin and theophylline. [Trade only: Tabs 10, 20 mg.] ▶L ♀B ▶– $$$$

ZILEUTON (*Zyflo CR*) 1200 mg PO two times per day. Take within 1 h after morning and evening meals. Hepatotoxicity, potentiates warfarin, theophylline, and propranolol. [Trade only: Tabs extended-release 600 mg.] ▶L ♀C ▶? $$$$$

Other Pulmonary Medications

ACETYLCYSTEINE-INHALED (*Mucomyst*) <u>Mucolytic:</u> 3 to 5 mL of 20% or 6 to 10 mL of 10% soln nebulized three to four times per day. [Generic/Trade: Soln for inhalation 10, 20% in 4, 10, 30 mL vials.] ▶L ♀B ▶? $

AMINOPHYLLINE <u>Acute asthma:</u> Loading dose: 6 mg/kg IV over 20 to 30 min. Maintenance 0.5 to 0.7 mg/kg/h IV. [Generic only: Tabs 100, 200 mg. Oral liquid 105 mg/5 mL.] ▶L ♀C ▶? $

CROMOLYN-INHALED (*Intal, Gastrocrom, ✦Nalcrom*) <u>Asthma:</u> 2 to 4 puffs four times per day or 20 mg nebs four times per day. <u>Prevention of exercise-induced bronchospasm:</u> 2 puffs 10 to 15 min prior to exercise. <u>Mastocytosis:</u> Oral concentrate 200 mg PO four times per day for adults, 100 mg four times per day in children 2 to 12 yo. [Trade only: MDI 800 mcg/actuation, 112, 200/canister. Oral concentrate 100 mg/5 mL in 8 amps/foil pouch (Gastrocrom). Generic/Trade: Soln for nebs: 20 mg/2 mL.] ▶LK ♀B ▶? $$$

DORNASE ALFA (*Pulmozyme*) <u>Cystic fibrosis:</u> 2.5 mg nebulized daily to two times per day. [Trade only: Soln for inhalation: 1 mg/mL in 2.5 mL vials.] ▶L ♀B ▶? $$$$$

EPINEPHRINE RACEMIC (*S-2*) <u>Severe croup:</u> 0.05 mL/kg/dose diluted to 3 mL w/NS. Max dose 0.5 mL. [Trade only: Soln for inhalation: 2.25% epinephrine in 15, 30 mL.] ▶Plasma ♀C ▶- $

IPRATROPIUM-INHALED (*Atrovent, Atrovent HFA*) 2 puffs four times per day, or one 500 mcg vial neb three to four times per day. Contraindicated with soy or peanut allergy (Atrovent MDI only). [Trade only: Atrovent HFA MDI: 17 mcg/actuation, 200/canister. Generic/Trade: Soln for nebulization: 0.02% (500 mcg/vial) in unit dose vials.] ▶Lung ♀B ▶? $$$$

KETOTIFEN (*✦Zaditen*) Canada only. For age 6 mo to 3 yo: give 0.05 mg/kg PO two times per day. Age older than 3 yo: give 1 mg PO two times per day. [Generic/Trade: Tabs 1 mg. Syrup 1 mg/5 mL.] ▶L ♀C ▶- $$

ROFLUMILAST (*Daliresp, ✦Daxas*) <u>Severe COPD due to chronic bronchitis:</u> 500 mcg PO daily with or without food. [Trade: Tabs 500 mcg.] ▶L - ♀C ▶- $$$$

THEOPHYLLINE (*Elixophyllin, Uniphyl, Theo-24, T-Phyl, ✦Theolair*) 5 to 13 mg/kg/day PO in divided doses. Max dose 900 mg/day. Peds dosing variable. [Generic/Trade: Elixir 80 mg/15 mL. Trade only: Caps: Theo-24: 100, 200, 300, 400 mg. T-Phyl: 12 h SR tabs 200 mg. Theolair: Tabs 125, 250 mg. Generic only: 12 h tabs 100, 200, 300, 450 mg, 12 h caps 125, 200, 300 mg.] ▶L ♀C ▶+ $

TIOTROPIUM (*Spiriva*) <u>COPD:</u> Handihaler: 18 mcg inhaled daily. [Trade only: Caps for oral inhalation 18 mcg. To be used with "Handihaler" device only. Packages of 5, 30, 90 caps with Handihaler device.] ▶K ♀C ▶- $$$$

TOXICOLOGY

Toxicology

ACETYLCYSTEINE (*N-acetylcysteine, Mucomyst, Acetadote, ♦Parvolex*) <u>Contrast nephropathy prophylaxis:</u> 600 mg PO two times per day on the day before and on the day of contrast. <u>Acetaminophen toxicity:</u> Mucomyst: Loading dose 140 mg/kg PO or NG, then 70 mg/kg q 4 h for 17 doses. May be mixed in water or soft drink diluted to a 5% soln. Acetadote (IV): Loading dose 150 mg/kg in 200 mL of D5W infused over 60 min; maintenance dose 50 mg/kg in 500 mL of D5W infused over 4 h followed by 100 mg/kg in 1000 mL of D5W infused over 16 h. [Generic/Trade: Soln 10%, 20%. Trade only: IV (Acetadote).] ▶L ♀B ▶? $$$$

CHARCOAL (*activated charcoal, Actidose-Aqua, CharcoAid, EZ-Char, ♦Charcodate*) 25 to 100 g (1 to 2 g/kg) PO or NG as soon as possible. May repeat q 1 to 4 h at doses equivalent to 12.5 g/h. When sorbitol is coadministered, use only with the first dose if repeated doses are to be given. [OTC/Generic/Trade: Powder 15, 30, 40, 120, 240 g. Soln 12.5 g/60 mL, 15 g/75 mL, 15 g/120 mL, 25 g/120 mL, 30 g/120 mL, 50 g/240 mL. Susp 15 g/120 mL, 25 g/120 mL, 30 g/150 mL, 50 g/240 mL. Granules 15 g/120 mL.] ▶Not absorbed ♀+ ▶+ $

DEFEROXAMINE (*Desferal*) <u>Chronic iron overload:</u> 500 to 1000 mg IM daily and 2 g IV infusion (no faster than 15 mg/kg/h) with each unit of blood or 1 to 2 g SC daily (20 to 40 mg/kg/day) over 8 to 24 h via continuous infusion pump. <u>Acute iron toxicity:</u> IV infusion up to 15 mg/kg/h (consult poison center). ▶K ♀C ▶? $$$$$

FLUMAZENIL (*Romazicon*) <u>Benzodiazepine sedation reversal:</u> 0.2 mg IV over 15 sec, then 0.2 mg q 1 min prn up to 1 mg total dose. <u>Overdose reversal:</u> 0.2 mg IV over 30 sec, then 0.3 to 0.5 mg q 30 sec prn up to 3 mg total dose. Contraindicated in mixed drug OD or chronic benzodiazepine use. ▶LK ♀C ▶? $$$$

HYDROXOCOBALAMIN (*Cyanokit*) <u>Cyanide poisoning:</u> 5 g IV over 15 min; may repeat prn. ▶K ♀C ▶? $$$$$

IPECAC SYRUP <u>Induce Emesis:</u> 30 mL PO for adults, 15 mL age 1 to 12 yo. [OTC Generic only: Syrup 30 mL.] ▶Gut ♀C ▶? $

ANTIDOTES

Toxin	Antidote/Treatment	Toxin	Antidote/Treatment
acetaminophen	N-acetylcysteine	digoxin	dig immune Fab
TCAs	sodium bicarbonate	ethylene glycol	fomepizole
		heparin	protamine
arsenic, mercury	dimercaprol (BAL)	iron	deferoxamine
benzodiazepine	flumazenil	lead	BAL, EDTA, succimer
beta-blockers	glucagon	methanol	fomepizole
calcium channel blockers	calcium chloride, glucagon	methemoglobin	methylene blue
		opioids/opiates	naloxone
cyanide	cyanide antidote kit, Cyanokit (hydroxocobalamin)	organophosphates	atropine+pralidoxime
		warfarin	vitamin K, FFP

METHYLENE BLUE (*Urolene blue*) Methemoglobinemia: 1 to 2 mg/kg IV over 5 min. Dysuria: 65 to 130 mg PO three times per day after meals with liberal water. May turn urine/contact lenses blue. [Trade only: Tabs 65 mg.] ▶K ♀C ▶? $

PRALIDOXIME (*Protopam, 2-PAM*) Organophosphate poisoning: consult poison center: 1 to 2 g IV infusion over 15 to 30 min or slow IV injection over 5 min or longer (max rate 200 mg/min). May repeat dose after 1 h if muscle weakness persists. High-dose regimen (unapproved): 2 g over 30 min, followed by 1 g/h for 48 h, then 1 g/h q 4 h until improved. Peds: 20 to 50 mg/kg/dose IV over 15 to 30 min. ▶K ♀C ▶? $$$$

SUCCIMER (*Chemet*) Lead toxicity in children 1 yo or older: Start 10 mg/kg PO or 350 mg/m² q 8 h for 5 days, then reduce the frequency to q 12 h for 2 weeks. [Trade only: Caps 100 mg.] ▶K ♀C ▶? $$$$$

UROLOGY

Benign Prostatic Hyperplasia

ALFUZOSIN (*UroXatral, ✦Xatral*) 10 mg PO daily after a meal. [Trade only: Tab extended-release 10 mg.] ▶KL ♀B ▶– $$$

DUTASTERIDE (*Avodart*) 0.5 mg PO daily. [Trade only: Caps 0.5 mg.] ▶L ♀X ▶– $$$$

FINASTERIDE (*Proscar, Propecia*) Proscar: 5 mg PO daily alone or in combination with doxazosin to reduce the risk of symptomatic progression of BPH. Androgenetic alopecia in men: Propecia: 1 mg PO daily. [Generic/Trade: Tabs 1 mg (Propecia), 5 mg (Proscar).] ▶L ♀X ▶– $$$

JALYN (dutasteride + tamsulosin) 0.5 mg dutasteride + 0.4 mg tamsulosin daily 30 minutes after a meal. [Trade only: Caps 0.5 mg dutasteride + 0.4 mg tamsulosin.] ▶LK– ♀X ▶– $$$$

SILODOSIN (*RAPAFLO*) 8 mg PO daily with a meal. [Trade: Caps 8 mg.] ▶LK – ♀B ▶– $$$$

TAMSULOSIN (*Flomax*) 0.4 mg PO daily, 30 min after a meal. Maximum 0.8 mg/day. [Generic/Trade: Caps 0.4 mg.] ▶LK ♀B ▶– $$$$

Bladder Agents—Anticholinergics and Combinations

DARIFENACIN (*Enablex*) Overactive bladder with symptoms of urinary urgency, frequency, and urge incontinence: 7.5 mg PO daily. May increase to max dose 15 mg PO daily in 2 weeks. Max dose 7.5 mg PO daily with moderate liver impairment or when coadministered with potent CYP3A4 inhibitors (ketoconazole, itraconazole, ritonavir, nelfinavir, clarithromycin, and nefazodone). [Trade only: Tabs extended-release 7.5, 15 mg.] ▶LK ♀C ▶– $$$$

FESOTERODINE (*Toviaz*) Overactive bladder: 4 to 8 mg PO daily. [Trade only: Tabs extended-release 4, 8 mg.] ▶plasma ♀C ▶– $$$$

OXYBUTYNIN (*Ditropan, Ditropan XL, Gelnique, Oxytrol, ✦Uromax*) Bladder instability: 2.5 to 5 mg PO two to three times per day, max 5 mg PO four times per day. Extended-release tabs: 5 to 10 mg PO daily, increase 5 mg/day q

(cont.)

week to 30 mg/day. Oxytrol: 1 patch two times per week on abdomen, hips, or buttocks. Gelnique: Apply gel once daily to abdomen, upper arms/shoulders, or thighs. [Generic/Trade: Tabs 5 mg. Syrup 5 mg/5 mL. Tabs extended-release 5, 10, 15 mg. Trade only: Transdermal patch (Oxytrol) 3.9 mg/day. Gelnique 10% gel, 1 g unit dose.] ▶LK ♀B ▶? $

PROSED/DS (methenamine + phenyl salicylate + methylene blue + benzoic acid + hyoscyamine) Bladder spasm: 1 tab PO four times per day with liberal fluids. May turn urine/contact lenses blue. [Trade only: Tabs (methenamine 81.6 mg/phenyl salicylate 36.2 mg/methylene blue 10.8 mg/benzoic acid 9.0 mg/hyoscyamine sulfate 0.12 mg).] ▶KL ♀C ▶? $$

SOLIFENACIN (VESIcare) Overactive bladder with symptoms of urinary urgency, frequency, or urge incontinence: 5 mg PO daily. Max dose: 10 mg daily (5 mg daily if CrCl less than 30 mL/min, moderate hepatic impairment, or concurrent ketoconazole or other potent CYP3A4 inhibitors). [Trade only: Tabs 5, 10 mg.] ▶LK ♀C ▶– $$$$

TOLTERODINE (Detrol, Detrol LA, ✦ Unidet) Overactive bladder: 1 to 2 mg PO two times per day (Detrol) or 2 to 4 mg PO daily (Detrol LA). [Trade only: Tabs 1, 2 mg. Caps extended-release 2, 4 mg.] ▶L ♀C ▶– $$$$

TROSPIUM (Sanctura, Sanctura XR, ✦ Trosec) Overactive bladder with urge incontinence: 20 mg PO two times per day; give 20 mg at bedtime if CrCl less than 30 mL/min. If age 75 yo or older may taper down to 20 mg daily. Extended-release: 60 mg PO q am, 1 h before food. [Trade only: Tabs 20 mg, Caps extended-release 60 mg.] ▶LK ♀C ▶– $$$$

URISED (methenamine + phenyl salicylate + atropine + hyoscyamine + benzoic acid + methylene blue) Dysuria. 2 tabs PO four times per day. May turn urine/contact lenses blue. Do not use with sulfa. [Trade only: Tabs (methenamine 40.8 mg/phenyl salicylate 18.1 mg/atropine 0.03 mg/hyoscyamine 0.03 mg/4.5 benzoic acid/5.4 mg methylene blue).] ▶K ♀C ▶? $

UTA (methenamine + sodium phosphate + phenyl salicylate + methylene blue + hyoscyamine) Bladder spasm: 1 cap PO four times per day with liberal fluids. [Trade only: Caps (methenamine 120 mg/sodium phosphate 40.8 mg/phenyl salicylate 36 mg/methylene blue 10 mg/hyoscyamine 0.12 mg).] ▶KL ♀C ▶? $

UTIRA-C (methenamine + sodium phosphate + phenyl salicylate + methylene blue + hyoscyamine) Bladder spasm: 1 cap PO four times per day with liberal fluids. [Trade only: Tabs (methenamine 81.6 mg/sodium phosphate 40.8 mg/phenyl salicylate 36.2 mg/methylene blue 10.8 mg/hyoscyamine 0.12 mg).] ▶KL ♀C ▶? $$

Bladder Agents—Other

BETHANECHOL (Urecholine, Duvoid) Urinary retention: 10 to 50 mg PO three to four times per day. [Generic/Trade: Tabs 5, 10, 25, 50 mg.] ▶L ♀C ▶? $$$$

PHENAZOPYRIDINE (Pyridium, Azo-Standard, Urogesic, Prodium, Pyridiate, Urodol, Baridium, UTI Relief) Dysuria: 200 mg PO three times per day for 2 days. May turn urine/contact lenses orange. [OTC Generic/Trade: Tabs 95, 97.2 mg. Rx Generic/Trade: Tabs 100, 200 mg.] ▶K ♀B ▶? $

Erectile Dysfunction

ALPROSTADIL (*Muse, Caverject, Caverject Impulse, Edex, Prostin VR Pediatric*, prostaglandin E1, ✦ *Prostin VR*) 1 intraurethral pellet (Muse) or intracavernosal injection (Caverject, Edex) at lowest dose that will produce erection. Onset of effect is 5 to 20 min. [Trade only: Syringe system (Edex) 10, 20, 40 mcg. (Caverject) 5, 10, 20, 40 mcg. (Caverject Impulse) 10, 20 mcg. Pellet (Muse) 125, 250, 500, 1000 mcg. Intracorporeal injection of locally compounded combination agents (many variations): "Bi-mix" can be 30 mg/mL papaverine + 0.5 to 1 mg/mL phentolamine, or 30 mg/mL papaverine + 20 mcg/mL alprostadil in 10 mL vials. "Tri-mix" can be 30 mg/mL papaverine + 1 mg/mL phentolamine + 10 mcg/mL alprostadil in 5, 10, or 20 mL vials.] ▶L ♀– ▶ $$$$

SILDENAFIL (*Viagra*) Start 50 mg PO 0.5 to 4 h prior to intercourse. Max 1 dose/day. Usual effective range 25 to 100 mg. Start at 25 mg if for age 65 yo or older or liver/renal impairment. Contraindicated with nitrates. [Trade only (Viagra): Tabs 25, 50, 100 mg. Unscored tab but can be cut in half.] ▶LK ♀B ▶– $$$$

TADALAFIL (*Cialis*) 2.5 to 5 mg PO daily without regard to timing of sexual activity. As needed dosing: Start 10 mg PO at least 30 to 45 min prn prior to sexual activity. May increase to 20 mg or decrease to 5 mg prn. Max 1 dose/day. Start 5 mg (max 1 dose/day) if CrCl is 31 to 50 mL/min. Max 5 mg/day if CrCl < 30 mL/min including patients on dialysis. Max 10 mg/day if mild to moderate hepatic impairment; avoid in severe hepatic impairment. Max 10 mg once in 72 h if concurrent potent CYP3A4 inhibitors. Contraindicated with nitrates and alpha-blockers (except tamsulosin 0.4 mg daily). Not FDA approved for women. [Trade only (Cialis): Tabs 2.5, 5, 10, 20 mg.] ▶L ♀B ▶– $$$$

VARDENAFIL (*Levitra*) Start 10 mg PO 1 h before sexual activity. Usual effective dose range 5 to 20 mg. Max 1 dose/day. Use lower dose (5 mg) if age 65 yo or older or moderate hepatic impairment (max 10 mg). Contraindicated with nitrates and alpha-blockers. Not FDA approved in women. [Trade only: Tabs 2.5, 5, 10, 20 mg.] ▶LK ♀B ▶– $$$$

YOHIMBINE (*Yocon, Yohimex*) 5.4 mg PO three times per day. Not FDA approved. [Generic/Trade: Tabs 5.4 mg.] ▶L ♀– ▶– $

Nephrolithiasis

CITRATE (*Polycitra-K, Urocit-K, Bicitra, Oracit, Polycitra, Polycitra-LC*) Urinary alkalinization: 1 packet in water/juice PO three to four times per day. [Generic/Trade: Polycitra-K packet 3300 mg potassium citrate/ea, Polycitra-K oral soln (1100 mg potassium citrate/5 mL, 480 mL). Oracit oral soln (490 mg sodium citrate/5 mL, 15, 30, 480 mL). Bicitra oral soln (500 mg sodium citrate/5 mL, 480 mL). Urocit-K wax (potassium citrate) Tabs 5, 10 mEq. Polycitra-LC oral soln (550 mg potassium citrate/500 mg sodium citrate per 5 mL, 480 mL). Polycitra oral syrup (550 mg potassium citrate/500 mg sodium citrate per 5 mL, 480 mL.] ▶K ♀C ▶? $$$

INDEX

PDA edition of the *Tarascon Pocket Pharmacopoeia* contains more than 6000 drug names, it is physically impossible to include all in pocket-sized manuals. Therefore, rarely used or specialized drugs appear in the PDA only (noted as "PDA" in the index) or in both the PDA and Deluxe edition (noted as "D" in the index).

15-methyl-prosta-
glandin F2
alpha 140
2-PAM 170
292 tab 10
3TC 22
5-Aspirin 110
5-FU
Dermatology 69
Oncology .... D
5-aminosalicylic
acid 110
6-MP .... D
8-MOP .... D

A

A-200 71
A-spaz. 106
A/T/S 68
A1C home
testing .... PDA
A1CNow .... PDA
abacavir 22
abacavir 21
abatacept .... D
ABC 22
abciximab 56
Abelcet 15
Abenol 12
Abilify 156
Abilify
Discmelt 156
abiraterone
acetate ....D
abobotulinum-
toxin A .... D
Abraxane ....D
Abreva 73
ACAM 2000 ....D
acamprosate 161
Acanya 67
acarbose 80
Accolate 167
Accu-Check
Advantage .....PDA
Accu-Check
Aviva ....PDA

Accu-Check
Compact ....PDA
Accu-Check
Compact Plus..PDA
Accu-Check
Complete ......PDA
Accu-Check
Voicemate .....PDA
Accu-Chek
Active ....PDA
Accu-Prep 108
AccuNeb 164
Accupril 42
Accuretic ....D
Accutane 68
acebutolol 57
acemannan ....D
Aceon 42
Acetadote 169
acetaminophen 12
acetaminophen
Analgesics 3,
.... 9–12, D
ENT ....D
Neurology 131
acetazolamide 61
acetic acid 98
acetohydroxamic
acid ....D
acetylcholine .... D
acetylcysteine 169
acetylcysteine........D
acetylcysteine
inhaled 168
acetylsalicylic
acid 4
acetylsalicylic acid
Analgesics 2, 3,
.... 10, 11
Cardiovascular
.... 56
Gastroenterology
.... 103
Acidophilus 121
AcipHex 106
acitretin 72
Aclasta 78
Aclovate ....D
acrivastine ....D
ActHIB 123

Acticin 72
Actidose-Aqua ... 169
Actifed Cold and
Allergy ....D
Actifed Cold and
Sinus ....D
Actigall 111
Actiq 7
Activase 64
Activase rt-PA 64
activated
charcoal 169
Activella 137
Actonel 78
Actonel Plus
Calcium 78
ACTOPLUS Met 80
Actos 85
Actron 5
Acular 150
Acular LS 150
Acutrim Natural
AM ....D
acyclovir 19
acyclovir - topical..72
Aczone 17
Adacel 123
Adalat 60
Adalat CC 60
Adalat PA 60
Adalat XL 60
adalimumab 1
adapalene 67
adapalene 68
Adcirca 64
Adderall 162
Adderall XR 162
adefovir 27
Adenocard 46
adenosine 46
ADH 94
Adipex-P. 164
Adoxa 38
adrenalin 63
Adriamycin ....D
Adrucil ....D
Advair 165
Advair HFA 165
Advate ....D
Advicor 50

Advil 5
Aerius 94
AeroBid 167
AeroBid-M 167
Aerospan 167
Aesculus hip-
pocastanum 120
Afeditab CR 60
Afinitor ....D
Afluria 123
African plum
tree. 121
Afrin 100
agalsidase
beta ....PDA
Aggrastat 57
Aggrenox 56
Agrylin ....D
Airomir 164
AK Tate 148
AK Tracin 146
AK-Con 144
AK-Dilate 149
AK-Mycin 146
AK-Pentolate 149
Akarpine 149
Akineton 132
Akten 150
Akurza 68
Alamast 145
Alavert 94
Alavert D-12 .... D
Alaway 144
Albalon 144
albendazole 18
Albenza 18
Albuminar 65
albumin 65
Albuminar 65
albuterol 164
albuterol 165
alcaftadine 144
Alcaine 150
alclometasone
dipropionate ......D
alcohol ....D
Aldactazide ....D
Aldactone 43
Aldara 73
aldesleukin ....D

Aldomet.............. 45
Aldoril.................D
Aldurazyme........PDA
AlphaNine SD ....D
alefacept 72
alemtuzumab ..... D
alendronate 77
Alertec............ 164
Aleve 6
Aleve Cold and
Sinus ....D
Alfenta ....D
alfentanil ....D
Alferon N.............D
alfuzosin 170
alglucerase ......PDA
alglucosidase
alfa ....PDA
Align................ 121
Alimta ....D
Alinia 18
aliskiren 35
aliskiren ....D
alitretinoin 75
Alka-Seltzer...... 103
Alkeran ....D
All Clear 144
Allegra............. 94
Allegra-D 12-hour ..D
Allegra-D 24-hour ..D
Aller-Chlor........ 95
Aller-Relief........ 95
Allerdryl............ 95
Allerfrim ....D
Allermax............ 95
AllerNaze........ 99
AlleRx ....D
Alli.................. 111
Allium sativum... 118
allopurinol 86
Alluna 122
Almora 88
almotriptan 131
Alocril ....D
Aloe vera ....D
Alomide 145
Aloprim 86
Alora 136
alosetron 110
Aloxi 101
alpha-1
antitrypsin ....D

Alpha-1 proteinase
inhibitor............D
alpha-
galactosidase...110
Alphagan........... 149
Alphagan P 149
Alphanate...........D
AlphaNine SD ......D
Alphatrex ....D
alprazolam 160
alprostadil 172
Alrex 147
Alsoy 89
Alsuma 131
Altabax 70
Altace 43
Altafrin 149
Alternagel......... 103
Altoprev 51
altretamine ....D
Alu-Cap............ 103
Alu-Tab............ 103
aluminum
acetate 98
aluminum
chloride 75
aluminum
hydroxide 103
aluminum hydroxide
Analgesics 2
Gastroenterology
.... 103, 104
Alvesco 166
alvimopan 110
amantadine 25
Amaryl 84
Amatine 63
ambenonium ......PDA
Ambien 161
Ambien CR 161
AmBisome 15
ambrisentan ....PDA
amcinonide ....D
Amerge 131
Amethia 139
amethocain........PDA
Amethyst 139
Amevive 72
Amicar 115
Amidate ....D
Amidrine 131
amifostine ....D
Amigesic 4
amikacin 13
Amikin 13
amiloride.............D
amiloride.............D

aminocaproic
acid 115
aminoglutethimide..D
aminohippurate....D
aminolevulinic
acid ....D
aminophylline ... 168
aminosalicylic
acid ....PDA
amiodarone 46
Amitiza 109
amitriptyline 151
amitriptyline.........D
amlexanox 98
amlodipine 59
amlodipine 59
Ammonul ....PDA
amobarbital ....PDA
amoxapine ....D
amoxicillin........ 35
amoxicillin........ 105
amoxicillin-
clavulanate 35
Amoxil 35
Amphadase ....D
amphetamine ... 162
Amphojel 103
Amphotec ....D
amphotericin B
deoxycholate... 15
amphotericin B
lipid
formulations... 15
ampicillin 36
ampicillin 36
ampicillin-
sulbactam 36
Ampyra 132
Amrix................. 2
amyl nitrite ....PDA
Anacin 4
Anadrol-50 76
Anafranil 151
anagrelide ....D
anakinra ....D
Analpram-HC ......D
Anaprox 6
Anaspaz 106
anastrozole ....D
Ancef 29
Ancobon 15
and Bisacodyl
Tablet Kit 108
Andriol ....D
andro...................D

Androderm........ 77
AndroGel 77
Android................D
Androstenedione...D
Androxy................D
Anectine 13
Anexsia 9
Angelica
sinensis 118
Angeliq 137
Angiomax 112
anhydrous
glycerins 98
anidulafungin 15
Ansaid 5
Antabuse 161
Antara 53
antazoline 144
Anthemis
nobilis - Roman
chamomile ... 117
anthralin 72
anti-inhibitor
coagulant
complex ....D
Antilirium ....D
antipyrine 96
antivenin-
crotalidae immune
Fab ovine
polyvalent 124
antivenin-crotalidae
polyvalent ....D
antivenin-
latrodectus
mactans ....PDA
Antivert 95
Antizol ....D
Anusol-HC ....D
Anzemet 101
Aphthasol 98
Apidra 83
Aplenzin 154
Aplisol 126
Apo-Bicalutamide...D
Apokyn 1
apomorphine 1
apraclonidine ....D
aprepitant 102
Apresazide ....D
Apresoline 55
Apri 139
Apriso 110
Aprodine.............D
Aptivus 25
Aquachloral
Suprettes...... 160

AquaMephyton..... 92
Aquasol E........... 92
AraC.....................D
Aralast..................D
Aralen............... 16
Aranelle 139
Aranesp............. 115
Arava 1
Arcalyst............PDA
Aricept............. 127
Arimidex..............D
Aredia 78
arformoterol 164
argatroban ....D
Aricept............. 127
Arimidex..............D
aripiprazole 156
Aristolochia ....D
aristolochic acid...D
Aristospan....... 80
Arixtra 112
armodafinil..........D
Armour Thyroid....D
arnica 116
Arnica montana..116
Aromasin...............D
Aromaticum..........D
Arranon ....D
arsenic trioxide.....D
Artane 132
artemether 16
Arthrotec 4
articaine.......... 13
artichoke leaf
extract 116
artificial tears ... 150
Arzerra ....D
Asacol 110
Asaphen 4
Asarum ....D
ascorbic acid...... 90
ascorbic acid....... 91
Ascriptin............... 2
asenapine 156
Aslera 118
Asmanex
Twisthaler 167
Asmavent 164
asparaginase .... D
Aspir-Mox 2
Aspirin................... 4
Assalix 122
Astelin 99
Astepro 99
astragalus......... 116
Astragalus mem-
branaceus 116
Atacand..................D
Atacand HCT ....D

Atacand Plus........D
Atarax............... 95
Atasol............... 12
Atasol 8, 15, 30,..11
atazanavir........ 23
Atelvia 78
atenolol 57
atenolol ....D
Atgam 125
Ativan 160
atomoxetine 162
atorvastatin 50
atorvastatin 51
atovaquone 18
atovaquone 16
atracurium .... D
Atripla 20
atropine............. 46
atropine................ 46
atropine-
ophthalmic 149
Atropine Care 149
atropine-
ophthalmic 149
Atrovent 168
Atrovent HFA 168
Atrovent Nasal
Spray 100
Attenuvax ....PDA
ATV.................... 23
augmented
betamethasone
dipropionate ....D
Augmentin 35
Augmentin
ES-600 35
Augmentin XR ... 35
Auralgan 96
auranofin..............D
Avage 69
Avalide ....D
Avandamet.......... 80
Avandaryl........... 85
Avandia 85
Avapro................ 43
Avastin..................D
Avaxim 123
Aventyl 151
avian influenza
vaccine H5N1-
inactivated
injection 123

Aviane 139
Avinza 8
Avodart............ 170
Avonex 132
Axert.................. 131
Axid 104
Axid AR............ 104
Axiron................ 77
Aygestin 140
azacitidine ....D
Azactam 39
Azasan ....D
Azasite 146
azathioprine 1
azelaic acid....... 67
azelastine-nasal..99
azelastine-
ophthalmic 144
Azelex 67
Azilect 134
azilsartan........... 43
azithromycin...... 31
azithromycin-
ophthalmic 146
Azmacort 167
Azo-Standard ... 171
Azopt 148
Azor ....D
aztreonam 39
Azulfidine 110
Azulfidine
EN-tabs 110
Azurette........... 139

B

B&O suppretes ....D
B-D Glucose 85
BabyBIG 125
Bacid................ 121
Bacillus of Calmette
& Guerin.............D
bacitracin......... 69
bacitracin
Dermatology ... 70
Ophthalmology..146
bacitracin-
ophthalmic 146
baclofen 2
Bactocill 35
Bactrim............. 38
Bactroban 70
BAL in oil............D
balsalazide 109
Balziva 139

banana bag....... 89
Banophen 95
Banzel 130
Baraclude 28
Baridium 171
barium sulfate ... 67
Basagel............ 103
basiliximab 126
Bayer..................... 4
Baygam 125
BayJet................D
BCG.......................D
BCG vaccine ... 123
BCNU...................D
Beano 110
becaplermin 75
beclomethasone .. 99
beclomethasone-
inhaled 165
Beconase AQ 99
belatacept....... 126
belimumab ....D
belladonna
Gastroenterology..D
Urology ....D
Bellergal
Spacetabs .....D
Bellergal-S ....D
Benadryl............ 95
Benadryl Allergy
and Cold ....D
Benadryl-D Allergy
and Sinus ....D
benazepril 41
benazepril ....D
bendamustine.....D
bendroflumethiaz-
ide ....D
DeneTin 122
Benefix.................D
Benicar.............. 44
Benicar HCT ....D
Benlysta ....D
Benoquin 76
Benoxyl 68
Bentyl 106
Bentyol 106
Benylin 96
Benzac 68
BenzaClin 68
Benzagel 10%.... 68
Benzamycin....... 68

Gastroenterology
... 100, 101, 106
Toxicology ....D
Urology 171

bicarbonate..... 103
Bicillin C-R..... 34
Bicillin L-A..... 34
Bicitra..... 172
BiCNU..... D
BiDil..... 65
Biest..... PDA
Bifantis..... 121
Bifidobacteria..... 121
bilberry..... 117
Biltricide..... 18
bimatoprost..... 149
Bionect..... 75
BioRab..... 124
biotin..... 91
biperiden..... 132
Biphentin..... 163
Biquin durules..... 49
bisacodyl..... 108
bismuth subcitrate potassium..... 105
bismuth subsalicylate..... 100
bismuth subsalicylate..... 104
bisoprolol..... 58
bisoprolol..... D
bitter melon..... 117
bitter orange..... 117
bivalirudin..... 112
black cohosh..... 117
Blenoxane..... D
Bleph-10..... 146
Blephamide..... 146
Blocadren..... D
blood transfusion..... PDA
bocepravir..... 27
Bonamine..... 95
Bonine..... 95
Boniva..... 78
Bontril..... D
Bontril Slow Release..... D
Boostrix..... 123
boric acid..... 141
bortezomib..... D
bosentan..... D
Botox..... D
Botox Cosmetic..... D
botulinum toxin type B..... D
botulism immune globulin..... 125
Bragantia..... D
Bravelle..... D

Brilinta..... 56
Brevibloc..... 58
Brevicon..... D
Brevicon 1/35.....D
Brevital..... 12
brimonidine..... 149
brimonidine..... 148
brinzolamide..... 148
bromazepam..... 159
Bromday..... D
bromfenac-ophthalmic..... 150
Bromfenex..... D
Bromfenex PD..... D
bromocriptine..... 93
brompheniramine..D
Brovana..... 164
Brovana..... D
buckeye..... 120
budesonide..... 110
budesonide..... D
budesonide-inhaled..... 166
budesonide-nasal..99
Bufferin..... 3
bumetanide..... 61
Bumex..... 61
Buminate..... 65
bupivacaine..... 13
bupivacaine..... 13
Buprenex..... D
buprenorphine..... D
buprenorphine..... 162
Buproban..... 154
bupropion..... 154
Burinex..... 61
burn plant..... D
BuSpar..... 160
buspirone..... 160
busulfan..... D
Busulfex..... D
butabarbital..... D
butalbital..... 3, 10
butamben..... 13
butenafine..... 70
Butisol..... D
butoconazole..... 141
butorphanol..... 6
Butrans..... D
butterbur..... 117
Byetta..... 82
Bystolic..... 59

C

C.E.S..... 137
cabazitaxel..... D

cabergoline..... 93
Caduet..... 51
Caelyx..... D
Cafcit..... 162
Cafergot..... 131
Caffedrine..... 162
caffeine..... 162
caffeine
  Analgesics..... 3,
  ..... 10, 11
  Neurology..... 131
calamine..... 75
Calan..... 60
Calcibind..... D
Calciferol..... 91
Calcijex..... 90
Calcimar..... 93
calcipotriene..... 72
calcipotriene..... 72
calcitonin..... 93
calcitriol..... 90
calcium acetate..86
calcium
  carbonate..... 86
calcium carbonate
  Analgesics..... 2, 3
  Gastroenterology
  104
  OB/GYN..... 142
calcium chloride..87
calcium citrate..... D
calcium gluconate
  87
Caldolor..... 5
calfactant..... D
CalMist..... 91
Calsan..... 86
Caltine..... 93
Caltrate..... 86
Cambia..... 4
Camellia sinensis
  119
Camila..... 140
Campath..... D
Campral..... 161
Camptosar..... D
Canasa..... D
Cancidas..... 15
candesartan..... D
candesartan..... D
Candistatin
  Antimicrobials..16
  Dermatology..... 71
Canesten
  Antimicrobials..14
  OB/GYN..... 141
Cankermelt..... 120

cannibis sativa L. extract .... D
Cantil 107
Capastat .... PDA
capecitabine .... D
Capex .... D
Capital with Codeine suspension 9
Capoten 41
Capozide 41
capreomycin ...... PDA
Caprex .... D
capsaicin 75
captopril 41
captopril .... D
Carac 69
Carafate 107
carbachol .... D
Carbaglu .... PDA
carbamazepine ... 127
carbamide peroxide 96
Carbatrol 127
carbidopa .... D
carbidopa 133
carbidopa/ levodopa .... D
carbinoxamine ...... D
carbinoxamine .... D
Carbocaine 13
Carbodec DM .... D
carboplatin .... D
carboprost 140
Cardene 59
Cardene SR 59
Cardizem 60
Cardizem CD 60
Cardizem LA 60
Cardura 45
Cardura XL 45
carglumic acid .. PDA
Carimune 125
carisoprodol 2
carisoprodol 3, 11
Carmol 40 .... D
Carmol HC .... D
carmustine .... D
Carnitor 89
carteolol- ophthalmic 148
Cartia XT 60
Cartilade 122
carvedilol 58
cascara .... D
Casodex .... D
caspofungin 15

castor oil 109
Cataflam 4
Catapres 44
Catapres-TTS 44
Cathflo 64
Caverject 172
Caverject Impulse 172
Cayston 39
Caziant 139
CCNU .... D
Ceclor 30
Cedax 30
Cedocard SR .... D
CeeNu .... D
cefaclor 30
cefadroxil 29
cefazolin 29
cefdinir 30
cefditoren 30
cefepime 31
cefixime 30
Cefizox 30
cefotaxime 30
cefotetan .... D
cefoxitin 30
cefpodoxime 30
cefprozil 30
ceftaroline 31
ceftazidime .... D
ceftibuten 30
Ceftin 30
ceftizoxime 30
ceftriaxone 30
cefuroxime 30
Cefzil 30
Celebrex 4
celecoxib 4
Celestone 78
Celestone Soluspan 78
Celexa 152
Cellcept 126
cellulose sodium phosphate .... D
Celontin .... PDA
Cena-K 89
Cenestin 137
Centany 70
cephalexin 29
Ceprotin .... D
Ceptaz 30
Cerebyx 128
Ceredase .... PDA
Cerefolin .... D
Cerefolin NAC .... D
Cerezyme .... D

Certain Dri............. 75
certolizumab 110
Cerubidine .... D
Cervidil 138
Cesamet 102
Cesium chloride...117
Cetacaine 13
cetirizine 95
cetirizine .... D
Cetraxal 96
cetrorelix acetate... D
Cetrotide .... D
cetuximab .... D
cevimeline 98
chamomile 117
Chantix 162
CharcoAid 169
Charcoal 169
Charcoal .... D
Charcodate 169
chasteberry 117
Chemet 170
Cheracol D Cough... D
Cheratussin AC .... D
Cheratussin DAC ... D
Children's Advil
Cold .... D
ChiRhoStim 111
Chlor-Trimeton 95
chloral hydrate ... 160
chlorambucil .... D
chloramphenicol ... 39
chlordiazepoxide.159
chlordiazepoxide... D
chlordiazepoxide-
clidinium 110
Chlordrine SR .... D
chlorhexidine gluconate 98
chlorodeoxyadenos-
ine .... D
Chloromycetin ... 39
chlorophyllin copper complex..76
chloroprocaine.... PDA
chloroquine 16
chlorothiazide........ D
chlorpheniramine...95
chlorpheniramine... D
chlorpromazine.... 1
chlorpropamide.... D
chlorthalidone 62
chlorthalidone........ D
chlorzoxazone 2
cholecalciferol...... 93
CholeRx 121
Cholestin 121
cholestyramine.... 49

choline magnesium trisalicylate 4
chondroitin 117
Choriogonadotropin alfa..........................D
Chorionic gonadotropin .... D
Chrysanthemum parthenium.......118
Ci-wu-jia 119
Cialis 172
ciclesonide 99
ciclesonide-
inhaled 166
ciclopirox 70
Cidecin 39
cidofovir 19
cigarette............ PDA
cilazapril 41
cilazapril .... D
cilostazol 66
Ciloxan 145
cimetidine 104
Cimicifuga racemosa.............D
Cimzia 110
cinacalcet .... D
Cinnamomum Cassia ....D
cinnamon .... D
Cipro 37
Cipralex 152
Cipro 37
Cipro HC Otic 96
Cipro XR 37
Ciprodex Otic 96
ciprofloxacin Antimicrobials .. 37
ciprofloxacin ENT 96
ciprofloxacin-
ophthalmic 145
cisapride .... D
cisatracurium 13
cisplatin .... D
citalopram 152
Citanest .... PDA
Citracal 87
citrate 172
citrate 103
Citri Lean 118
Citrocarbonate ... 103
Citrucel 107

Citrus aurantium...D
cladribine...D
Claforan...30
Claravis...68
Clarinex...94
Clarinex-D 12 hour..D
Clarinex-D 24 hour..D
Claripel...76
clarithromycin...34
clarithromycin...105
Claritin...94
Claritin Hives
Relief...94
Claritin RediTabs..94
Claritin-D 12 hr...D
Claritin-D 24 hr...D
Clarus...68
Clavulin...35
Clear Eyes...144
Clearasil...68
Clearasil
Cleanser...68
clemastine...95
Clenia...68
Cleocin
Antimicrobials ..39
OB/GYN...141
Cleocin T...68
clevidipine...59
Cleviprex...59
Climara...136
Climara Pro...137
Clindagel...68
ClindaMax...68
clindamycin...39
clindamycin...67–69,
............................D
clindamycin -
topical...68
clindamycin-
vaginal...141
Clindesse...141
Clindoxyl...68
Clinoril...9
clobazam...128
clobetasol...D
Clobex...D
clocortolone
pivalate...D
Cloderm...D
clodronate...D
clofarabine...D

clofazimine...D
Clolar...D
Clomid...138
clomiphene...138
clomipramine...151
Clonapam...159
clonazepam...159
clonidine...44
clonidine...D
clonidine -
epidural...PDA
clopidogrel...56
cloquinol...D
Clorpres...D
Clotrimaderm
Antimicrobials ..14
OB/GYN...141
clotrimazole...14
clotrimazole...73
clotrimazole -
topical...70
clotrimazole-
vaginal...141
clozapine...156
Clozaril...156
coal tar...D
Coartem...16
Coartemether...16
cobalamin...PDA
cocaine...PDA
codeine...7
codeine
Analgesics...9–11, D
ENT...D
coenzyme Q10 ...117
Cogentin...132
Cognex...PDA
Colace...109
Colazal...109
ColBenemid...86
colchicine...86
colchicine...86
Colcrys...86
Cold-fX...119
colesevelam...49
Colestid...49
Colestid Flavored..49
colestipol...49
colistimethate...PDA
colistin...98
*Coly-Mycin M
Parenteral*...PDA
Colyte...108
Combantrin...18
Combigan...148
CombiPatch...137

Combivent...165
*Combivent
inhalation soln*..165
Combivir...21
Combunox...9
Commit...161
Compazine...102
Complera...21
Comtan...1
Comvax...123
Concerta...163
Condyline...73
Condylox...73
cone flower...D
Congest...137
conivaptan...PDA
Conray...67
Copaxone...132
Copegus...28
copper gluconate...D
CoQ-10...117
Cordarone...46
Cordran...D
Cordran SP...D
Coreg...58
Coreg CR...58
Corgard...58
Coricidin HBP
Congestion and
Cough...D
Coricidin HBP
Cough and cold ...D
Corlopam...55
Cormax...D
Coronex...D
Correctol...108
Cortaid...D
Cortamed...D
Cortate...D
Cortef...79
Cortenema...79
Corticaine...D
corticotropin...D
Cortifoam...D
cortisone...78
Cortisporin...73
Cortisporin Otic...98
Cortisporin TC
Otic...98
Cortisporin-
ophthalmic...147
Cortizone...D
Cortoderm...D
Cortone...78
Cortrosyn...D

Corvert...48
*Corynanthe
yohimbe*...122
Corzide...D
Cosamin DS...119
Cosmegen...D
Cosopt...148
cosyntropin...D
Cotazym...111
cotrimoxazole...38
Coumadin...114
Covera-HS...60
Coversyl...42
Cozaar...44
Cranactin...117
cranberry...117
*Crataegus
laevigata*...120
creatine...D
Creon...111
Crestor...51
Crinone...140
Crixivan...24
CroFab...124
Crolom...145
cromolyn-
inhaled...168
cromolyn-nasal...100
cromolyn-
ophthalmic...145
crotamiton...71
Cryselle...139
*crystalline
DMSO2*...120
Cubicin...39
Culturelle...121
Cuprimine...D
Curosurf...D
Cutar...75
Cutivate...D
Cutter...D
Cuvposa...111
cyanocobalamin...91
cyanocobalamin
ENDOCRINE AND
METABOLIC 91
OB/GYN...142
Cyanokit...169
Cyclen...D
Cyclessa...139
cyclobenzaprine...2
Cyclocort...D
Cyclogyl...149
Cyclomen...142
cyclopentolate..149
cyclophosphamide...D
cycloserine ...PDA

Cycloset 93
cyclosporine 126
cyclosporine-
  ophthalmic ...116
Cyklokapron .... D
Cymbalta 153
Cynara scolymus ...116
cyproheptadine ... 95
cyproterone .... D
cyproterone 68
Cystadane ....PDA
Cystografin .... D
Cystospaz 106
Cytadren 67
cytarabine .... D
Cytogam ....PDA
cytomegalovirus
  immune globulin
  human ....PDA
Cytomel 90
Cytosar-U .... D
Cytotec
  Gastroenterology
  107
  OB/GYN 138
Cytovene .... D
Cytoxan .... D

D

d-biotin ....PDA
D.H.E. 45 131
D2T5 123
D4T .... D
dabigatran 112
dacarbazine .... D
daclizumab 126
Dacogen .... D
dactinomycin .... D
Dalacin 141
Dalacin C 39
Dalacin T 68
dalfampridine 132
dalfopristin 40
Daliresp 168
Dalmane 160
dalteparin 112
danazol 142
Danocrine 142
danshen .... D
Dantrium .... D
dantrolene .... D
dapsone 17
Daptacel 123
daptomycin 39
Daraprim 19

darbepoetin 115
darifenacin 170
darunavir 23
Darvocet .... D
Darvon
  Pulvules .... D
Darvon-N .... D
dasatinib .... D
daunorubicin .... D
DaunoXome .... D
Daxas 168
Daypro 6
Daytrana 163
DDAVP 93
DDI 22
DDrops 93
Debacterol 98
Debrox 96
Decadron 78
decitabine .... D
Declomycin 38
Deconamine .... D
Deconsal II .... D
DEET .... D
deferasirox 115
deferoxamine 169
degarelix .... D
dehydroepiandros-
  terone 118
Delatestryl 77
delavirdine ....PDA
Delestrogen 136
Delsym 96
Deltasone 80
Demadex 61
demeclocycline ... 38
Demerol 7
Demser .... D
Demulen .... D
Denavir 73
denileukin .... D
denosumab 93
Denticare 98
Depacon 130
Depade 161
Depakene 130
Depakote
  Neurology 130
  Psychiatry 155
Depakote ER
  Neurology 130
  Psychiatry 155
Depen .... D
Depo-Cyt .... D
Depo-Estradiol .. 136
Depo-Medrol 79
Depo-Provera ..... D

depo-subQ
  provera 104 .... D
Depo-Testosterone ...77
DepoDur 8
Deproic
  Neurology ....PDA
  Psychiatry 1
Derma-
  Smoothe/FS ..... D
Dermalac .... D
Dermasone .... D
Dermatop .... D
Dermazin .... D
Dermolate .... D
DermOtic 98
Desferal 169
desflurane ....PDA
desipramine 151
desirudin 112
desloratadine 94
desloratadine .... D
desmopressin 93
Desogen 139
desogestrel .... D
Desonate .... D
desonide .... D
DesOwen .... D
Desoxi .... D
desoximetasone ... D
Desoxyn ....PDA
Desquam 68
desvenlafaxine .. 153
Desyrel 154
Detrol 171
Detrol LA 171
devil's claw 118
Dex-4 85
dexamethasone ... 78
dexamethasone ... 96
dexamethasone -
  ophthalmic 147
Dexasone 78
Dexatrim Natural
  Ephedrine Free ...D
dexbrompheni-
  ramine .... D
dexchlorpheni-
  ramine 95
dexchlorphen-
  iramine .... D
Dexedrine 163
DexFerrum 88
Dexiron 88
dexlansoprazole ...105
dexmedetomidine
  12

dexmethylpheni-
  date 163
Dexpak 78
dexrazoxane .... D
dextran 65
dextroamphet-
  amine 163
dextroamphet-
  amine 162
dextromethorphan
  96
dextromethorphan ..D
dextromethorphan/
  quinidine .... D
Dextrose 85
dextrose .... D
DHEA 118
Diabeta 85
Diabinese .... D
Diamorphine .....PDA
Diamox 61
Diamox Sequels .. 61
Diane-35 68
Diarr-eze 101
Diastat 159
Diastat AcuDial ..159
diatrizoate 67
Diatx Zn ....PDA
Diazemuls 159
diazepam 159
diazoxide .... D
Dibenzyline .... D
dibucaine 75
Dicel .... D
dichloral-
  phenazone 131
Diclectin 102
diclofenac 4
diclofenac 4
diclofenac -
  topical 69
diclofenac-
  ophthalmic 150
dicloxacillin 35
dicyclomine 106
didanosine 22
Didrex .... D
Didronel 78
diethylpropion ..... D
difenoxin 101
Differin 67
Dificid 34

180
Index
D,PDA = see page 173

diflorasone .... D
Diflucan 14
diflunisal 4
difluprednate 147
Digibind 47
DigiFab 47
Digitek 46
digoxin 46
digoxin immune
Fab 47
dihydrocodeine ... 11
dihydroergotamine
.... 131
diiodohydroxyquin
.... PDA
Dilacor XR 60
Dilantin 129
Dilatrate-SR .... D
Dilaudid 7
Dilaudid-5 7
Diltia XT 60
diltiazem 60
Diltiazem CD 60
Diltzac 60
dimenhydrinate ... 102
Dimetane-DX
Cough Syrup .... D
Dimetapp Cold
and Allergy ...... D
Dimetapp Cold
and Cough ...... D
Dimetapp
Decongestant
Infant Drops 96
Dimetapp
Nighttime Cold
and Congestion .. D
dimethyl sulfone .. 120
dimethyl sulfoxide..D
dinoprostone 138
Diocarpine 149
Diodoquin .... PDA
Diogent 145
Diopred .... D
Dioscorea villosa..122
Diovan 44
Diovan HCT .... D
Dipentum 110
Diphen 95
Diphenhist 95
diphenhydramine..95

diphenhydramine
.... 99
diphenoxylate 100
diphenhydramine... D
diphtheria tetanus
and acellular
pertussis
vaccine 123
diphtheria tetanus
and acellular
pertussis
vaccine 124
diphtheria-tetanus
toxoid 123
dipivefrin .... D
Diprivan 13
Diprolene .... D
Diprolene AF .... D
Diprosone .... D
dipyridamole 56
dipyridamole 56
Disalcid 4
Diskets 7
disopyramide 47
DisperMox.......... 35
disulfiram 161
Ditropan 170
Ditropan XL 170
Diuril .... D
divalproex
Neurology 130
Psychiatry 155
Divigel 136
Dixarit 44
DLV .... PDA
DMSO .... D
dobutamine 63
Dobutrex 63
docetaxel .... D
docosanol 73
docusate 109
docusate 109
dofetilide 47
dolasetron 101
Dolobid .... D
Dolophine 7
Doloteffin 118
Domeboro otic 98
domperidone 102
Dona 119
donepezil 127
dong quai 118
Donnatal 106
dopamine 63
Dopram .... D
Doribax 29
doripenem 29

dornase alfa 168
Doryx 38
dorzolamide 148
dorzolamide 148
Dostinex 93
doxapram .... D
doxazosin 45
doxepin 151
doxepin - topical ..75
doxercalciferol 91
Doxil .... D
doxorubicin
liposomal .... D
doxorubicin
non-liposomal .... D
Doxycin 38
doxycycline 38
doxylamine 102
doxylamine
Analgesics 10
Gastroenterology
.... 102
Dramamine 102
Drisdol 91
Dristan 12 Hr
Nasal 100
Drithocreme 72
Drixoral Cold and
Allergy .... D
dronabinol 102
dronedarone 47
droperidol 102
drospirenone 137
drotrecogin 39
Droxia 115
DRV 23
Dry Eyes 150
Drysol 75
DT 123
DTaP 123
DTIC-Dome .... D
Duac 68
Duetact 81
Dulcolax 108
Dulera 165
duloxetine 153
Duocaine 13
Duodote .... D
Duolube 150
DuoNeb 165
Duoneb UDV .... D
Duragesic 7
Duralast .... D
Duratuss .... D
Duratuss GP .... D
Duratuss HD .... D

Durdrin 131
Durezol 147
Duricef 29
dutasteride 170
dutasteride 170
Duvoid 171
Dyazide .... D
Dynacin 38
DynaCirc 59
DynaCirc CR 59
Dynapen 35
Dyrenium .... D
DYSPORT .... D
Dytan 95

E

E Pam 159
E-mycin 34
E. angustifolia.... D
E. pallida .... D
E. purpurea .... D
Ebixa 127
EC-Naprosyn 6
echinacea .... D
Echinacin Madaus..D
EchinaGuard .... D
echothiophate
iodide .... D
econazole 70
Econopred Plus.. 148
Ecotrin 4
Ecstacy .... PDA
eculizumab.......... PDA
ED Spaz 106
Edarbi 43
Edecrin 61
edetate .... D
Edex 172
Edluar 161
edrophonium 132
EDTA .... D
Edurant 23
EES .... D
efavirenz 21
efavirenz 20
Effer-K 89
Effexor 153
Effexor XR 153
Effient 56
Efidac/24 96
eflornithine 75
Efudex 69
EFV 21
EGb 761 119
Egrifta .... PDA

Elaprase............PDA
Elavil.................151
Eldepryl............134
elderberry.........118
Eldopaque.........76
Eldoquin............76
Eldoquin Forte....76
Electropeg.........108
Elestat...............144
Elestrin............136
eletriptan...........D
Eleutherococcus
  senticosus......119
Elidel...................D
Eligard................D
Elimite...............72
Eliphos...............86
Elitek..................D
Elixophyllin.......168
Ella....................D
Ellence................D
Elmiron...............D
Elocom................D
Clocon................D
Eloxatin...............D
Elspar.................D
eltrombopag....PDA
Eltroxin.............90
Emadine............144
Emcyt.................D
emedastine........144
Emend...............102
Emetrol..............D
EMLA..................75
Emo-Cort............D
Empirin................4
Empirin with
  Codeine...........10
Emsam..............152
emtricitabine..21, 22
emtricitabine....20,
...................21
Emtriva..............22
Enablex............170
enalapril.............41
enalapril..............D
enalaprilat..........41
Enbrel..................1
Enca..................38
Endantadine......25
Endocet.............10
Endocodone........D
Endodan.............10
Endometrin.......140
Endrate..............D
Enduron...............D
Enemeez...........109

Enemol..............108
Enfamil..............89
enflurane.......PDA
enfuvirtide..........D
Engerix-B...........123
Enjuvia.............137
Enlon................132
enoxaparin.......113
Enpresse..........139
entacapone...........1
entacapone.......133
entecavir...........28
Entereg.............110
Entex LA.............D
Entex Liquid........D
Entex PSE............D
Entocort EC.......110
Entonox.........PDA
Entozyme..........111
Entrophen............1
Entsol................100
Enulose.............107
Epaxal..............123
ephedra................D
Ephedra sinica.....D
ephedrine............63
Epiduo................68
Epifoam................D
Epiject.................1
epinastine.........144
epinephrine.........63
epinephrine
  racemic...........168
EpiPen................63
EpiPen Jr............63
EpiQuin Micro......76
epirubicin............D
Epitol................127
Epival...................1
Epivir..................22
Epivir-HBV..........22
eplerenone..........43
epoetin alfa..........D
epoetin beta........D
Epogen.................D
epoprostenol.......43
eprosartan..........43
eprosartan...........D
eptifibatide.........56
Epzicom.............21
Equalactin..........107
Equetro.............127
Eraxis.................15
Erbitux.................D
Ergocalciferol.....91

Ergomar...........PDA
ergotamine.....PDA
ergotamine
  Gastroenterology..D
  Neurology.......131
Eribulin................D
erlotinib...............D
Errin.................140
Ertaczo..............71
ertapenem.........29
Ery-Tab..............34
Erybid................34
Eryc...................34
Erycette..............68
Eryderm.............68
Erygel.................68
Eryped.................D
Erysol..................68
Erythrocin IV.......34
Erythromid.........34
erythromycin -
  topical.............68
erythromycin base..34
erythromycin base...68
erythromycin ethyl
  succinate...........D
erythromycin ethyl
  succinate..........34
erythromycin
  lactobionate.....34
erythromycin-
  ophthalmic......146
erythropoietin
  alpha - Eprex, D
erythropoietin
  beta..................D
escitalopram 152
Fsclim...............136
Esgic...................3
Esidrix................62
Eskalith...............1
Eskalith CR..........1
esmolol..............58
esomeprazole 105
Esoterica............76
Estalis...............137
estazolam.........160
esterified
  estrogens........136
esterified
  estrogens.........137
Estrace..............136
Estraderm.........136
estradiol............136
estradiol.............137
estradiol
  acetate............136

estradiol acetate
  vaginal ring.....136
estradiol
  cypionate........136
estradiol gel......136
estradiol topical
  emulsion..........136
estradiol transder-
  mal patch........136
estradiol transder-
  mal spray........136
estradiol vaginal
  ring.................136
estradiol
  vaginal tab.......136
estradiol
  valerate...........136
estradiol valerate
  and estradiol
  valerate/
  dienogest...........D
Estradot............136
estramustine.......D
Estrasorb..........136
Estratest...........137
Estratest H.S.....137
Estring..............136
estriol...............PDA
Estrogel............136
estrogen vaginal
  cream.............136
estrogens
  conjugated.....137
estrogens conju-
  gated......137, 138
estrogens
  synthetic
  conjugated A ..137
estrogens
  synthetic
  conjugated B ..137
estrone............PDA
estropipate.......137
Estrostep Fe.....139
eszopiclone.......160
etanercept...........1
ethacrynic acid....61
ethambutol........17
Ethanol................D
ethinyl estradiol
  Dermatology.....68
  OB/GYN...........137

182
Index
D,PDA = see page 173

ethinyl estradiol
transdermal.... 135
ethinyl estradiol
vaginal ring.... 135
ethionamide......... PDA
ethosuximide...... 128
ethotoin............ PDA
Ethrane............. PDA
ethynodiol.............D
Ethyol..................D
Etibi................. 17
etidronate.......... 78
etodolac.............. 5
etomidate.............D
etonogestrel..........D
etonogestrel...... 135
Etopophos............D
etoposide.............D
ETR................. 21
etravirine.......... 21
Euflex.................D
Euglucon........... 85
Eulexin...............D
Eurax............... 71
Euthyrox........... 90
Evamist........... 136
evening primrose
oil................ 118
everolimus...........D
Evista............. 140
Evithrom.............D
Evoclin............ 68
Evoxac............. 98
Evra............... 135
Ex-Lax............ 109
Exalgo.............. 7
Excedrin
Migraine........... 3
Exelon............ 127
Exelon Patch..... 127
exemestane..........D
exenatide.......... 82
Exforge............ 59
Exforge HCT.........D
Exjade............ 115
Exsel............. 76
Extina............ 70
EZ-Char........... 169
ezetimibe.......... 53
ezetimibe.......... 52
Ezetrol............ 53

F

Fabrazyme......... PDA
Factive............ 37
factor IX............D
factor VIIa..........D
factor VIII..........D
famciclovir........ 20
famotidine........ 104
famotidine........ 104
Famvir............ 20
Fanapt............ 156
Fangchi..............D
Fansidar.............D
Fareston.............D
Faslodex.............D
Fasturtec............D
fat emulsion...... 89
FazaClo ODT...... 156
febuxostat......... 86
Feen-a-Mint...... 108
Feiba NF.............D
Feiba VH.............D
Feiba VH Immuno..D
felbamate......... 128
Felbatol.......... 128
Feldene............. 6
felodipine......... 59
felodipine...........D
Femara...............D
Femcon Fe........ 139
Femhrt............ 137
Femizol-M........ 141
FemPatch......... 136
Femring........... 136
Femtrace......... 136
fenofibrate........ 53
fenofibric acid.... 53
fenoldopam........ 55
fenofenol............D
fenoterol............D
fentanyl............. 7
Fentora............. 7
fenugreek......... 118
Feosol............. 88
Fer-in-Sol......... 88
Feraheme.......... 88
Fergon..............D
Feridex............ 67
Ferodan............ 88
Ferrex 150........ 88
ferric gluconate
complex.......... 87
Ferrlecit.......... 87

ferrous fumarate...D
ferrous gluconate..D
ferrous sulfate.... 88
Fertinex.............D
ferumoxides....... 67
ferumoxsil......... 67
ferumoxytol....... 88
fesoterodine...... 170
feverfew.......... 118
Fexicam............. 6
Fexmid.............. 2
fexofenadine...... 94
fexofenadine.........D
fiber - dietary... PDA
Fiberall.............D
FiberCon.......... 107
Fibricor............ 53
fidaxomicin....... 34
Fidelin............ 118
filgrastim......... 115
Finacea............ 67
finasteride........ 170
Finevin............ 67
fingolimod........ 132
Fioricet............. 3
Fioricet with
Codeine.......... 10
Fiorinal............. 3
Fiorinal C-1/2..... 10
Fiorinal C-1/4..... 10
Fiorinal with
Codeine.......... 10
fish oil............ 89
FK 506............ 126
Flagyl............. 39
Flagyl ER.......... 39
Flamazine.......... 70
Flarex............ 147
flavocoxid........... 6
flavoxate...........D
Flebogamma...... 125
flecainide.......... 48
Flector.............. 4
Fleet........ 107, 108
Fleet enema...... 108
Fleet EZ-Prep..... 108
Fleet Mineral
Oil Enema....... 109
Fleet Pain Relief.. 75
Fleet Phospho-
Soda............ 108
Fletcher's
Castoria......... 109
Flexeril............. 2
Flixonase...........D
Flixotide............D
Flo-Pred........... 79

Flolan..............D
Flomax............ 170
Flonase............ 99
Florastor.......... 121
Florazole ER....... 39
Florinef............ 79
Flovent Diskus... 167
Flovent HFA...... 167
Floxin............. 37
Floxin Otic........ 98
floxuridine..........D
Fluanxol............D
Fluanxol Depot.....D
Fluarix........... 123
fluconazole........ 14
flucytosine........ 15
Fludara.............D
fludarabine.........D
fludrocortisone.... 79
FluLaval.......... 123
Flumadine......... 25
flumazenil........ 169
flumethasone.......D
FluMist........... 123
flunarizine....... 131
flunisolide........ 99
flunisolide-
inhaled.......... 167
fluocinolone.........D
fluocinolone...... 77
fluocinolone -
ophthalmic..... PDA
fluocinolone-otic.. 98
fluocinonide.........D
Fluor-A-Day....... 88
Fluor-I-Strip..... PDA
Fluor-I-Strip AT.. PDA
fluorescein....... PDA
fluoride........... 88
fluorometholone..147
Fluoroplex........ 69
fluorouracil.........D
fluorouracil -
topical.......... 69
Fluothane........ PDA
Fluotic............ 88
fluoxetine........ 152
fluoxetine........ 161
fluoxymesterone....D
Flupenthixol........D
flupentixol..........D
fluphenazine..... 155
flurandrenolide.....D
flurazepam....... 160
flurbiprofen........ 5
flurbiprofen-
ophthalmic.........D

flutamide.............D
fluticasone - inhaled 165
fluticasone - topical .... D
fluticasone-inhaled...... 167
fluticasone-nasal..99
fluvastatin.......... 51
Fluviral 123
Fluvirin 123
Fluzone 123
FML 147
FML Forte........... 147
FML-S liquifilm......D
Focalin 163
Focalin XR 163
folate Folvite....... 91
Folgard ....D
Folgard Rx.........D
folic acid 91
folic acid
 ENDOCRINE AND
 METABOLIC ... 91
 OB/GYN 142
folinic acid ....D
Follistim AQ ....D
follitropin alfa......D
follitropin beta .....D
Folotyn ....D
Foltx ....D
fomepizole...........D
fondaparinux 112
food .... PDA
Foradil 164
Forane .... PDA
formoterol......... 164
formoterol......... 165
formulas - infant..89
Formulex 106
Fortamet 85
Fortaz 30
Forteo 94
Fortical 93
Fosamax 77
Fosamax Plus D... 77
foscarnet........... 19
Foscavir 19
fosfomycin........ 39
fosinopril............ 42
fosinopril ....D

fosphenytoin...... 128
fospropofol......... 12
Fosrenol 90
FPV 23
Fragmin 112
FreeStyle Flash .... PDA
FreeStyle Freedom .... PDA
FreeStyle Freedom Lite .... PDA
FreeStyle Lite... PDA
French maritime
 pine tree bark..121
Frova 131
frovatriptan....... 131
FSH ....D
FSH and LH.......D
FTC 22
Fucidin H......... 73
FUDR ....D
Ful-Glo .... PDA
fulvestrant..........D
Fulvicin ....D
Fungizone 15
Furadantin 39
furosemide......... 61
fusidic acid 73
fusidic acid - topical 69
fusidic acid- ophthalmic .... PDA
Fusilev ....D
Fuzeon ....D

G

G-CSF 115
G115 119
gabapentin........ 128
Gabitril 130
gadobenate 66
gadodiamide 66
gadopentetate... 66
gadoteridol........ 66
gadoversetamide
 66
galantamine...... 127
gallium..............D
gadsulfase....... PDA
Galzin ....D
Gamastan 125
gamma hydroxybu-
 tyrate............ 135
Gammagard 125
Gammaplex 125

Gamunex........... 125
ganciclovir
 Antimicrobials .. 19
 Ophthalmology..146
Gani-Tuss NR ....D
ganirelix ....D
Ganite ....D
Garamycin
 Antimicrobials .. 14
 Dermatology 69
 Ophthalmology
 145
garcinia............ 118
Garcinia cambogia ... 118
Gardasil 123
garlic
 supplements... 118
Gas-X............ 107
Gastrocrom........ 168
Gastrografin 67
GastroMARK 67
gatifloxacin-
 ophthalmic 145
Gaviscon ....D
gefitinib..............D
Gelclair 98
Gelnique 170
gemcitabine ......D
gemfibrozil 54
gemifloxacin 37
gemtuzumab .....D
Gemzar ....D
Generess Fe....... 139
Gengraf 126
Genisoy............ 122
Genoptic 145
Genotropin....... 94
Gentak............ 145
gentamicin 14
gentamicin........ 147
gentamicin -
 topical 69
gentamicin-
 ophthalmic 145
GenTeal 150
Gentran 65
Geodon 159
GHB............... 135
GI cocktail 106
Gianvi............. 139
Gilenya 132
ginger.............. 118
ginkgo biloba ... 119
Ginkgold.......... 119
Ginkoba 119
Ginsana 119

183
Index
D,PDA = see page 173

ginseng-American
 119
ginseng-Asian... 119
ginseng-Siberian
 119
glatiramer 132
Gleevec ....D
Gliadel ....D
gliclazide 84
glimepiride........ 84
glimepiride... 80, 81
glipizide 84
glipizide............ 82
GlucaGen 85
glucagon 85
Glucobay 80
Gluconorm.........D
Glucophage 85
Glucophage XR.... 85
glucosamine..... 119
glucose home
 testing........ PDA
Glucotrol........... 84
Glucotrol XL....... 84
Glucovance 81
Glumetza 85
glutamine........ PDA
Glutose 85
glyburide 85
glyburide............ 81
glycerin 107
GlycoLax 108
glycopyrrolate.... 111
Glycyrrhiza glabra 120
Glycyrrhiza uralensis 120
Glynase PresTab.. 85
Glyquin 76
Glysennid 109
Glyset 80
GM-CSF 115
gold sodium
 thiomalate .....D
goldenseal........ 119
GoLytely 108
Gonadotropins......D
Gonal-F ....D
Gonal-F RFF Pen...D
Goody's Extra
 Strength Headache
 Powder 3

goserelin .... D
Gralise 128
gramicidin 146
granisetron 101
grape seed
extract 119
grapefruit juice ..PDA
Gravol 102
green goddess 106
green tea 119
Grifulvin V .... D
Gris-PEG .... D
griseofulvin .... D
griseofulvin
ultramicrosize....D
guaiacolsulfonate..D
guaifenesin 96
guaifenesin .... D
Guaifenex DM .... D
Guaifenex PSE ...... D
Guaitex ii SR/PSE ..D
guanabenz .... D
guanfacine
Cardiovascular ...45
Psychiatry 163
guarana 119
guggul 120
guggulipid 120
Guiatuss 96
Guiatuss AC .... D
Guiatuss PE .... D
Guiatussin DAC ....D
Gynazole 141
Gyne-Lotrimin 141
Gynodiol 136

H

H-BIG 125
H.P. Acthar Gel......D
Habitrol 162
haemophilus B
vaccine 123
haemophilus B
vaccine ... 123, 124
Halaven .... D
halcinonide .... D
Halcion 160
Haldol 155
HalfLytely 108
Halfprin 4

halobetasol
propionate .... D
halofantrine ...... PDA
Halog .... D
haloperidol 155
Halotestin .... D
halothane .... PDA
Halotussin AC......D
Halotussin DAC ....D
Harpadol 118
Harpagophytum
procumbens.... 118
Havrix 123
hawthorn 120
HCE50 120
hCG .... D
HCTZ 62
Healthy Woman..122
HeartCare 120
Hectorol 91
Helidac 104
Helixate .... D
Hemabate 140
Hemofil M............ D
heparin 113
hepatitis A
vaccine 123
hepatitis A
vaccine 124
hepatitis B immune
globulin 125
hepatitis B
vaccine 123
hepatitis B
vaccine ... 123, 124
Hepsera 27
Heptovir 22
Herceptin .... D
heroin .... PDA
Hespan 65
hetastarch 65
Hexabrix 67
Hexalen .... D
Hextend 65
HibTITER 123
Hicon 90
Hiprex .... PDA
Histinex HC .... D
histrelin .... D
Histussin D........... D
Histussin HC .... D
Hizentra 125
homatropine 149
homatropine..........D
honey 120
Horizant 128

horse chestnut
seed extract.... 120
HP-Pac 105
huang qi 116
huckleberry 117
Humalog 83
Humalog Mix
50/50.............. 84
Humalog Mix
75/25.............. 84
human growth
hormone 94
human papilloma-
virus recombinant
vaccine 123
Humate P .... D
Humatrope 94
Humibid DM .... D
Humibid LA........... D
Humira 1
Humulin 50/50.... 84
Humulin 70/30.... 84
Humulin N 83
Humulin R 83
Hyalgan .... D
hyaluronate .... D
hyaluronic acid.... 75
hyaluronidase....PDA
Hycamtin .... D
Hycoclear Tuss.....D
Hycodan .... D
Hycotuss.............. D
Hyderm .... D
hydralazine 55
hydralazine 65
HydraSense 100
Hydrastis
canadensis 119
Hydrea 115
hydrochlorothiazide
.... 62
hydrochlorothiazide
.... 62
Hydrocil .... D
Hydrocortisone
Dermatology ... 73,
.... 76
ENT 96, 98

hydrocortisone -
ophthalmic 147
hydrocortisone -
topical .... D
hydrocortisone
acetate .... D
hydrocortisone
acetate .... D
hydrocortisone
butyrate .... D
hydrocortisone
probutate .... D
hydrocortisone
valerate .... D
HydroDiuril 62
Hydromorph
Contin............... 7
hydromorphone...... 7
hydroquinone 76
hydroquinone....... 77
Hydroval .... D
hydroxocobalamin
.... 169
hydroxychloroquine
.... 1
hydroxyprogesterone
caproate 138
hydroxypropyl
cellulose 150
hydroxyurea 115
hydroxyzine 95
hylan GF-20.......... D
hymenoptera
venom 126
hyoscine 106
hyoscyamine 106
hyoscyamine
Gastroenterology
.... 106
Urology 171
Hyosol 106
Hyospaz 106
Hypaque 67
HyperHep B......... 125
Hypericum
perforatum 122
HyperRAB S/D.... 126
HyperRHO S/D.... 142
Hyperstat .... D
Hyphanox 14
Hypocol 121
Hypotears 150
Hytone .... D
Hytrin 46
Hytuss 96
Hyzaar .... D

I

ibandronate.........78
ibritumomab ....D
Ibudone.........10
ibuprofen.........5
ibuprofen
Analgesics...9–11, 5
ENT.........5
ibutilide.........48
Idamycin.........D
idarubicin.........D
idursulfase.........PDA
IDV.........24
Ifex.........D
ifosfamide.........D
iloperidone.........156
iloprost.........156
Ilotycin.........146
imatinib.........D
Imdur.........62
imiglucerase.........PDA
imipenem-
  cilastatin.........29
imipramine.........151
imiquimod.........73
Imitrex.........131
Immucyst
  Immunology.........123
  Oncology.........D
immune globulin-
  intramuscular.........125
immune globulin-
  intravenous.........125
immune globulin
  subcutaneous.........125
Immunine VH.........D
Immunoprin.........130
Imodium.........101
Imodium AD.........101
Imodium Multi-
  Symptom
  Relief.........100
Imogam
  Rabies-HT.........126
Imovax Rabies.........124
Implanon.........D
Imuran.........1
inamrinone.........63
Inapsine.........102
Incivek.........29
incobotulinum-
  toxin A ....D
Increlex.........PDA
indapamide.........62
Inderal.........59

Inderal LA.........59
Inderide.........D
Indigo Carmine..PDA
indigotindisul-
  fonate ....PDA
indinavir.........24
Indium DTPA.........PDA
Indocid-P.D.A.........5
Indocin.........5
Indocin IV.........5
indomethacin.........5
Infanrix.........123
Infasurf.........D
InFed.........88
Infergen.........PDA
Inflamase Forte..148
infliximab.........1
influenza vaccine-
  inactivated
  injection 123
influenza
  vaccine-live
  intranasal.........123
Infufer.........88
INH.........17
Inhibace.........41
Inhibace Plus.........D
Innohep.........113
InnoPran XL.........59
INOmax.........D
Inspra.........43
Insta-Glucose.........85
insulin - injectable
  intermediate/
  long-acting.........83
insulin - injectable
  short/rapid-
  acting.........83
insulin injectable
  combinations.........84
Intal.........168
Integrilin.........56
Intelence.........21
interferon alfa-2a..D
interferon alfa-2b..D
interferon alfa-n3..D
interferon
  alfacon-1.........PDA
interferon
  beta-1A 132
interferon
  beta-1B 132
interleukin-2 ....D
IntestiFlora.........121
Intralipid.........89
Intron A.........28

Intropin.........63
Intuniv.........163
Invanz.........29
Invega.........157
Invega
  Sustenna.........157
Inversine.........D
Invirase.........24
iodixanol.........67
iodoquinol.........PDA
Iodotope.........90
iohexol.........67
Ionamin.........164
IONSYS.........7
iopamidol.........67
Iopidine.........D
iopromide.........67
Iosat.........D
iothalamate.........67
ioversol.........67
ioxaglate.........67
ioxilan.........67
ipecac syrup.........169
Ipilimumab.........D
IPOL.........124
ipratropium.........165
ipratropium-
  inhaled.........168
ipratropium-
  nasal.........168
Iprivask.........112
Iquix.........145
irbesartan.........43
irbesartan.........D
Iressa.........D
irinotecan.........D
iron dextran.........88
iron
  polysaccharide..88
iron sucrose.........88
Isentress.........21
ISMO.........D
isocarboxazid 152
isoflurane.........PDA
Isomil.........89
isometheptene.........131
isoniazid.........17
isoniazid.........17
isopropyl alcohol..98
isoproterenol.........48
Isoptin SR.........60
Isopto Atropine.149
Isopto Carbachol..D
Isopto Carpine.149
Isopto
  Homatropine.149
Isordil.........D

isosorbide
  dinitrate.........D
isosorbide
  dinitrate.........65
isosorbide
  mononitrate.........62
isosulfan blue ...PDA
Isotamine.........17
isotretinoin.........68
Isovue.........67
isoxsuprine.........D
isradipine.........59
Istalol.........148
Istodax.........D
Isuprel.........48
itraconazole.........14
ivermectin.........18
ixabepilone.........D
Ixempra.........D

J

Jalyn.........170
Jantoven.........114
Janumet.........82
Januvia.........82
japanese
  encephalitis
  vaccine.........D
JE-Vax.........D
Jenloga.........44
Jevtana.........D
Jin Fu Kang.........116
Jolivette.........140
Junel.........D
Junel Fe.........D

K

K+10.........89
K+8.........89
K+Care.........89
K+Care ET.........89
K-Dur.........89
K-G Elixir.........89
K-Lease.........89
K-Lor.........89
K-Lyte.........89
K-Lyte Cl.........89
K-Norm.........89

K-Phos 89
K-Tab 89
K-vescent 89
Kabikinase 65
Kadian 8
Kaletra 24
kanamycin .... PDA
Kantrex .... PDA
Kaochlor 89
Kaon 89
Kaon Cl. 89
Kaopectate 100
Kaopectate
Stool Softener ..109
Kapidex 105
Kapvay 44
karela 117
Kariva 139
kava .... D
Kay Ciel 89
Kayexalate 93
Kaylixir 89
Keflex 29
Kelnor .... D
Kemstro 2
Kenalog
Dermatology .... D
ENDOCRINE AND
METABOLIC ... 80
Kenalog in
Orabase .... D
Kepivance .... D
Keppra 129
Keppra XR 129
Kerlone 57
Ketalar 12
ketamine 12
Ketek 40
ketoconazole 14
ketoconazole -
topical 70
Ketoderm 70
ketoprofen 5
ketorolac 5
ketorolac-
ophthalmic 150
ketotifen 168
ketotifen-
ophthalmic 144
Kidrolase .... D
Kineret 1
Kinlytic 65

Kira 122
Klaron 69
Klean-Prep 108
Klonopin 159
Klonopin
Wafer 159
Klor-con 89
Klorvess
Effervescent 89
Klotrix 89
Koate .... D
Kogenate .... D
Kolyum 89
Kombiglyze XR 82
kombucha tea .... D
Kondremul 109
Konsyl .... D
Konsyl Fiber 107
Korean red
ginseng 119
Kristalose 107
Krystexxa 86
Ku-Zyme 111
Ku-Zyme HP 111
Kuvan .... PDA
Kwai 118
Kwellada-P 72
Kyolic 118
Kytril 101

L

L-glutamine .... PDA
L-methylfolate ... PDA
L-Thyroxine 90
labetalol 58
Lac-Hydrin .... D
lacosamide 128
Lacrilube 150
Lacrisert 150
Lactaid 111
lactase 111
lactic acid .... D
Lactinex 121
Lactobacillus 121
lactulose 107
Lamical
Neurology 128
Psychiatry 154
Lamical CD
Neurology 128
Psychiatry 154
Lamical ODT
Neurology 128
Psychiatry 154
Lamical XR 154

Lamisil
Antimicrobials ... 16
Dermatology 71
Lamisil AT 71
lamivudine 22
lamivudine 21
lamotrigine
Neurology 128
Psychiatry 154
Lamprene .... D
Lanoxicaps 46
Lanoxin 46
lanreotide .... PDA
lansoprazole 105
lansoprazole 105
Lansoyl 109
lanthanum
carbonate 90
Lantus 83
Lanvis .... D
lapatinib .... D
Lariam 16
laronidase .... PDA
Lasix 61
Lastacaft 144
latanoprost 149
Latisse 149
Latuda 156
Leena 139
leflunomide 1
Legalon 120
lenalidomide .... D
leopard's
bane 116
lepirudin 112
Lescol 51
Lescol XL 51
Lessina 139
Letairis .... PDA
letrozole .... D
leucovorin .... D
Leukeran .... D
Leukine 115
leuprolide .... D
Leustatin .... D
levalbuterol 164
Levaquin 37
Levatol 57
Levbid 106
Levemir 83
levetiracetam 129
Levitra 172
Levo-Dromoran 7
Levo-T 90
levobunolol 148
levocabastine-
nasal 100

levocabastine-
ophthalmic 144
levocarnitine 89
levocetirizine 95
levodopa 133
levofloxacin 37
levofloxacin-
ophthalmic 145
Levolet 90
levoleucovorin ...... D
levonorgestrel ... 135
levonorgestrel ... 137
levonorgestrel
IS 135
Levophed 64
Levora 139
levorphanol 7
Levothroid 90
levothyroxine 90
levothyroxine .... D
Levoxyl 90
Levsin 106
Levsinex 106
Levulan
Kerastick .... D
Lexapro 152
Lexiva 23
Lexxel .... D
LI-160 122
Lialda 110
Librax 110
Librium 110
licorice 120
Lidemol .... D
Lidex .... D
Lidex-E .... D
lidocaine 48
lidocaine - local
anesthetic 13
lidocaine -
topical 76
lidocaine -
topical 75, 77
lidocaine—local
anesthetic 13
lidocaine-
ophthalmic 150
lidocaine-viscous ..99
Lidoderm 76
Limbitrol .... D
Limbitrol DS .... D
Limbrel 118
linagliptin .... D
Lincocin .... PDA
lincomycin .... PDA
lindane 71
linezolid 39

Lioresal 2
liothyronine 90
liothyronine .... D
Liotrix .... D
Lipidil EZ 53
Lipidil Micro 53
Lipidil Supra 53
Lipitor 50
Lipofen 53
Lipolysar 121
Liposyn 89
Liqui-Doss 109
liraglutide 82
lisdexamfetamine
  163
lisinopril 42
lisinopril .... D
Lithane 1
lithium 1
Lithobid 1
Lithostat .... D
Livalo 51
LiveBac 121
Livostin 144
LMX 76
Lo/ovral 139
Locacorten
  Vioform .... D
LoCHOLEST 49
LoCHOLEST
  Light 49
Locoid .... D
Locoid Lipocream .... D
Lodosyn .... D
Lodoxamide 145
Loestrin .... D
Loestrin 24 Fe 139
Loestrin Fe .... D
Lomine 106
Lomotil 100
lomustine .... D
Loniten .... D
Loperacap 101
loperamide 101
loperamide .... D
Lopid 54
lopinavir-ritonavir ... 24
Lopressor 58
Lopressor HCT .... D
Loprox 70
loratadine 94
loratadine .... D
lorazepam 160
Lorcet 10
Lortab 10
losartan 44
losartan .... D

Loseasonique 139
Losec 106
Lotemax 147
Lotensin 41
Lotensin HCT .... D
loteprednol 147
loteprednol .... D
Lotrel .... D
Lotriderm 73
Lotrimin AF 70
Lotrimin Ultra 70
Lotrisone 73
Lotronex 110
lovastatin 51
lovastatin 50
Lovaza 89
Lovenox 113
Low-ogestrel 139
Loxapac .... D
loxapine .... D
Loxitane .... D
Lozide 62
Lozol 62
lubiprostone 109
Lucentis .... D
Ludiomil .... PDA
lumefantrine .... D
Lumigan 149
Luminal 129
Lunesta 160
Lupron .... D
Lupron Depot .... D
Lupron Depot-Ped ... D
lurasidone 156
Luride 88
Lusedra 17
Lustra 76
Lutera 139
lutropin alfa .... D
Luveris .... D
Luvox 153
Luvox CR 153
Luxiq foam .... D
Lybrel 139
Lymphazurin .... PDA
lymphocyte immune
  globulin 125
Lyrica 129
Lysodren .... D
Lysteda .... D

M

M-M-R II 123
M-Zole 141

M.O.S. 8
ma huang .... D
Maalox 103
MabCampath .... D
Macrobid 39
Macrodantin 39
Macrodex 65
Macugen .... D
mafenide 69
Mag-200 88
Mag-Ox 400 88
magaldrate 104
Maganate .... D
Magic
  mouthwash 99
Maglucate 88
Magnacet .... D
magnesium
  carbonate
  Analgesics 3
  Gastroenterology .. D
magnesium
  chloride 88
magnesium
  citrate 108
magnesium
  gluconate 88
magnesium
  hydroxide 108
magnesium
  hydroxide
  Analgesics 2
  Gastroenterology
  .... 103, 104
magnesium oxide... 88
magnesium oxide... 3
magnesium
  sulfate 89
magnesium
  sulfate .... D
Magnevist 66
Magtrate 88
Makena 138
Malarone 16
malathion 72
maltodextrin 98
Manchurian or
  Kargasok tea ..... D
Mandelamine .... PDA
mangafodipir 67
mannitol 135
Mantoux 126
maprotiline .... PDA
maraviroc 20
Marcaine 13
marijuana .... PDA
Marinol 102

Marplan 152
Marvelon .... D
Matricaria
  recutita – German
  chamomile 117
Matulane .... D
Mavik 43
Maxair Autohaler .. 164
Maxalt 131
Maxalt MLT 131
Maxeran 102
Maxidone 10
Maxiflor .... D
Maxilene 76
Maximum Strength
  Pepcid AC 104
Maxipime 31
Maxitrol 147
Maxivate .... D
Maxzide .... D
Maxzide-25 .... D
MD-Gastroview 67
MDMA .... PDA
measles mumps &
  rubella
  vaccine 123
measles mumps &
  rubella
  vaccine 124
measles vaccine ... PDA
Mebaral .... PDA
mebendazole 18
mecamylamine ...... D
mecasermin .... PDA
mechlorethamine ... D
Meclicot 95
meclizine 95
meclofenamate 5
Medihoney 120
Medispaz 106
Medivert 95
Medrol 79
medroxyprogester-
  one 138
medroxyprogester-
  one 137, 138
medroxyprogester-
  one-injectable .... D
mefenamic acid 5
mefloquine 16
Mefoxin 30
Megace 140

Megace ES...........140
Megacillin............34
megestrol...........140
Melaleuca
  alternifolia......122
melaleuca oil......122
Melanex..............76
Mellaril.............156
meloxicam............6
melphalan.............D
memantine...........127
Membrane Blue........D
Menactra............123
Menest..............136
Meni-D...............95
meningococcal
  vaccine...........123
Menjugate...........123
Menofem.............123
Menomune-
  A/C/Y/W-135.....123
Menopur..............D
Menostar............136
menotropins..........D
Mentax..............70
Mentha x piperita
  oil...............120
mepenzolate........107
meperidine............7
mephobarbital.....PDA
Mephyton............92
mepivacaine.........13
Mepron..............18
mequinol.............76
mercaptopurine......D
Meridia.............164
meropenem...........29
Merrem IV...........29
Mersyndol with
  Codeine...........10
Meruvax II.........PDA
mesalamine.........110
Mesasal.............110
mesna................D
Mesnex...............D
Mestinon............132
Mestinon
  Timespan.........132
mestranol............D
Metadate CD........163
Metadate ER........163

Metadol..............7
Metaglip............82
Metamucil............D
Metanx.............PDA
Metastron............D
metaxalone...........2
metformin...........85
metformin.......80–82
methacholine.........D
methadone............7
Methadose............7
methamphetamine
  ....PDA
methazolamide......148
methenamine........171
methenamine
  hippurate.......PDA
methenamine
  mandelate.......PDA
Methergine.........140
methimazole.........90
Methitest............D
methocarbamol.......2
methohexital........12
methotrexate.........1
methotrimeprazine...D
methoxsalen..........D
methscopolamine......D
methscopolamine......D
methsuximide......PDA
methyclothiazide.....D
methylaminolevuli-
  nate..............69
methylcellulose....107
methylcobalamin
  ....PDA
methyldopa..........45
methyldopa...........D
methylene blue....170
methylene blue.......D
methylene-
  dioxymethamphet-
  amine...........PDA
methylergonovine
 140
Methylin............163
Methylin ER........163
methylnaltrexone....D
methylphenidate....163
methylprednisolone
 79
methylsulfonyl-
  methane..........120
methyltestosterone..D
methyltestosterone
 137

metipranolol.......148
metoclopramide...102
metolazone..........62
Metopirone..........D
metoprolol..........58
metoprolol...........D
Metozolv ODT.....102
MetroCream..........69
MetroGel............69
MetroGel-Vaginal
 141
MetroLotion.........69
metronidazole.......39
metronidazole...104,
 105
metronidazole -
  topical...........69
metronidazole-
  vaginal..........141
Metvix..............69
Metvixia............69
metyrapone...........D
metyrosine...........D
Mevacor.............51
mexiletine..........48
Mexitil.............48
Miacalcin...........93
micafungin..........15
Micardis............44
Micardis HCT.........D
Micardis Plus........D
Micatin..............D
miconazole.........141
miconazole -
  buccal............14
miconazole -
  topical............D
miconazole -
  topical...........77
Micort-HC
  Lipocream.........D
Micozole............D
MICRhoGAM........142
Micro-K.............89
Micro-K LS..........89
Microgestin Fe......D
Micronor...........140
Microzide...........62
Midamor.............D
midazolam...........13
midodrine...........63
Midrin.............131
Mifeprex...........142
mifepristone.......142
MIG-99.............118
miglitol............80
miglustat.........PDA

Migquin............131
Migra-Lief.........118
Migranal...........131
MigraSpray.........118
Migratine..........131
Migrazone..........131
mild and strong
  silver protein.....D
Milk of Magnesia
 108
milk thistle.......120
milnacipran........135
milrinone...........63
Min-Ovral............D
mineral oil........109
Minestrin 1/20.......D
Minipress...........45
Minirin.............93
Minitran............63
Minizide.............D
Minocin.............38
minocycline.........38
minoxidil............D
minoxidil - topical..76
Minoxidil for Men...76
Miochol-E............D
Miostat..............D
MiraLax............108
Mirapex............133
Mirapex ER.........133
Mircera..............D
Mircette...........139
mirtazapine........154
misoprostol........107
misoprostol..........4
misoprostol- OB..138
mitomycin............D
Mitomycin-C..........D
mitotane.............D
mitoxantrone.........D
MMRV...............124
Moban................D
Mobic................6
Mobicox..............6
moclobemide.........D
modafinil..........164
Modecate...........155
Modeten............155
Modicon............139
Moduret..............D
Moduretic............D
moexipril...........42
moexipril............D
molindone............D
mometasone -
  inhaled..........165

mometasone - topical ....D
mometasone - inhaled 167
mometasone - nasal 99
Momordica charantia...117
Monarc-M.........D
Monascus purpureus ...121
Monazole 141
Monistat 141
Monistat 1-Day...142
monobenzone 76
Monoclate P.......D
Monocor 58
Monodox 38
monogyna...........120
Monoket 62
MonoNessa 139
Mononine ....D
Monopril 42
Monopril HCT.......D
montelukast ...16/17
Monurol 39
Morinda citrifolia...120
morphine 8
Motofen 101
Motrin...........5
Movana 122
Moviprep 108
Moxatag 35
Moxeza 145
moxifloxacin 37
moxifloxacin - ophthalmic 145
Mozobil...........D
MS Contin...........8
MSIR...........8
MSM...........120
Mu Tong ....D
Mucaine 103
Mucinex 96
Mucinex D...........D
Mucinex DM........D
Mucomyst Pulmonary ...168
  Toxicology ...169
Multaq 47
MultiHance 66
multivitamins 91
mumps vaccine..PDA
Mumpsvax.........PDA
mupirocin 70
Murine Ear...........96

Muse 172
Mustargen...........D
Mutamycin...........D
MVC...........20
MVI...........D
Myambutol...........17
Mycamine...........15
Mycelex
  Antimicrobials ...14
  Dermatology 70
Mycelex 7...........141
Mycelex-3...........141
Mycobutin...........17
Mycolog II 73
mycophenolate mofetil 126
Mycostatin
  Antimicrobials ...16
  Dermatology 71
  OB/GYN 142
Mydfrin 149
Mydriacyl 150
Myfortic 126
Mylanta 104
Mylanta 99
Mylanta Children's 86
Myleran ....D
Mylicon 107
Mylotarg...........D
Myobloc ....D
Myochrysine....D
Myotonachol ...171
Myozyme...........PDA
Mysoline 130
Mytelase.........PDA

N

N-acetyl-5-methoxytryptamine 120
N-acetylcysteine...169
n-n-diethyl-m-toluamide 120
NABI-HB...........125
nabilone 102
nabumetone 6
nadolol 58
nadolol...........D
Nadopen-V...........35
nafarelin 35
nafcillin...........35
naftifine 71
Naftin...........71

Naglazyme.........PDA
nalbuphine 7
Nalcrom 168
Nalfon ....PDA
naloxone 11
naloxone 162
naltrexone 161
Namenda...........127
Namenda XR 127
naphazoline 144
naphazoline 144
Naphcon 144
Naphcon-A 144
NapraPac 6
Naprelan 6
Naprosyn 6
naproxen 6
naproxen
  ENT...........D
Neurology 131
naratriptan 131
Narcan 11
Nardil 152
Naropin ....PDA
Nasacort AQ 99
Nasacort HFA.....99
NaSal 100
NasalCrom 99
Nasalide 99
Nasarel 99
Nascobal 91
Nasonex 99
natalizumab ......D
Natazia 139
nateglinide 84
Natrecor 66
Natroba 72
Navane 156
Navelbine ....D
nebivolol 59
Nebcin 14
NebuPent 18
Necon 14
Necon 1/50 139
Necon 10/11......D
Necon 7/7/7 139
nedocromil - inhaled ....D
nedocromil - ophthalmic ....D
nefazodone ....D
nelarabine ....D
nelfinavir 24
Nemasol Sodium ....PDA
Nembutal 13
Neo-Fradin 111

189
Index
D,PDA = see page 173

Neo-Synephrine
  Cardiovascular...64
  ENT...........D
neomycin
  Dermatology...70, 73
  ENT...........98
  Ophthalmology 146, 147
neomycin-oral ...111
NeoProfen 5
Neoral 126
Neosar...........D
Neosporin cream...70
Neosporin ointment 70
Neosporin ointment - ophthalmic 146
Neosporin solution - ophthalmic 146
neostigmine 132
Neovisc...........D
nepafenac...........D
Nephrocap 91
Nephrovite 91
Neptazane 148
Nesacaine ......PDA
nesiritide 66
NESP 115
Nettle root 120
Neulasta...........115
Neumega 115
Neupogen 115
Neurontin 128
Neutra-Phos 89
Nevanac...........D
nevirapine 21
Nexavar...........D
Nexium 105
NFV...........24
niacin 91
niacin
  Cardiovascular 50, 51
  ENDOCRINE AND METABOLIC ...91
niacinamide ....PDA
Niacor 91
Niaspan...........91
Niastase...........D
nicardipine 59

NicoDerm CQ...... 162
Nicolar.............. 91
Nicorette........... 161
Nicorette DS...... 161
Nicorette inhaler.. 161
nicotine gum 161
nicotine inhalation
system............ 161
nicotine lozenge... 161
nicotine nasal
spray.............. 162
nicotine patches.. 162
nicotinic acid...... 91
Nicotrol............ 162
Nicotrol inhaler... 161
Nicotrol NS........ 162
Nidazol.............. 39
nifedipine........... 60
Niferex.............. 88
Niferex-150........ 88
Nilandron............ D
nilotinib..............D
Nilstat
Antimicrobials.. 16
Dermatology.... 71
OB/GYN......... 142
nilutamide...........D
Nimbex.............. 13
nimodipine........ 135
Nimotop..............D
Nipent................D
Niravam........... 160
nisoldipine........ 135
nitazoxanide...... 18
nitisinone......... PDA
Nitoman........... 135
nitrazepam...........D
nitric oxide...........D
Nitro-BID............ 62
Nitro-Dur............ 63
nitrofurantoin...... 39
nitroglycerin
intravenous
infusion.......... 62
nitroglycerin
ointment.......... 62
nitroglycerin
spray.............. 63
nitroglycerin
sublingual........ 63
nitroglycerin sus-
tained release.... D

nitroglycerin
transdermal...... 63
Nitrolingual........ 63
NitroMist........... 63
Nitropress...........D
nitroprusside........D
NitroQuick......... 63
Nitrostat............ 63
nitrous oxide.... PDA
nizatidine.......... 104
Nizoral
Antimicrobials.. 14
Dermatology.... 70
NoDoz.............. 162
Nolvadex......... 140
none.............. 117
noni................ 120
Nor-Q.D............ 140
Nora-BE........... 140
Norco................ 10
Norcuron........... 13
Nordette.......... 139
Norditropin........ 94
NordiFlex........... 94
norelgestromin... 135
norepinephrine.... 64
norethindrone... 140
norethindrone... 137
Norflex............... 2
norfloxacin......... 37
Norgesic............. 3
norgestimate..... 137
norgestrel............D
Norinyl 1+35..... 139
Norinyl 1+50..... 139
Noritate............ 69
Noroxin............. 37
Norpace............. 47
Norpace CR........ 47
Norpramin......... 151
Nortrel................D
Nortrel 7/7/7..... 139
nortriptyline...... 151
Norvasc............ 59
Norvir.............. 24
Nostrilla........... 100
Not yet determined..D
Novafed A............D
Novamoxin......... 35
Novantrone..........D
Novarel...............D
Novasen.............. 4
Novocain........ PDA
Novolin 70/30..... 84

Novolin N............ 83
Novolin R............ 83
NovoLog............ 83
Novolog Mix
50/50.............. 84
Novolog Mix
70/30.............. 84
NovoRapid......... 83
NovoSeven...........D
NovoSeven RT......D
Novothyrox......... 90
Noxafil.............. 14
Nplate................D
Nu-Iron 150........ 88
Nubain................ 7
Nucynta............ 12
Nuedexta............D
NuLev.............. 106
Nulojix............. 126
NuLytely........... 108
Numby Stuff....... 76
Nupercainal........ 75
Nuprin................ 5
Nursoy............. 89
Nutramigen
Lipil............... 89
NutreStore....... PDA
Nutropin........... 94
Nutropin AQ........ 94
Nutropin Depot.... 94
NuvaRing.......... 135
Nuvigil................D
NVP.................. 21
Nyaderm
Antimicrobials.. 16
Dermatology.... 71
OB/GYN......... 142
nystatin............ 16
nystatin............ 73
nystatin - topical.. 71
nystatin-vaginal.. 142
Nytol................. 95

O

oatmeal............. 76
Ocean.............. 100
Octagam........... 125
Octostim............ 93
octreotide........ 111
Ocufen................D
Ocuflox...............D
Ocupress.......... 148

ofatumumab ....D
Off.....................D
ofloxacin–........... 37
ofloxacin–
ophthalmic..........D
ofloxacin-otic.... 98
Ogen................ 137
Ogestrel........... 139
olanzapine........ 156
olanzapine........ 161
Oleptro............ 154
olmesartan......... 44
olmesartan...........D
olopatadine....... 144
olopatadine-
nasal.............. 100
olsalazine......... 110
Olux....................D
omalizumab..........D
omega 3 fatty
acids.............. 89
omega-3-acid
ethyl esters...... 89
omeprazole....... 106
omeprazole...........D
Omnaris............ 99
Omnicef............. 30
Omnipaque........ 67
Omniscan.......... 66
Omnitrope......... 94
onabotulinum
toxin type A........D
Oncaspar............D
Oncotice
Immunology.... 123
Oncology.............D
Oncovin...............D
ondansetron...... 101
OneTouch Ultra.. PDA
OneTouch
UltraMin....... PDA
Onglyza............ 82
Ontak..................D
Onxol..................D
Opana................. 9
Ophthaine........ 150
Ophthetic......... 150
opium.............. 101
opium tincture... 101
oprelvekin........ 115
Oprisine........... 130
Opticrom.......... 145
OptiMARK.......... 66
Optipranolol...... 148
Optiray............. 67
Optivar............ 144

Oracea................38
Oracit................172
Oracort................D
OraDisc A................98
Oramorph SR................8
Orap................156
Orapred................79
Orapred ODT................79
Oraqix................14
Orazinc................89
Orencia................D
Oretic................62
Orfadin................PDA
Orgalutran................D
orlistat................111
orphenadrine................2
orphenadrine................3
Ortho Evra................135
Ortho Tri-Cyclen................139
Ortho Tri-Cyclen
Lo................139
Ortho-Cept................139
Ortho-Cyclen................139
Ortho-Est................137
Ortho-Novum
1/35................139
Ortho-Novum
7/7/7................139
Orthovisc................D
Orudis................5
Orudis KT................5
Oruvail................5
Orvaten................63
Os-Cal................86
oseltamivir................25
Osmitrol................135
Osmoprep................108
Osteoforte................91
others................D
Ovcon-35................139
Ovcon 50................139
Ovide................72
Ovidrel................D
Ovol................107
oxacillin................35
oxaliplatin................D
Oxandrin................77
oxandrolone................77
oxaprozin................6
oxazepam................160
oxcarbazepine................D
Oxeze Turbuhaler................164
oxiconazole................71
Oxilan................71
Oxistat................71
Oxizole................71

oxprenolol................59
Oxsoralen-Ultra................D
oxyacantha................120
oxybate................135
Oxybutyn................170
oxybutynin................170
Oxycocet................10
Oxycodan................10
oxycodone................8
oxycodone................9-11, 8
OxyContin................8
OxyFAST................8
OxyIR................8
oxymetazoline................100
oxymetholone................PDA
oxymorphone................8
oxytocin................138
Oxytrol................170
Oyst-Cal................86

P

P.C.E.................34
Pacerone................46
Pacis................D
paclitaxel................D
PAH................D
Palgic................D
Palgic DS................D
palifermin................D
paliperidone................157
palivizumab................D
palonosetron................101
pamabrom................12
Pamelor................151
pamidronate................78
Pamine................D
Pamine Forte................D
Panadol................12
Panafil................76
Panax ginseng................119
Panax quinquefo
lius L.................119
Pancrease................111
pancreatin................111
Pancreaze................111
Pancrecarb................111
pancrelipase................111
pancuronium................D
Pandel................D
panitumumab................D
Panixine
DisperDose................29
Panretin................75
Pantoloc................106
pantoprazole................106

pantothenic acid................91
papain................76
papaverine................D
para-aminosalicylic
acid................PDA
paracetamol................12
Parafon Forte DSC................2
Paraplatin................D
Parcopa................D
paregoric................101
paricalcitol................92
Pariet................106
Parlodel................93
Parnate................152
paromomycin................18
paroxetine................153
Parvolex................169
PAS................PDA
Paser................PDA
Pataday................144
Patanase................100
Patanol................144
Paullinia
cupana................119
Pausinystalia
yohimbe................122
Pavulon................D
Paxil................153
Paxil CR................153
pazopanib................D
PCO................119
PediaCare Infants'
Decongestant
Drops................96
Pediapred................79
Pediarix................124
Pediatrix................12
Pediazole................34
Pediotic................98
PodvaxHIB................123
PEG-Intron................28
Peg-Lyte................108
Peganone................PDA
pegaptanib................D
pegaspargase................D
Pegasys................28
pegfilgrastim................115
peginterferon
alfa-2a................28
peginterferon
Alfa-2b................D
peginterferon
alfa-2b................28
peglotlcase................86
pegvisomant................PDA
pemetrexed................D
pemirolast................145

191
Index
D, PDA = see page 173

Penbritin................36
penbutolol................D
penciclovir................73
penicillamine................D
penicillin G................34
penicillin V................35
Penlac................70
Pentam................18
pentamidine................18
Pentasa................110
pentazocine................7
pentazocine................11
pentetate
indium................PDA
pentobarbital................13
Pentolair................149
pentosan................D
pentostatin................D
Pentothal................D
pentoxifylline................66
Pepcid................104
Pepcid AC................104
Pepcid
Complete................104
peppermint oil................120
Peptic Relief................104
Pepto-Bismol................100
peramivir................D
Percocet................10
Percocet-demi................10
Percodan................10
Percolone................8
Performist................164
Pergonal................D
Peri-Colace................109
Periactin................95
Peridex................98
perindopril................42
Periogard................98
Periostat................38
Perlane................75
permethrin................72
perphenazine................155
perphenazine................D
Persantine................56
Petadolex................117
Petaforce................117
Petasites
hybridus................117
pethidine................7
petrolatum................150
Pexeva................153

PGE1
Gastroenterology
............................107
OB/GYN 138
PGE2 138
Pharmorubicin......D
Phazyme.............107
Phenazo...............171
phenazopyridine.171
phendimatrizine...D
phenelzine 152
Phenergan.............D
Phenergan VC ......D
Phenergan VC
w/codeine ....D
Phenergan with
codeine 1
Phenergan/dex-
tromethorphan...D
pheniramine........144
phenobarbital......129
phenobarbital.......106
phenoxybenzamine.D
phentermine 164
phentolamine 56
phenyl salicylate...171
phenylephrine...... 96
phenylephrine.......D
phenylephrine-
intravenous 64
phenylephrine-
nasal....................D
phenylephrine-
ophthalmic 149
Phenytek..............129
phenytoin 129
Phoslax...............108
PhosLo.................. 86
Phospholine Iodide...D
phosphorated
carbohydrates..102
phosphorus 89
Photofrin 3
Phrenilin 3
physostigmine ...... D
Phyto Joint...........118
Phytosoya............122
Phytonadione...... 92
pilocarpine 99
pilocarpine-
ophthalmic 149
Pilopine HS.........149

pimecrolimus ....D
pimozide..............156
Pin-X.....................18
pinaverium 111
pindolol 59
Pinworm...............18
pioglitazone........ 85
pioglitazone... 80, 81
Piper methysticum..D
piperacillin-
tazobactam 36
piperonyl
butoxide...... 71, 72
pirbuterol 164
piroxicam 51
pitavastatin 51
Pitocin.................138
Pitressin 94
plague vaccine ..124
Plan B 1
Plan B One-Step..135
Plaquenil 1
Plasbumin........... 65
plasma protein
fraction............. 65
Plasmanate......... 65
Plasmatein.......... 65
Platinol-AQ...........D
Plavix.................. 56
Plenaxis................D
Plendil 59
plerixafor...............D
Pletal.................. 66
Pliagis..................D
Pneumo 23.........124
pneumococcal
23-valent
vaccine 124
pneumococcal
7-valent
conjugate
vaccine 124
Pneumovax..........124
Podocon-25........ 73
Podofilm 73
podofilox 73
Podofin............... 73
podophyllin......... 73
Polaramine......... 65
policosanol 121
polio vaccine 124
polio vaccine 124
Polocaine............. 13
poly-L-lactic acid ..D
polycarbophil......107

Polycitra 172
Polycitra-K..........172
Polycitra-LC........172
polyethylene
glycol 108
polyethylene glycol
with electrolytes
............................108
polymyxin
Dermatology..70, 73
ENT 98
Ophthalmology
............146, 147
Polyphenon E..... 119
Polysporin 70
Polysporin-
ophthalmic 146
Polytar.................. 75
polythiazide..........D
Polytopic............. 70
Polytrim-
ophthalmic 146
Ponstan 5
Ponstel 5
Pontocaine
Anesthesia........PDA
Ophthalmology...150
poractant ....D
porfimer 3
Portia 139
posaconazole...... 14
Potaba...............PDA
potassium 89
potassium iodide...D
potassium
p-aminobenzoate
............................PDA
potassium sulfate..D
Power-Dophilus..121
PPD 126
Pradax ....D
Pradaxa..............112
pralatrexate...........D
pralidoxime 170
pralidoxime...........D
pramipexole........133
pramlintide.......... 85
Pramosone.......... 76
Pramox HC.......... 76
pramoxine 75
pramoxine 76
pramoxine—
topical..................D
Prandimet 82
Prandin.................D
Prasterone.........118
prasugrel............. 56

Pravachol............. 51
pravastatin 51
praziquantel........ 18
prazosin 45
prazosin.................D
Precedex.............. 12
Precose............... 80
Pred Forte.........148
Pred G 147
Pred Mild.............148
prednicarbate.......D
prednisolone....... 79
prednisolone -
ophthalmic ..146,
............................147
prednisolone-
ophthalmic 148
prednisone 80
Prefest................137
Prelone 79
Premarin .. 136, 137
Premesis-Rx........142
Premphase 137
Premplus............138
Prempro...............138
Prepidil...............138
Pressyn AR 94
Pretz..................100
Prevacid
Analgesics........... 6
Gastroenterology
............................105
Prevalite.............. 49
Prevex-HC............D
Previfem 139
Prevnar 124
PrevPac 105
Prezista 23
Priait.................PDA
Priftin 18
prilocaine ....PDA
prilocaine
Anesthesia..........D
Dermatology..... 75
Prilosec 106
Primacor 63
Primadophilus...121
primaquine 17
Primaxin 29
primidone 130
Primsol 41
Principen 36
Prinivil 42
Prinzide..............D
Priorix................123

Pristiq 153
Privigen 125
Pro-Banthine 107
Pro-Fast 164
ProAir HFA 164
ProAmatine 63
probenecid 86
probenecid 86
Probiotica 121
probiotics 121
procainamide 48
procaine .... PDA
procaine
  penicillin 35
procaine
  penicillin 34
procarbazine 60
Procardia 60
Procardia XL 60
Prochieve 140
prochlorperazine... 102
Procrit .... D
Proctocream HC.... D
Proctofoam HC ..... D
ProctoFoam NS ... 75
procyanidolic
  oligomers 119
Prodium 171
Piodium Plain..... D
Progest .... PDA
progesterone gel.. 140
progesterone in
  oil .... D
progesterone
  micronized 140
progesterone
  micronized
  gel .... PDA
progesterone
  vaginal insert...140
Prnglycem.......... D
Prngraf 126
proguanil 16
Prohance 66
Prolastin .... D
Proleukin .... D
Prolia 93
Prolixin 155
Proloprim............ 41
Promacta .... PDA
Promensil 121
promethazine ...... D
promethazine ...... D
Prometrium 140
Pronestyl 48
Propaderm.......... D
propafenone........ D

Propanthel......... 107
propantheline...... 107
proparacaine 150
Propasi HP.......... D
Propecia 170
propofol 13
propoxyphene...... D
propoxyphene ..... D
propranolol 59
propranolol......... D
Propulsid........... D
Propyl Thyracil.... 90
propylene glycol... 98
propylthiouracil... 90
ProQuad 123
ProQuin XR 37
Proscar 170
Prosed/DS.......... 171
ProSobee 89
ProSom 160
prostaglandin
  E1 172
Prostep............. 162
Prostigmin......... 132
Prostin E2.......... 172
Prostin VR 172
Prostin VR
  Pediatric 172
protamine.......... 116
protein C
  concentrate ....PDA
Protenate.......... 65
Protonix 106
Protopam........... 170
Protopic............ 73
protriptyline....... 151
Protropin 94
Protylol 106
Provenge........... D
Proventil HFA 164
Provera 138
Provigil............. 164
Provocholine....... D
Prozac 152
Prozac Weekly.... 152
prussian blue.....PDA
Pseudo-chlor...... D
pseudoephedrine.. 96
pseudoephedrine.. D
Pseudofrin......... 96
Psorcon E.......... D
psyllium............ D
PTU 90
Pulmicort
Flexhaler 166

Pulmicort
  Respules 166
Pulmozyme 168
Puregon............. D
Purinethol......... D
PVF-K 35
pycnogenol 121
pygeum
  africanum 121
Pylera 105
pyrantel 18
pyrazinamide 17
pyrazinamide....... D
pyrethrins..... 71, 72
Pyridiate 171
Pyridium 171
pyridostigmine ... 132
pyridoxal
  phosphate ......PDA
pyridoxine 92
pyridoxine
ENDOCRINE AND
  METABOLIC 91
Gastroenterology
  102
OB/GYN 142
pyrilamine........... D
pyrimethamine ... 19
pyrimethamine..... D
PZA 17

Q

Quadramet.......... D
Qualaquin 17
Quasense 139
Quelicin........... 13
Questran 49
Questran Light ... 49
quetiapine 157
Quick-Pep......... 162
quinapril 42
quinapril............. D
quinidine 49
quinine 17
quinine............... D
quinupristin........ 40
Quixin 145
QVAR 165

R

R&C 71
RabAvert 124
rabeprazole 106

rabies immune
  globulin
  human 126
rabies vaccine.... 124
Rabies Vaccine
  Adsorbed 124
Radiogardase....PDA
RAL 21
rally pack .... D
raloxifene 140
raltegravir 21
ramelteon 160
ramipril 43
Ranexa 66
ranibizumab....... D
Ranicor............. 30
ranitidine 104
ranolazine 66
RAPAFLO........... 170
Rapamune 126
rasagiline 134
rasburicase .... D
Razadyne 127
Razadyne ER 127
Reaclive 95
Rebetol 28
Rebif 132
Reclast 78
Reclipsen 139
Recombinate...... D
Recombivax HB..123
Recothrom......... D
Red clover 121
red clover
  isoflavone
  extract 121
red wine ....PDA
red yeast rice..... 121
Redoxon 90
ReFacto .... D
Refludan 112
Refresh 149
Refresh PM........ 150
Refresh Tears 150
Regitine 56
Reglan.............. 102
Regonal............ 132
Regranex 75
Rejuva-A 69
Relafen 6
Relenza 25

Relistor............111
Relpax.............131
Remeron............154
Remeron
   SolTab...........154
Remicade............1
Remifemin............D
remifentanil.........D
Reminyl............127
Remodulin..........160
Renagel............90
Renedil............59
Reno-60.............67
Reno-DIP............67
RenoCal.............67
Renografin.........67
Renova.............90
Renvela............90
ReoPro.............56
repaglinide..........D
repaglinide.........82
Repel................D
Repronex............D
Requip.............133
Requip XL..........133
Rescriptor..........PDA
Resectisol...........D
reserpine..........135
RespiGam..........126
Restasis...........150
Restoril...........160
Restylane...........75
retapamulin..........70
Retavase............65
reteplase............65
Retin-A.............D
Retin-A Micro........D
Retisert...........PDA
Retisol-A...........69
Retrovir............22
Revatio
   Cardiovascular
  64
   Urology..........172
ReVia.............161
Revlimid.............D
Reyataz.............23
Rheomacrodex........65
Rheumatrex...........1
Rhinalar.............99
Rhinocort Aqua......99

RHO immune
   globulin.........142
RhoGAM............142
Rhophylac..........142
Rhotral.............57
Ribasphere..........28
ribavirin -
   inhaled...........28
ribavirin - oral.......28
riboflavin...........92
riboflavin...........91
RID.................72
Ridaura..............D
Rideril............156
rifabutin............17
Rifadin.............17
Rifamate............17
rifampin............17
rifampin............18
rifapentine..........18
Rifater.............18
rifaximin............40
rilonacept.........PDA
rilpivirine..........21
Rilutek............135
riluzole...........135
rimantadine..........25
rimexolone.........148
Rimostil...........121
Rimso-50............D
Risperdal..........158
Risperdal
   Consta..........158
risperidone........158
Ritalin............163
Ritalin LA..........163
Ritalin SR..........163
ritonavir...........24
Rituxan..............D
rituximab............D
rivaroxaban........112
rivastigmine.......127
Rivotril...........159
rizatriptan........131
Robaxin..............2
Robaxin-750..........2
Robinul..............D
Robinul Forte.......111
Robitussin.........96
Robitussin AC........D
Robitussin CF........D
Robitussin
   Cough...........96
Robitussin DAC.......D

Robitussin DM.......D
Rocaltrol...........90
Rocephin............30
rocuronium..........13
Rofact..............18
Roferon-A............D
roflumilast........168
Rogaine.............76
Rogaine Extra
   Strength.........76
Rogitine............56
Rolaids............104
Romazicon..........169
romidepsin...........D
romiplostin..........D
Rondec...............D
Rondec DM............D
Rondec infant
   drops.............D
ropinirole.........133
ropivacaine........PDA
Rosanil.............69
rosiglitazone.......85
rosiglitazone.......80
Rosula...............D
Rosula NS...........69
rosuvastatin........51
Rotarix...........124
RotaTeq...........124
rotavirus
   vaccine.........124
Rowasa.............110
Roxanol..............8
Roxicet.............11
Roxicodone...........8
Rozerem............160
RPV.................21
RSV immune
   globulin.........126
RTV.................24
RU-486............142
rubella
   vaccine.........PDA
Rubex...............D
Rubini.............118
Rufen................5
rufinamide.........130
Rylosol.............49
Ryna-12 S............D
Rynatan..............D
Rynatan pediatric
   suspension........D
Rythmodan...........47
Rythmodan-LA........47
Rythmol..............D
Rythmol SR...........D
Ryzolt..............12

S-2...............168
s-adenosylmethion-
   ine.............122
S.A.S..............110
Saccharomyces
   boulardii.......121
Safyral...........139
Saint John's wort...122
Saizen..............94
Salagen.............99
Salazopyrin
   En-tabs.........110
salbutamol.........164
Salflex..............4
salicin............122
Salicis cortex......122
salicylic acid.......68
saline nasal
   spray...........100
Salix alba.........122
salmeterol.........165
salmeterol.........165
Salofalk...........110
salsalate............4
Salvia miltiorrhiza...D
SAM-e.............122
samarium 153.........D
Sambucol...........118
Sambucus nigra......118
sammy..............122
Samsca..............D
Sanctura...........171
Sanctura XR........171
Sancuso............101
Sandimmune........126
Sandostatin........111
Sandostatin LAR....111
Sans-Acne...........68
Saphris............156
sapropterin........PDA
saquinavir..........24
Sarafem............152
sargramostim.......115
Sativex..............D
Savella............135
saxagliptin.........82
saxagliptin.........82
Scopace............103
scopolamine........103
scopolamine........106
Sculptra.............D
SeaMist............100
Seasonale..........139

Seasonique........ 139
secobarbital........PDA
secobarbital........PDA
Seconal........PDA
SecreFlo........ 111
secretin........ 111
Sectral........ 57
Sedapap........ 3
Select 1/35........D
selegiline........ 134
selegiline-
    transdermal........ 152
selenium sulfide... 76
Selsun........ 76
Selzentry........ 20
Semprex-D........ 21
senna........ 109
senna........ 109
sennosides........ 109
Senokot........ 109
Senokot-S........ 109
SenokotXTRA... 109
Sensipar........ 138
Sensorcaine.... 13
Septocaine........ 13
Septra........ 38
Serax........ 160
Serenoa repens.. 122
Serevent Diskus.. 165
Seromycin........PDA
Serophene........ 138
Seroquel........ 157
Seroquel XR..... 157
Serostim........ 94
Serostim LQ..... 94
Serpasil........D
sertaconazole.... 71
sertraline........ 160
sevelamer........ 90
Seville orange....... D
sevoflurane........ D
Sevorane........PDA
shark cartilage.. 122
sibutramine........ 164
Siladryl........ 95
sildenafil
    Cardiovascular..64
    Urology........ 172
Silenor........ 151
silodosin........ 170
Silvadene........ 70
silver ion........D
silver sulfadiazine
    70
Silver-colloidal... D
Silybum
    marianum........ 120

silymarin........ 120
Simcor........ 51
simethicone.... 107
simethicone.... 100,
    104
Similac........ 89
Simulect........ 126
simvastatin..... 51
simvastatin..... 51, 52
sinecatechins.... 73
Sinemet........D
Sinemet CR......D
Sinequan........ 151
Singulair........ 167
Sinupret........ 118
sipuleucel-T........D
sirolimus........ 126
sitagliptin........ 82
sitagliptin........ 82
Skelaxin........ 2
Skelid........PDA
SI........ 89
Slo-Niacin........ 91
Slow-FE........ 88
Slow-Fe........ 88
Slow-Mag........ 88
Slow-Trasicor.... 59
smallpox vaccine..D
smoking........PDA
sodium
    benzoate........PDA
sodium iodide
    I-131........ 90
Sodium Iodide I-131
    Therapeutic.... 90
sodium phenylac-
    etate........PDA
sodium phosphate
    108
sodium phosphate
    171
sodium polystyrene
    sulfonate........ 93
sodium sulfate.....D
sodium valproate
    130
Solag........ 76
Solage........ 76
Solaquin........ 76
Solaraze........ 69
solifenacin........ 171
Soliris........PDA
Solodyn........ 38
Soltamox........ 140
Solu-Cortef........ 79
Solu-Medrol........ 79
Solugel........ 68

Soma........ 2
Soma Compound .. 3
Soma Compound
    with Codeine... 11
Somatropin........ 94
Somatuline
    Depot........PDA
Somavert........PDA
Sominex........ 95
Somnote........ 160
Sonata........ 122
sorafenib........D
sorbitol........ 108
Soriatane........ 72
Sorilux........ 72
sotalol........ 49
Sotret........ 68
soy........ 122
Soyalac........ 89
Spacol........ 106
Spasdel........ 106
Spectracef........ 30
spinosad........ 74
Spiriva........ 168
spironolactone.... 43
spironolactone......D
Sporanox........ 14
Sprintec........D
Sprycel........D
SQV........ 24
SSD........ 70
SSKI........D
Stadol........ 6
Stadol NS........ 6
Stalevo........ 133
standardized
    extract WS
    1442 - Crataegutt
    novo........ 120
starch........ 75
Starlix........ 84
Starnoc........ 161
stavudine........D
Stavzor
    Neurology........D
    Psychiatry..... 155
Stay Awake... 162
Stelara........ 72
Stelazine........D
Stemetil........ 102
Sterapred........ 80
stevia........ 122
Stevia
    rebaudiana... 122
Stieprox
    shampoo........ 70

Stieva-A........ 69
Stimate........ 93
stinging nettle... 120
Strattera........ 162
Streptase........ 65
streptokinase.... 65
streptomycin.... 14
streptozocin........D
Striant........ 77
Stridex Pads... 68
Stromectol........ 18
strontium-89......D
Sublimaze........ 7
Suboxone........ 162
Subutex........D
succimer........ 170
succinylcholine... 13
sucralfate........ 107
sucralfate........ 99
Sudafed........ 96
Sudafed 12 Hour.. 96
Sudafed PE....... 96
Sufenta........D
sufentanil........D
Sular........D
Sulcrate........ 107
Sulf-10........ 146
Sulfacet-R........ 68
sulfacetamide
    Dermatology.... 68
    Ophthalmology
    .... 146, 147
sulfacetamide -
    lupical........ 69
sulfacetamide-
    ophthalmic.... 146
sulfadiazine........ 37
sulfadoxine........D
Sulfamylon........ 69
sulfasalazine.... 110
Sulfatrim........ 38
sulfisoxazole.... 34
sulfonated
    phenolics........ 98
sulfur........ 68
sulfuric acid..... 98
sulindac........ 6
sumatriptan..... 131
sumatriptan..... 131
Sumycin........ 38
sunitinib........D
sunscreen........PDA

Supartz.................D
Supeudol................8
Supprelin LA............D
Suprane..............PDA
Suprax.................30
Suprep.................D
Supro.................122
Surfak................109
Surgam..................6
Surgam SR...............6
Surmontil............PDA
Surpass................86
Survanta...............D
Sustiva................21
Sutent.................D
Swim-Ear...............98
Sylatron...............D
Symax.................106
Symbicort.............165
Symbyax...............161
Symlin.................85
Symlinpen..............85
Symmetrel..............25
Synacort...............D
Synacthen..............D
Synagis................D
Synalar................D
Synalgos-DC............11
Synarel.................D
Synera.................77
Synercid...............40
Synphasic..............D
Syntest D.S............D
Syntest H.S............D
Synthroid..............90
Synvisc................D
Syprine..............PDA
Systane...............150

T

T-20....................D
t-PA...................64
T-Phyl................168
T3.....................90
T4.....................90
Tabloid................D
Taclonex...............72
tacrine..............PDA
tacrolimus............126
tacrolimus -
    topical............73
tadalafil
    Cardiovascular.....64
    Urology...........172
Tagamet...............104
Tagamet HB............104
Talacen................11
Talwin NX...............7
Tambocor...............48
Tamiflu................25
Tamone................140
Tamofen...............140
tamoxifen.............140
tamsulosin............170
tamsulosin............170
Tanacetum parthe-
    nium L.............118
Tanafed DMX............D
Tapazole...............90
tapentadol.............12
Tarabine...............D
Tarceva................D
Targretin..............D
TARO-sone..............D
Tarsum.................75
Tarka..................D
Tasigna................D
Tasmar.................D
Tavist ND..............94
Tavist-1...............95
Taxol..................D
Taxotere...............D
tazarotene.............69
Tazicef................30
Tazocin................36
Tazorac................69
Taztia XT..............60
Td....................123
Tdap..................123
TDF....................22
Tea tree oil..........122
Tears Naturale........150
Tecnal..................3
Tecnal C-1/2...........10
Tecnal C-1/4...........10
Teflaro................31
tegaserod..............D
Tegens................117
Tegretol..............127
Tegretol XR...........127
Tegrin.................75
Tegrin-HC..............D
Tekamlo................D
Tekturna...............55
Tekturna HCT...........D

telaprevir.............29
telavancin.............40
telbivudine............29
telithromycin..........40
telmisartan............44
telmisartan............D
Telzir.................23
temazepam............160
Temodal................D
Temodar................D
Temovate...............D
temozolomide...........D
Tempra.................12
temsirolimus...........D
tenecteplase...........65
Tenex..................45
teniposide.............D
tenofovir..........21, 22
tenofovir..........20, 21
Tenoretic..............D
Tenormin...............57
Tensilon..............132
Tenuate................D
Tenuate Dospan.........D
Terazol................D
terazosin..............46
terbinafine............16
terbinafine -
    topical............71
terconazole............D
teriparatide...........94
Tesalin...............117
tesamorelin..........PDA
Teslascan..............67
Tessalon...............95
Tessalon Perles........95
Testim.................77
Testopel...............77
testosterone...........77
Testred................D
Testro AQ..............77
tetanus immune
    globulin...........126
tetanus toxoid........124
tetrabenazine.........135
tetracaine...........PDA
tetracaine
    Dermatology........77
    ENT................13
tetracaine-
    ophthalmic........150
tetracycline...........38
tetracycline...104, 105
Tev-Tropin.............94
Teveten................43
Teveten HCT............D
thalidomide............D

Thalitone..............62
Thalomid...............D
Theo-24..............168
Theo-Dur.............168
Theolair.............168
theophylline.........168
TheraCys...............D
Theroxidil Extra
    Strength...........76
thiamine...............92
thiamine...............91
thiethylperazine......103
thioguanine............D
Thiola...............PDA
thiopental.............D
Thioplex...............D
thioridazine..........156
thiotepa...............D
thiothixene...........156
Thisylin..............120
thonzonium.............98
Thorazine...............1
thrombin - topical.....D
Thrombin-JMI...........D
Thyro-Tabs.............90
Thyrogen.............PDA
Thyroid USP............D
thyroid-desiccated.....D
Thyrolar...............D
Thyrosafe..............D
Thyroshield............D
thyrotropin alfa.....PDA
tiagabine.............130
Tiamol.................D
tiaprofenic acid........6
Tiazac.................60
ticagrelor.............56
ticarcillin-
    clavulanate........36
Tice BCG
    Immunology........123
    Oncology...........D
Ticlid.................57
ticlopidine............57
Tigan.................103
tigecycline............41
Tikosyn................47
Tilade.................D
tiludronate..........PDA
Timentin...............36
timolol................D
timolol...............148
timolol-ophthalmic
   148
Timoptic..............148
Timoptic Ocudose.....148
Timoptic XE...........148

Tinactin 71
Tindamax 19
tinidazole 19
tinzaparin 113
tioconazole 142
tiopronin .... PDA
tiotropium 168
tipranavir 25
tirofiban 57
Tirosint .... D
tizanidine 2
TNKase 65
Tobacco .... PDA
TOBI 14
Tobradex 147
Tobradex ST 147
tobramycin 14
tobramycin-
   ophthalmic 145
Tobrex 145
Tocopherol 92
Tofranil 151
Tofranil PM 151
tolazamide .... D
tolbutamide .... D
tolcapone .... D
Tolectin 6
Tolinase .... D
tolmetin 6
tolnaftate 71
tolterodine 171
tolvaptan .... D
Topamax
   Neurology 130
   Psychiatry 1
Topicort .... D
Topicort LP .... D
Topilene Glycol ...... D
topiramate
   Neurology 130
   Psychiatry 1
Toposar .... D
topotecan .... D
Toprol-XL 58
Topsyn .... D
Toradol 5
Torecan 103
toremifene .... D
Torisel .... D
torsemide 61
tositumomab .... D
Totect .... D
Toviaz 170
tpa 64
TPV 25
Tracleer .... D

Tracrium .... D
Tradjenta 82
Tramacet 3
tramadol 12
tramadol 3
Trandate 58
trandolapril 43
trandolapril .... D
tranexamic acid ...... D
Transderm-Scop...103
Transderm-V 103
Tranxene 159
Tranxene SD 159
tranylcypromine ...152
Trasicor 59
trastuzumab .... D
Travatan 149
Travatan Z 149
travoprost 149
trazodone 154
Treanda .... D
Trecator .... PDA
trefoil 121
Trelstar .... D
Trelstar Depot .... D
Trental 66
treprostinil .... D
treprostinil sodium ..D
tretinoin 69, 76, 77
tretinoin - topical ...69
Trexall 1
Treximet 131
Tri-Cyclen .... D
Tri-Legest 139
Tri-Legest Fe....... 139
Tri-Luma .... D
Tri-Nasal 99
Tri-Norinyl 139
Tri-Previfem 139
Tri-Sprintec 139
Triaderm .... D
triamcinolone 80
triamcinolone 73
triamcinolone -
   topical .... D
triamcinolone -
   vitreous .... PDA
triamcinolone-
   inhaled 167
triamcinolone-
   nasal 99
Triaminic Chest
   and Nasal
   Congestion .... D
Triaminic Cold
   and Allergy .... D

Triaminic Cough and
   Sore Throat .... D
Triaminic Day Time
   Cold and Cough ..D
Triaminic Flu
   Cough and
   Fever .... D
Triaminic Night
   Time Cold and
   Cough .... D
Triaminic Oral
   Infant Drops 96
triamterene .... D
triamterene .... D
Trianal 3
Triatec 11
Triavil .... D
Triazide .... D
triazolam 160
Tribenzor .... D
TriCor 53
Tridesilon .... D
Tridil 62
trientine .... PDA
Trifolium
   pratense 121
Triglide 53
Trigonelle foenum-
   graecum 118
trihexyphenidyl ... 132
TriHibit 124
Trikacide 39
Trileptal .... D
TriLipix 53
Trilisate 4
Trilyte 108
trimethobenzamide
   103
trimethoprim 41
trimethoprim 146
trimethoprim-
   sulfamethoxazole
   38
trimipramine ..... PDA
Trimox 35
Trinessa 139
Trinipatch 63
Trinovin 121
Triostat 90
Tripacel 123
Tripedia 123
triprolidine .... D
triptorelin .... D

197
Index
D,PDA = see page 173

Triquilar .... D
Trisenox .... D
Trivaris 80
Trivora-28 139
Trizivir 21
Tropicacyl 150
tropicamide 150
Trosec 171
trospium 171
Trusopt 148
Truvada 21
trypan blue .... D
tryptophan .... D
tuberculin PPD 126
Tubersol 126
Tucks 75
Tucks Hemorrhoidal
   Ointment 75
Tucks Suppositories
   75
Tuinal .... PDA
Tums 86
Tuss-HC .... D
Tussicaps .... D
Tussin .... D
Tussionex .... D
Twinject 63
Twinrix 124
Twynsta .... D
Tygacil 41
Tykerb .... D
Tylenol 12
Tylenol with
   Codeine 11
Tylox 11
Typherix 124
typhim Vi............. 124
typhoid vaccine-
   inactivated
   injection 124
typhoid vaccine-live
   oral 124
tyramine-rich
   foods .... PDA
Tysabri .... D
Tyvaso .... D
Tyzeka 29

U

ubiquinone 117
Ulesfia 71

ulipristal acetate... D
Uloric.................. 86
Ultane.............. PDA
Ultiva................... D
Ultracet................. 3
Ultram................. 12
Ultram ER............. 12
Ultraquin............. 76
Ultrathon.............. D
Ultravate............... D
Ultravist............... 67
Unasyn................ 36
Unidet................ 171
Uniphyl............. 168
Uniretic................ D
Unisom Nighttime
  Sleep Aid....... 102
Unithroid............. 90
Univasc............... 42
UP446................. D
urea..................... D
urea..................... 76
Urecholine......... 171
Urex................ PDA
Urised................ 171
Urispas................. D
Urocit-K............. 172
Urodol................ 171
urofollitropin....... 65
Urogesic............ 171
urokinase............. 65
Urolene blue....... 170
Uromax.............. 170
Uromitexan........... D
Uroquid-acid No. 2..D
UroXatral........... 170
URSO................. 111
URSO Forte....... 111
ursodiol............. 111
Urtica dioica
  radix............... 120
ustekinumab....... 72
UTA.................... D
UTI Relief........... 171
Utira-C.............. 171

V

Va-Zone............ 131
vaccinia vaccine ...D

Vaccinium macro-
  carpon.......... 117
Vaccinium
  myrtillus........ 117
Vagifem............ 136
Vagistat-1.......... 142
valacyclovir........ 20
Valcyte............... 19
valerian............. 122
Valeriana
  officinalis....... 122
valganciclovir...... 19
Valium............... 159
valproic acid
  Neurology....... 130
  Psychiatry...... 155
valrubicin............ D
valsartan............ 44
valsartan.............. D
Valstar................ D
Valtaxin............... D
Valtrex................ 20
Valtropin............ 94
Valturna.............. D
Vancenase........... 99
Vancenase AQ
  Double
  Strength......... 99
Vancocin............. 41
vancomycin......... 41
Vandazole.......... 141
Vandetanib........... D
Vaniqa................ 75
Vanos................... D
Vanspar............. 160
Vantas................. D
Vantin................ 30
Vaponefrin......... 168
Vaprisol........... PDA
Vaqta................ 123
vardenafil.......... 170
varenicline......... 162
varicella vaccine..124
varicella vaccine..124
varicella-zoster
  immune
  globulin......... 126
Varilrix.............. 124
Varivax.............. 124
VariZIG............. 124
Vascoray............. 67
Vaseretic.............. D
Vasocidin........... 147
Vasocon-A......... 144
Vasodilan.............. D
vasopressin......... 94
Vasotec............... 41

Vaxigrip............ 123
VCR..................... D
Vectibix................ D
vecuronium.......... 13
Veetids............... 35
Velban.................. D
Velcade................ D
Velivet.............. 139
Veltin.................. 69
Venastat............ 120
venlafaxine........ 153
Venofer.............. 88
Ventavis............... D
Ventolin HFA...... 164
VePesid................ D
Veramil.............. 60
Veramyst............ 99
verapamil............ 60
verapamil.............. D
Verdeso................ D
Veregen.............. 73
Verelan............... 60
Verelan PM......... 60
Vermox............... 18
Versed................ 13
Versel................. 76
versenate.............. D
verteporfin........... D
Vesanoid............. D
VESIcare........... 171
vetch................ 116
Vexol................ 148
Vfend................. 15
Viactiv............... 86
Viagra............... 172
Vibativ............... 40
Vibra-Tabs.......... 38
Vibramycin......... 38
Vick's 44 Cough... 96
Vicks Sinex.......... D
Vicks Sinex 12
  Hr............... 100
Vicodin.............. 11
Vicoprofen.......... 11
Victoza.............. 82
Victrelis............. 27
Vidaza................. D
Videx.................. 22
Videx EC............. 22
vigabatrin............. D
Vigamox............ 145
Viibryd.............. 151
vilazodone......... 151
Vimpat............. 128
vinblastine........... D
Vincasar.............. D
vincristine............ D

vinorelbine .... D
Viokase............. 111
Viola-A................ D
Viracept............. 24
Viramune............ 21
Viramune XR....... 21
Virazole.............. 28
Viread................ 22
Virilon................. D
Viroptic............. 146
Visicol.............. 108
Visine-A............ 144
Vision Blue........... D
Visipaque............ 67
Visken................ 59
Vistaril.............. 95
Vistide............... 19
Visudyne.............. D
vitamin A............. 92
Vitamin A Acid
  Cream............ 69
vitamin B1.......... 92
vitamin B12........ 91
vitamin B2.......... 92
vitamin B3.......... 91
vitamin B6.......... 92
vitamin C........... 90
vitamin D2.......... 91
vitamin D3.......... 93
vitamin E............ 92
vitamin K............ 92
Vitex agnus
  castus fruit
  extract.......... 117
Vitis vinifera L....119
Vivactil............ 151
Vivaglobulin...... 125
Vivarin............. 162
Vivelle.............. 136
Vivelle Dot........ 136
Vivitrol............ 161
Vivol................ 159
Vivotif Berna..... 124
VLB..................... D
VM-26................. D
VMA extract...... 117
Voltaren
  Analgesics........ 4
  Dermatology..... 69
  Ophthalmology..150
Voltaren Ophtha..150
Voltaren Rapide.... 4
Voltaren XR......... 4
voriconazole....... 15
vorinostat............ D
VoSol HC............ 98
VoSpire ER........ 164
Votrient.............. D

VP-16	D	
VSL#3	121	
Vumon	D	
Vusion	77	
Vytorin	52	
Vyvanse	163	
VZIG	126	

W

warfarin	114	
Wartec	73	
Welchol	49	
Wellbutrin	154	
Wellbutrin SR	154	
Wellbutrin XL	154	
Wellcovorin	D	
Westcort	D	
white petrolatum	77	
wild yam	122	
willow bark extract	122	
Winpred	80	
WinRho SDF	142	
witch hazel	75	
wolf's bane	116	
Women's Tylenol Menstrual Relief	12	
Women.s Rogaine	76	
Wycillin	35	
Wygesic	11	
Wytensin	D	

X

Xalatan	149	
Xanax	160	
Xanax XR	160	
Xarelto	112	
Xatral	170	
Xeloda	D	
Xenazine	135	
Xenical	111	
Xeomin	D	

Xgeva	D	
Xifaxan	40	
Xodol	11	
Xolair	D	
Xolegel	70	
Xopenex	164	
Xopenex HFA	164	
Xuezhikang	121	
Xylocaine Anesthesia	13	
Cardiovascular	48	
Dermatology	76	
ENT	99	
Xylocard	48	
Xyntha	D	
Xyrem	135	
Xyzal	95	

Y

Yasmin	139	
Yaz	139	
yellow fever vaccine	124	
Yervoy	D	
YF-Vax	124	
Yocon	172	
Yodoxin	PDA	
yohimbine	122	
yohimbine	172	
Yohimex	172	

Z

Zaditor	144	
zafirlukast	167	
zaleplon	161	
Zanaflex	2	
zanamivir	25	
Zanosar	D	
Zantac	104	
Zantac 150	104	
Zantac 75	104	
Zantac Efferdose	104	
Zarah	139	
Zarontin	128	

Zaroxolyn	62	
Zavesca	PDA	
ZDV	22	
ZE 339	117	
ZeaSorb AF	D	
Zebeta	58	
Zegerid	D	
Zelapar	134	
Zelnorm	D	
Zemaira	D	
Zemplar	92	
Zemuron	13	
Zenapax	126	
Zenhale	165	
Zenpep	111	
Zeosa	139	
Zephrex-LA	D	
Zerit	D	
Zestoretic	D	
Zestril	42	
Zetia	53	
Zevalin	D	
Zhibituo	121	
Ziac	59	
Ziagen	22	
Ziana	D	
ziconotide	PDA	
zidovudine	22	
zidovudine	21	
zileuton	168	
Zinacef	30	
zinc acetate	D	
zinc oxide Dermatology	77	
ENDOCRINE AND METABOLIC	PDA	
zinc sulfate	89	
Zincate	89	
Zinecard	D	
Zingiber officinale	118	
Zingo	76	
ziprasidone	159	
Zipsor	4	
Zirgan	146	
Zithromax	31	
Zmax	31	
Zocor	51	
Zofran	101	

Zoladex	D	
zoledronic acid	78	
Zolinza	D	
zolmitriptan	131	
Zoloft	D	
zolpidem	161	
Zolpimist	161	
Zometa	78	
Zomig	131	
Zomig ZMT	131	
Zonalon	75	
Zonegran	130	
zonisamide	130	
zopiclone	161	
Zorbtive	94	
Zorcaine	13	
Zorprin	4	
Zostavax	124	
zoster vaccine-live	124	
Zostrix	75	
Zostrix-HP	75	
Zosyn	36	
Zovia	D	
Zovirax Antimicrobials	19	
Dermatology	72	
zuclopenthixol	D	
Zyban	154	
Zydone	11	
Zyflo CR	168	
Zylet	147	
Zyloprim	86	
Zymaxid	145	
Zyprexa	156	
Zyprexa Relprevv	156	
Zyprexa Zydis	156	
Zyrtec	95	
Zyrtec-D	D	
Zytiga	D	
Zyvox	39	
Zyvoxam	39	

APPENDIX

ADULT EMERGENCY DRUGS (selected)

ALLERGY	diphenhydramine (*Benadryl*): 50 mg IV/IM. epinephrine: 0.1–0.5 mg IM (1:1000 solution), may repeat after 20 minutes. methylprednisolone (*Solu-Medrol*): 125 mg IV/IM.
HYPERTENSION	esmolol (*Brevibloc*): 500 mcg/kg IV over 1 minute, then titrate 50–200 mcg/kg/min. fenoldopam (*Corlopam*): Start 0.1 mcg/kg/min, titrate up to 1.6 mcg/kg/min. labetalol (*Normodyne*): Start 20 mg slow IV, then 40–80 mg IV q10 min prn up to 300 mg total cumulative dose. nitroglycerin (*Tridil*): Start 10–20 mcg/min IV infusion, then titrate prn up to 100 mcg/min. nitroprusside (*Nipride*): Start 0.3 mcg/kg/min IV infusion, then titrate prn up to 10 mcg/kg/min.
DYSRHYTHMIAS / ARREST	adenosine (*Adenocard*): PSVT (not A-fib): 6 mg rapid IV & flush, preferably through a central line or proximal IV. If no response after 1–2 minutes, then 12 mg. A third dose of 12 mg may be given prn. amiodarone (*Cordarone, Pacerone*): V-fib or pulseless V-tach: 300 mg IV/IO; may repeat 150 mg just once. Life-threatening ventricular arrhythmia: Load 150 mg IV over 10 min, then 1 mg/min × 6 h, then 0.5 mg/min × 18 h. atropine: 0.5 mg IV, repeat prn to maximum of 3 mg. diltiazem (*Cardizem*): Rapid A-fib: bolus 0.25 mg/kg or 20 mg IV over 2 min. May repeat 0.35 mg/kg or 25 mg 15 min after 1st dose. Infusion 5–15 mg/h. epinephrine: 1 mg IV/IO q 3–5 minutes for cardiac arrest. [1:10,000 solution]. lidocaine (*Xylocaine*): Load 1 mg/kg IV, then 0.5 mg/kg q 8–10 min prn to max 3 mg/kg. Maintenance 2 g in 250 mL D5W (8 mg/mL) at 1–4 mg/min drip (7–30 mL/h).
PRESSORS	dobutamine (*Dobutrex*): 2–20 mcg/kg/min. 70 kg: 5 mcg/kg/min with 1 mg/mL concentration (eg, 250 mg in 250 mL D5W) = 21 mL/h. dopamine (*Intropin*): Pressor: Start at 5 mcg/kg/min, increase prn by 5–10 mcg/kg/min increments at 10 min intervals, max 50 mcg/kg/min. 70 kg: 5 mcg/kg/min with 1600 mcg/mL concentration (eg, 400 mg in 250 mL D5W) = 13 mL/h. Doses in mcg/kg/min: 2–4 = (traditional renal dose, apparently ineffective) dopaminergic receptors; 5–10 = (cardiac dose) dopaminergic and beta1 receptors; >10 = dopaminergic, beta1, and alpha1 receptors. norepinephrine (*Levophed*): 4 mg in 500 mL D5W (8 mcg/mL) at 2–4 mcg/min. 22.5 mL/h = 3 mcg/min. phenylephrine (*Neo-Synephrine*): Infusion for hypotension: 20 mg in 250 mL D5W (80 mcg/mL) at 40–180 mcg/min (35–160 mL/h).
INTUBATION	etomidate (*Amidate*): 0.3 mg/kg IV. methohexital (*Brevital*): 1–1.5 mg/kg IV. propofol (*Diprivan*): 2.0–2.5 mg/kg IV. rocuronium (*Zemuron*): 0.6–1.2 mg/kg IV. succinylcholine (*Anectine*): 1 mg/kg IV. Peds (<5 yo): 2 mg/kg IV. thiopental (*Pentothal*): 3–5 mg/kg IV.
SEIZURES	diazepam (*Valium*): 5–10 mg IV, or 0.2–0.5 mg/kg rectal gel up to 20 mg PR. fosphenytoin (*Cerebyx*): Load 15–20 "phenytoin equivalents" per kg either IM, or IV no faster than 100–150 mg/min. lorazepam (*Ativan*): 0.05–0.15 mg/kg up to 3–4 mg IV/IM. phenobarbital: 200–600 mg IV at rate ≤60 mg/min; titrate prn up to 20 mg/kg. phenytoin (*Dilantin*): 15–20 mg/kg up to 1000 mg IV no faster than 50 mg/min.

CARDIAC DYSRHYTHMIA PROTOCOLS (for adults and adolescents)

Chest compressions ~100/min. Ventilations 8-10/min if intubated; otherwise 30:2 compression/ventilation ratio. Drugs that can be administered down ET tube (use 2–2.5 × usual dose): epinephrine, atropine, lidocaine, naloxone, vasopressin*.

V-Fib, Pulseless V-Tach

Airway, oxygen, CPR until defibrillator ready
Defibrillate 360 J (old monophasic), 120–200 J (biphasic), or with AED
Resume CPR × 2 min (5 cycles)
Repeat defibrillation if no response
Vasopressor during CPR:
• Epinephrine 1 mg IV/IO q 3–5 minutes, or
• Vasopressin* 40 units IV to replace 1 * or 2nd dose of epinephrine
Rhythm/pulse check every ~2 minutes
Consider antiarrhythmic during CPR:
• Amiodarone 300 mg IV/IO; may repeat 150 mg just once
• Lidocaine 1 0–1 5 mg/kg IV/IO, then repeat 0.5–0.75 mg/kg to max 3 doses or 3 mg/kg
• Magnesium sulfate 1–2 g IV/IO if suspect torsades de pointes

Asystole or Pulseless Electrical Activity (PEA)

Airway, oxygen, CPR
Vasopressor (when IV/IO access):
• Epinephrine 1 mg IV/IO q 3–5 min, or
• Vasopressin* 40 units IV/IO to replace 1 * or 2nd dose to epinephrine
Consider atropine 1 mg IV/IO for asystole or slow PEA. Repeat q 3–5 min up to 3 doses.
Rhythm/pulse check every ~2 minutes
Consider 6 H's: hypovolemia, hypoxia, H+acidosis, hyper/ hypokalemia, hypoglycemia, hypothermia
Consider 5 T's: Toxins, tamponade-cardiac, tension pneumothorax, thrombosis (coronary or pulmonary), trauma

Bradycardia, <60 bpm and Inadequate Perfusion

Airway, oxygen, IV
Prepare for transcutaneous pacing; don't delay if advanced heart block
Consider atropine 0.5 mg IV; may repeat q 3–5 min to max 3 mg
Consider epinephrine (2–10 mcg/min) or dopamine(2–10mcg/kg/min)
Prepare for transvenous pacing

Tachycardia with Pulses

Airway, oxygen, IV
If unstable and heart rate >150 bpm, then synchronized cardioversion
If stable narrow-QRS (<120 ms):
• Regular: Attempt vagal maneuvers, If no success, adenosine 6 mg IV
• Irregular: Control rate with diltiazem or beta blocker (caution in CHF or severe obstructive disease).
If stable wide-QRS (>120 ms):
• Regular and suspect V-tach: Amiodarone 150 mg IV over 10 min; repeat prn to max 2.2 g/24 h. Prepare for elective synchronized cardioversion.
• Regular and suspect SVT with aberrancy: adenosine as per narrow-QRS above.
• Irregular and A-fib: Control rate with diltiazem or beta blocker (caution in CHF/ severe obstructive pulmonary disease).
• Irregular and A-fib with pre-excitation (WPW): Avoid AV nodal blocking agents; consider amiodarone 150 mg IV over 10 min,
• Irregular and torsades de pointes: magnesium 1–2 g IV load over 5–60 min, then infusion.

bpm=beats per minute; CPR=cardiopulmonary resuscitation; ET=endotracheal; IO=intraosseous; J=Joules; ms=milliseconds; WPW=Wolff-Parkinson-White. Sources: *Circulation* 2005; 112, suppl IV; *NEJM* 2008;359:21–30 (demonstrated no benefit over epinephrine and worse long-term neurological outcomes).

ANTIVIRAL DRUGS FOR INFLUENZA	Treatment* (Duration of 5 days)	Prevention (Duration of 7 to 10 days post-exposure)†
OSELTAMIVIR *(Tamiflu)*		
Adults and adolescents age 13 years and older		
	75 mg PO bid	75 mg PO once daily
Children, 1 year of age and older‡		
Body weight ≤15 kg	30 mg PO bid	30 mg PO once daily
Body weight >15 to 23 kg	45 mg PO bid	45 mg PO once daily
Body weight >23 to 40 kg	60 mg PO bid	60 mg PO once daily
Body weight >40 kg	75 mg PO bid	75 mg PO once daily
Infants, newborn to 11 months of age‡¶		
Age 3 to 11 months old	3 mg/kg/dose PO bid	3 mg/kg/dose PO once daily
Age younger than 3 months old§	3 mg/kg/dose PO bid	Not for routine prophylaxis in infants <3 mo
ZANAMIVIR *(Relenza)* **		
Adults and children (age 7 years and older for treatment, age 5 years and older for prophylaxis)		
	10 mg (two 5-mg inhalations) bid	10 mg (two 5-mg inhalations) once daily

Adapted from http://www.cdc.gov/mmwr/pdf/rr/rr6001.pdf

*Start treatment as soon as possible; benefit is greatest when started within 2 days of symptom onset. Consider longer treatment for patients who remain severely ill after 5 days of treatment.

†Duration is 10 days after household exposure, and 7 days after most recent known exposure in other situations. For long-term care facilities and hospitals, prophylaxis should last a minimum of 14 days and up to 7 days after the most recent known case was identified.

‡In July 2011, the concentration of Tamiflu suspension was changed from 12 mg/mL to 6 mg/mL. Tamiflu prescribing information contains instructions for pharmacists to compound a 6 mg/mL suspension when Tamiflu suspension is not available. The new Tamiflu suspension is provided with a 10 mL oral dispenser measured in mL rather than mg. Capsules can be opened and mixed with sweetened fluids to mask bitter taste. Make sure units of measure on dosing instructions match dosing device provided.

¶Oseltamivir is not FDA-approved for use in infants less than 1 year old. An Emergency Use Authorization for use in infants expired in June 2010.

§This dose is not intended for premature infants. Immature renal function may lead to slow clearance and high concentrations of oseltamivir in this age group.

**Zanamivir should not be used by patients with underlying pulmonary disease. Do not attempt to use *Relenza* in a nebulizer or ventilator; lactose in the formulation may cause the device to malfunction.

bid=two times per day.

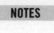